Handbook of Frontal Lobe Assessment

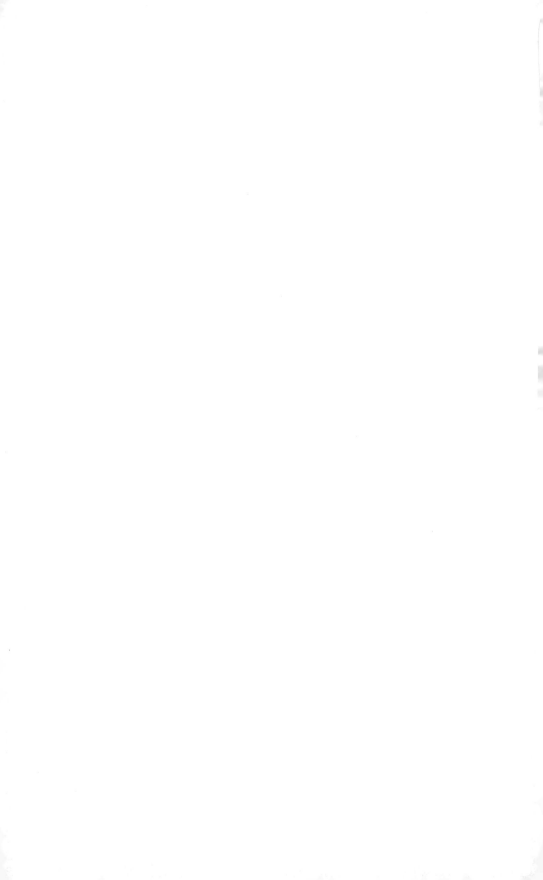

Handbook of Frontal Lobe Assessment

Sarah E. MacPherson
Sergio Della Sala

with

Simon R. Cox
Alessandra Girardi
Matthew H. Iveson

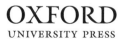

OXFORD
UNIVERSITY PRESS

OXFORD
UNIVERSITY PRESS

Great Clarendon Street, Oxford, OX2 6DP,
United Kingdom

Oxford University Press is a department of the University of Oxford.
It furthers the University's objective of excellence in research, scholarship,
and education by publishing worldwide. Oxford is a registered trade mark of
Oxford University Press in the UK and in certain other countries

First Edition published in 2015

Impression: 1

Published in the United States of America by Oxford University Press
198 Madison Avenue, New York, NY 10016, United States of America

British Library Cataloguing in Publication Data

Data available

Library of Congress Control Number: 2014953106

ISBN 978–0–19–966952–3

Printed in Great Britain by
Clays Ltd, St Ives plc

Oxford University Press makes no representation, express or implied, that the
drug dosages in this book are correct. Readers must therefore always check
the product information and clinical procedures with the most up-to-date
published product information and data sheets provided by the manufacturers
and the most recent codes of conduct and safety regulations. The authors and
the publishers do not accept responsibility or legal liability for any errors in the
text or for the misuse or misapplication of material in this work. Except where
otherwise stated, drug dosages and recommendations are for the non-pregnant
adult who is not breast-feeding

Links to third party websites are provided by Oxford in good faith and
for information only. Oxford disclaims any responsibility for the materials
contained in any third party website referenced in this work.

To Sophie and Joseph
and
To Emma and Marta
who will eventually develop their frontal lobes!

Acknowledgments

First, we wish to express our gratitude to Charlotte Green, Senior Assistant Commissioning Editor for Psychology and Social Work at Oxford University Press, who supported us throughout. We are also thankful to a number of clinicians and researchers working in the area of frontal lobe functions who offered their advice on the tests we included in the book: Professor Sharon Abrahams, Professor Shelly Channon, Professor Jordan Grafman, Professor Tim Shallice, and Professor Donald Stuss. We are particularly grateful to Dr Jennifer Foley who kindly gave her time to read through and comment on all chapters in this book. Her careful and constructive comments and suggestions were invaluable. Her willingness to give her time so generously has been very much appreciated.

Sarah E. MacPherson and Sergio Della Sala
August 2014

Contents

Figures

Boxes

Tables

Advance Praise

The effects of lesions to the frontal lobes on cognition, emotion, and personality are among the most difficult to assess in all of neuropsychology. Many very different tests have been proposed, but the utility of quite a number has been questioned, and the literature on their application is complex and diffusely located. This Handbook is therefore enormously valuable in synthesizing a vast amount of material on the 30 most widely used different types of test. The Handbook will prove an essential resource for anyone involved in the assessment of the behavioural consequences of frontal lobe lesions.

Professor Tim Shallice, University College London, UK

Clear and insightful chapters detailing convergent evidence on the usefulness of the tests currently used to assess frontal lobe functional domains will enable you to become familiar with the costs and benefits of using both classic and novel, state-of-the-art, test instruments including commentary on each test's validity and reliability. If you evaluate or study patients with frontal lobe lesions or dysfunction, you must have this book in easy reach as it is a one-stop shop designed to simplify your decision making about which frontal lobe tests are right for your clinical patients or research participants. There is simply no substitute for it.

Professor Jordan Grafman, Ph.D., Rehabilitation Institute of Chicago, USA

This is an excellent, much-needed resource. If evidence were needed of the richness and variety of frontal lobe functions then readers need look no further than this text. The authors provide an accomplished account of the tools of frontal lobe assessment, their evidence-base and neural correlates that will be of immense value to clinicians and researchers alike.

Professor Julie S Snowden, Consultant Neuropsychologist,
Cerebral Function Unit, Greater Manchester Neuroscience Centre,
Salford Royal NHS Foundation Trust, UK

Chapter 1

Introduction: Fractionating the frontal lobe syndrome

1.1 Frontal lesions and behavior change

When one hears the term "frontal lobe function," even the most junior psychology student might think of the classic "crowbar" case of Phineas Gage (Harlow 1848; MacMillan 2002). Nowadays, it seems surprising that the accepted wisdom was once that this region was associated with few, if any, cognitive functions (e.g., Pfeifer 1910; Feuchtwanger 1923). Gage experienced severe personality changes as a result of a tamping iron penetrating his frontal lobes, and yet many medical textbooks published around that time, including the first five editions of Dalton's physiology textbook, *A Treatise on Human Physiology* (1859–1871), stated that Gage was, "in perfect health ... with the mental and bodily functions entirely unimpaired" (see Barker 1995). Paradoxically, the *American Phrenological Journal* reported in 1851 that the frontal lobes were not a monolithic entity and that a number of cognitive abilities would have been impaired by Gage's damage to the various phrenological organs (Anonymous 1851). Yet, it took John M. Harlow, Gage's physician, 20 years to report to the medical community that Phineas Gage was "no longer Gage" due to his frontal lobe damage (Harlow 1868; MacMillan 2002). Whereas accounts may vary of what happened that fateful afternoon in September 1848, this story has fuelled the interests of both scientists and laypeople alike (Kean 2014).

Delving a little deeper into the literature, a number of similar cases of behavior change had been reported in patients with frontal lobe damage. For example, one of the most prominent photographers of the nineteenth century, Eadweard J. Muybridge (Figures 1.1 and 1.2), suffered personality changes following head trauma from a stagecoach accident (see Shimamura 2002). These changes included becoming more eccentric, irritable, a riskier decision-maker, and often Muybridge was described as displaying uncontrollable outbursts. He was even acquitted of the murder of his wife Flora's lover and father of her son, after his friends testified that he was a different man post accident. Although the exact localization of his brain damage is unknown, Muybridge's symptoms were consistent with someone who had damage to the orbitofrontal cortex (Shimamura 2002).

In another example, in the early twentieth century, the Italian psychiatrist Cesare Agostini (1914) published a report describing the considerable

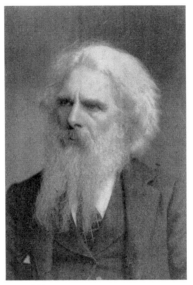

Fig. 1.1 Portrait of Eadweard J. Muybridge, Wm. Vick Studio, c.1881. © The Library of Congress.

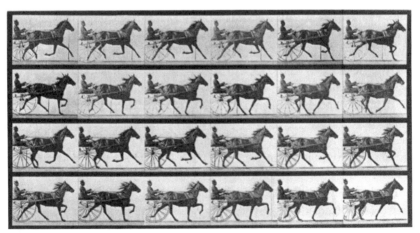

Fig. 1.2 Photograph by Eadweard J. Muybridge: Horse in Motion from Animal Locomotion, 1887. © The Library of Congress.

personality change experienced by one of his patients, P. Vincenzo, a 47-year-old laborer (Figure 1.3). The patient was described as having become irritable, quick- and bad-tempered, and had an inclination for criminal behavior. In 1907, Vincenzo stabbed a road worker to death after a minor row over a barrow. It was not until Vincenzo's death due to an epileptic seizure in 1909 that he was diagnosed as having a right orbital frontal lobe tumor. These patients, as well as other single-case examples reported in the eighteenth and early nineteenth centuries, consistently showed that orbital and medial prefrontal damage resulted in severe personality change.

It was therefore astonishing that damaging the frontal lobes would become a treatment for mental illness. Egas Moniz, the Portuguese neurologist and Nobel Prize winner in 1949, devised the infamous frontal lobotomy (Moniz 1936), later aggressively promoted in the USA by Walter Freeman (e.g., Freeman and Watts 1942), arguing that the benefits of this surgical procedure for reducing the symptoms of mental illness outweighed the acute personality changes that resulted (for scientific criticisms see Valenstein 1986; for literary criticisms read *Suddenly, Last Summer* by Tennessee Williams; for patients' stories see Raz 2013). The behavioral effects of frontal lesions are now laypeople parlance, and "frontal" has become a defining adjective. Indeed, even movies feature characters with behavioral changes due to lesions in the frontal lobes (Table 1.1 and Figure 1.4; for specific symptoms such as anarchic hand, see Della Sala 2009).

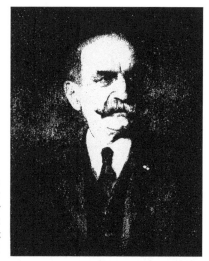

EMMA
DESSAU-GOITEIN
PORTRÄT
PROFESSORE
CESARE
AGOSTINI

Fig. 1.3 Portrait of Professor Cesare Agostini. © JCS Universitätsbibliothek Frankfurt am Main/Digitale Sammlung Judaica. http://sammlungen.ub.uni-frankfurt. de/2926241.

Table 1.1 Behavioral effects of frontal lesions as shown in movies

Movie	Character with frontal lobe lesion	Aetiology	Behaviour	Relevant sentence
A Fine Madness (1966)	Sean Connery (poet Samson Shillitoe)	Frontal lobotomy	Aggressive behaviour, social faux pas	Samson's wife: "Hey, Samson, Mr Butler's got some great news for you!" Samson: "Mister? When did he get the operation?"
Planet of the Apes (1968)	Robert Gunner (astronaut Landon)	Frontal lobotomy	Mutacism and abulia	Taylor, Landon's friend: "You cut up his brain, you bloody baboon!... You cut out his memory. You took his identity."
Night of the Living Dead (1968)	Zombie	Thin frontal lobe	Impulsivity	Scientist: "Kill the brain, and you kill the ghoul."
One Flew Over the Cuckoo's Nest (1975)	Jack Nicholson (anarchic criminal "Mac" McMurphy)	Frontal lobotomy	Catatonia	Martini (Danny DeVito) and Scanlon (Delos V. Smith Jr), Mac's fellow interns in the mental institution seeing him after surgery: "Nothing like him," "Sure," "Just like one of those store dummies ain't that right?," "Damn right. Whole thing you know, too blank."
Zelig (1983)	Woody Allen (common man Leonard Zelig)	Not specified	Environmental Dependency Syndrome	Zelig's conned victim (Louise Deitch): "He painted my house a disgusting colour. He said he was a painter. I couldn't believe the results."
Regarding Henry (1991)	Harrison Ford (attorney Henry Turner)	Gun shot in the right frontal lobe (though curiously with paralysis in the right limbs)	Childlike behaviour	Dr Sultan (James Rebhorn): "Mrs Turner, your husband, incredibly lucky. The bullet wound to the head caused minimum damage. See (pointing to scans) it hit the right frontal lobe, which is the only part of the brain which has redundant systems. I mean if you have to be shot in the head, that's the way to do it."
The Shadow (1994)	John Lone (warlord Shiwan Khan)	Glass shard head injury	Confusion and lack of mental power	Doctor (Aaron Lustig) to Khan: "Save your life, that's what. Of course we had to remove a section of your frontal lobes, but you'll never miss it, believe me. It's a part nobody ever uses."

Source	Character	Cause	Condition	Quote
A Life Less Ordinary (1997)	Stanley Tucci (dentist Elliot Zweikel)	Brain injury during a "William Tell" shooting game	Disinhibition and impulsiveness	Elliot (operating an injured leg without any surgical experience): "They wanted me to take a break you know, take a break. Go get counselling, you know. Fuck off.... The principles of surgery are the same above or below the neck!"
"My Sister, My Sitter," 17th episode, Season 8, The Simpsons (1997)	Bart Simpson	Fall downstairs and banging head against wall	Anosodiaphoria	Lisa: "Bart, are you okay?" Bart: "Yeah, I think so. It's just a bump on my head." Lisa: "Eww! Your arm! It's got extra corners!" Bart: "Oh, cool! It must be dislocated or something."
"HOMЯ," 9th episode, Season 12, The Simpsons (2001)	Homer Simpson	Crayon stuck in his frontal lobe	IQ boosted after removal	Scientist: "We could perform a surgery and remove the crayon from your brain. It could vastly increase your brain power. Or it could possibly kill you." Homer: "Hmm... increase my killing power, eh?"
"The Social Contract," 17th episode, Season 5, House (2009)	Jay Karnes (editor Nick Greenwald)	Doege–Potter syndrome	Disinhibition	Dr Lisa Cuddy: "I was paged." Nick: "I would do her in a minute with fudge and cherries on top..." Dr Remy "Thirteen" Hadley: "He has frontal lobe disinhibition."

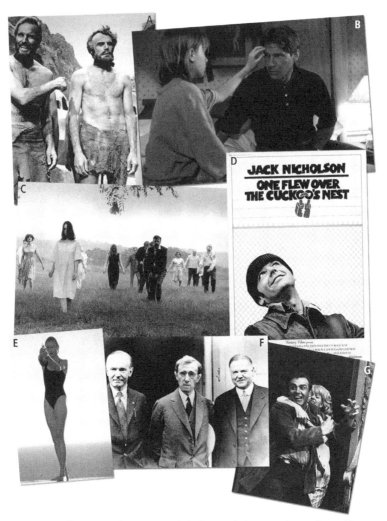

Fig. 1.4 Movies featuring characters with behavioral changes due to frontal lesions. (A) *Planet Of The Apes (1968)* (reproduced courtesy of 20th Century Fox/The Kobal Collection); (B) *Regarding Henry* (reproduced courtesy of Paramount/The Kobal Collection/Duhamel, Francois); (C) *Night Of The Living Dead (1968)* (reproduced courtesy of Image Ten/The Kobal Collection); (D) *One Flew Over The Cuckoo's Nest* (reproduced courtesy of United Artists/Fantasy Films/The Kobal Collection); (E) *A Life Less Ordinary* (reproduced courtesy of Polygram/The Kobal Collection); (F) *Zelig* (reproduced courtesy of Orion/Warner Bros/The Kobal Collection); (G) *A Fine Madness* (reproduced courtesy of Pan Arts/Warner Bros/The Kobal Collection).

1.2 **Neuroanatomy of the frontal lobes**

The writings of thirteenth-century Florentine writer and philosopher Brunetto Latini propose that different functions can be mapped on to distinct neuro-anatomical regions, including functions associated with the frontal lobes. His enchanting poem *Il Tesoretto* (Little Treasure), written *c*.1261–1266, declares, "Anterior is the lodging of all intellectual properties and the stamina to learn that which one could understand" (Figure 1.5).

The French physician and anatomist Félix Vicq d'Azyr referred to three brain regions within each hemisphere; the frontal, parietal, and occipital lobes (Vicq d'Azyr and Moreau de la Sarthe 1805), labels which are still used today. However, it was not until the nineteenth century that anatomists acknowledged that different gyri and sulci within the brain formed patterns. Within the frontal lobes, three gyri on the lateral surface (Ecker 1869, 1873) as well as gyri on the orbital and medial surfaces of the frontal lobes (Leuret 1839; Valentin 1841; Foville 1844; Gratiolet 1857) were illustrated. Further advancement in the early 1900s led cortical regions to be considered in terms of their differences in cellular structure and organization (Campbell 1905; Brodmann 1909; Vogt and Vogt 1919; Von Economo and Koskinas 1925). Whereas similar nomenclatures were

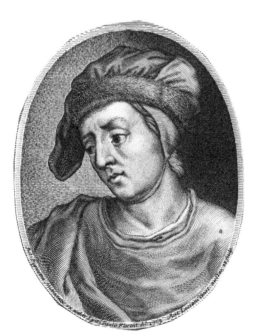

Il Tesoretto

Nel capo son tre celle
E io ti diro' di quelle.
Davanti e' lo ricetto,
di tutto lo intelletto
e la forza d'aprendere
quello che puoi intendere

Little Treasure

In the head there are three rooms
And I'll speak about those.
Anterior is the lodging,
of all intellectual properties
and the stamina to learn
that which one could understand

Fig. 1.5 Portrait of Brunetto Latini (© DeAgostini Picture Library/Scala, Florence) and *Il Tesoretto*, canto VII, by Brunetto Latini (c.1261–1266).

devised, anatomists most usually employed Brodmann's (1909) to differentiate regions by their cytoarchitectural differences—and still do so. This classification system has led to the identification of various frontal subregions, including the dorsolateral prefrontal cortex that comprises Brodmann's Areas (BAs) 9 and 46, the anterior cingulate cortex (BAs 24, 25, 32, and 33), the inferior frontal gyrus (BAs 44, 45, and dorsal parts of 47), the orbitofrontal cortex (BAs 11–14, and ventral parts of 47) and the frontal pole (BA 10) (Devinsky et al. 1995; Rajowska and Goldman-Rakic 1995; Pandya and Yeterian 1996; Uylings et al. 2010). The frontal lobes also include the primary motor (BA 4), supplementary motor regions (BA 6), and the frontal eye fields (BA 8), but these regions are not thought to play a relevant role in complex cognitive behavior, decision-making, nor in moderating social behavior.

It might be surprising for some to read that more than one hundred years ago, Jakob, a German neurobiologist working in Argentina, first advocated the importance of also studying the anatomical connectivity of the frontal lobes in order to understand its function (see Théodoridou and Triarhou 2012 for a translation). As Jakob's writings were in Spanish and German, they were largely ignored by English-speaking scientists. Yet, his view is still held today (cf. Catani and ffytche 2005; ffytche and Catani 2005; see Catani and Stuss 2012a, 2012b) and has led to the identification of a number of different cortico-cortical connections in relation to the subdivisions of the frontal lobes (Pandya and Yeterian 1996; Rolls 1996; Barbas 2000; Zald 2007; Rolls 2014a, 2014b). In terms of frontal intra-connectivity, short-range fiber anatomy and its functional significance are relatively underexplored in humans. The lateral prefrontal cortex is connected to premotor regions via the superior and inferior frontal portions of the longitudinal fasciculus, which run parallel to the superior and inferior frontal sulci (Catani et al. 2012). The anterior cingulate cortex is densely interconnected with most parts of the frontal cortex (Barbas 1995), although it has become clear that dorsal regions of the anterior cingulate preferentially connect with dorsal frontal cortex, that posterior regions are intimately associated with motor and premotor cortex, and that anterior ventral regions are associated with the orbitofrontal cortex (Beckmann et al. 2009; Yeterian et al. 2012). Other short-range tracts have recently been investigated: the fronto-orbitopolar tract connects orbitofrontal and frontopolar regions, medial and lateral frontal pole regions interconnect via the fronto-marginal tract, and a complex series of longitudinal and lateral tracts interconnect gyri along the walls of the frontal sulci (Catani et al. 2012). Thus, direct connectivity between dorsolateral and orbital frontal regions is minimal.

In relation to the frontal subregions and their differential connections with other brain regions, the branches of the superior and inferior frontal portions of the longitudinal fasciculus extend posteriorly to form long-range connections with the parietal lobe (Thiebaut de Schotten et al. 2012). Furthermore, the arcuate fasciculus is a dorsal projection which arcs around the sylvian fissure, connecting temporal, parietal, and lateral frontal regions. The orbitofrontal cortex receives inputs from the amygdala, hippocampus, olfactory cortex, and insula, along with auditory and visual information from temporal and occipital cortices via the uncinate and inferior fronto-occipital fasciculi (Petrides and Pandya 2004; Catani and Thiebaut de Schotten 2008; Catani et al. 2012; Yeterian et al. 2012). Via U-shaped fibers from the cingulum bundle that, like the cingulate cortex, loop around the corpus callosum, the anterior cingulate cortex is also connected to parietal, occipital, and temporal lobes, including radiations into the parahippocampal gyrus (Mufson and Pandya 1984; Catani and Thiebaut de Schotten 2008). The orbitofrontal cortex, anterior cingulate cortex, and lateral prefrontal cortex can also be differentiated on the basis of their distinct connections to the mediodorsal nucleus of the thalamus (Klein et al. 2010).

1.3 **Fractionation of frontal lobe functions**

Despite these developments over the past 150 years or so, in terms of neuroanatomical and histological research, fractionation of the frontal lobes into specific functional domains has made remarkably slow progress (Della Sala et al. 1998b; Frith 2000). In his 1966 book *Higher Cortical Functions in Man*, Alexander Luria proposed the existence of several "frontal lobe syndromes" in which distinct frontal regions are associated with different functional domains: the premotor area with the changing aspects of motor and skilled movements; the prefrontal convex division (which includes the dorsolateral prefrontal cortex) with planning and monitoring in goal-directed behavior; and the mediobasal or orbital prefrontal region with changes in personality (Della Sala et al. 1998a).

Almost 40 years later, Stuss and Knight (2002) predicted that the first decade of this millennium would provide us with a clearer sense of whether general versus multiple hypotheses would best explain the role of the frontal lobes. Yet, in the second edition of their *Principles of Frontal Lobe Function* book (2013), they admit that their prediction did not come true. Several theories within the frontal lobe literature have highlighted the role of the frontal lobes as a supervisory system or central executive that controls and regulates other cognitive domains such as language, memory, and attention (Norman and Shallice 1980, 1986; Baddeley 1996; Stuss et al. 2002). However, there remains a debate as to whether the functions of the frontal lobes can be fractionated into separate functions (Stuss and Benson 1986; Shallice 2002) or whether they are simply functions that overlap (Duncan and Miller 2002).

With the emergence of functional neuroimaging techniques in the late twentieth century that have come to dominate the frontal literature, researchers are now able to better understand the brain regions associated with different cognitive processes (Frackowiak et al. 1997; Rugg 1997; Gazzaniga 2000). On the basis of functional neuroimaging research, Duncan and Miller (2002) proposed the Adaptive Coding Model, which claims that the neurons within the prefrontal cortex do not have set functions; instead they contribute toward many functions. Functional neuroimaging studies have demonstrated the same "multiple-demand" pattern of frontal activity involving the inferior frontal sulcus, anterior insula/frontal operculum, dorso-medial prefrontal cortex, and the intraparietal sulcus, despite tasks requiring different cognitive demands (Duncan 2006, 2010). Similarly, Fuster (2013, p. 12) has proposed the Cognit Paradigm of Cognition, which claims that, "... all higher cognitive functions, like perception, use the same system of widely distributed, interconnected and overlapping cortical networks." Cognits or units of knowledge within networks of cell assemblies (Hebb 1949) are formed and distributed throughout the cortex. Cognits within the prefrontal cortex contain units of executive memories important for future goal-direction actions.

These global frontal theories suppose that it is not possible to ascribe different functions to distinct frontal subregions, given the flexibility of frontal neurons. Yet, it is not easy to reduce frontal functions to a single frontal process. In addition to the cytoarchitectural and hodological (i.e., the study of connectional anatomy; Catani 2007) differentiation of frontal lobe regions (which are likely to constrain the type of information processing each region performs; Barbas 2000; Zald 2007), lesion studies suggest that different frontal subregions are associated with a number of cognitive processes (Shallice and Burgess 1996; Shallice 2002; Stuss et al. 2002; Koechlin et al. 2003). Researchers have stressed the importance of not relying solely on neuroimaging evidence as the only source of data and have argued for the benefits of cross-method agreement (e.g., Duncan and Owen 2000; Burgess et al. 2005; Burgess 2011; Stuss and Alexander 2009). Functional neuroimaging studies simply indicate localized magnetic inhomogeneities due to metabolism of oxygen or glucose within certain brain areas during a particular cognitive task. Thus, they may be used to infer which brain regions may be *involved* in a particular cognitive task. By contrast, lesion studies provide information about the pattern of spared and impaired abilities among individuals with brain damage when compared with a control group, allowing inferences about which regions may be *necessary* for a particular cognitive task. For example, in neuroimaging studies, certain frontal regions such as the frontal pole are activated by a wide variety of tasks, yet patients with lesions in these same regions do not necessarily show impairments on these same tasks. Burgess et al. (2005) describe the case of patient AP who suffered a head injury resulting in his frontal pole being removed. AP showed significant multitasking difficulties in everyday situations but performed within normal limits on measures of frontal executive functions (Shallice and Burgess 1991; Metzler and Parkin 2000). Nonetheless, neuroimaging studies have suggested that the frontal pole is activated while performing these traditional frontal executive measures (e.g., Ramnani and Owen 2004). Neuroimaging alone cannot demonstrate brain regions that are necessary for a particular cognitive function.

Tsujimoto et al. (2011) recommended that neurophysiological studies of non-human primates should be considered as an additional source of information when attempting to understand the functions of frontal subregions (typically these involve rhesus macaques) as there are several similarities between monkey and human brains. First, the prefrontal cortex of a monkey brain, like the human brain, consists of regions that are segregated both in terms of cellular composition and implied function (Brodmann 1909). Furthermore, the broad anatomical layout of the regions within the frontal lobes is fairly similar between the two species (Brodmann 1909; Petrides and Pandya 1994; Pandya and Yeterian 1996), with the position of major prefrontal regions such as the dorsolateral prefrontal cortex, ventrolateral prefrontal cortex, ventromedial prefrontal cortex, the frontal pole, and anterior cingulate cortex showing rough correspondence in terms of cytoarchitecture between human and monkey brains (Figure 1.6). The distribution of myelinated cells is also similar between the corresponding regions of each species (Pandya and Yeterian 1996) and some have observed that the position and connections of the frontal areas are similar across species (Ulying and Van Eden 1990). However, it should also be noted that the anatomy of the monkey cortex differs from the human cortex in terms of the number of granular and agranular layers (Petrides and Pandya 1994). Neubert et al. (2014) used both structural and functional imaging to parcellate both human and monkey prefrontal cortex. Although the authors noted similarities in the cortico-cortical and subcortical connections of prefrontal regions in both species, they noted that the frontal pole in humans showed functional connections to other prefrontal regions and the inferior parietal lobule. By contrast, the frontal pole in the monkey brain showed functional connectivity with temporal regions and the amygdala. The frontal pole is significantly larger in proportion to brain and frontal lobe size in humans when compared with apes, and in humans it has increased connectivity with higher-order association areas when compared with any other primate (Semendeferi et al. 2001). Moreover, the human anterior cingulate cortex is thought to have undergone recent neocortical specialization that allows a

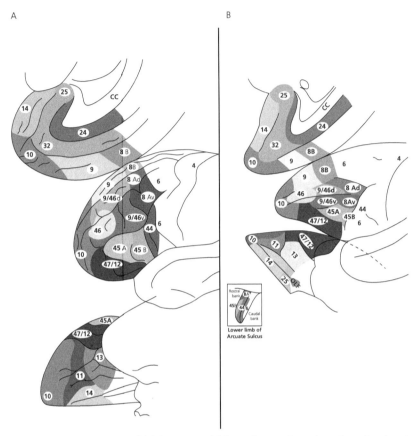

Fig. 1.6 Cytoarchitecture of (A) human and (B) monkey prefrontal cortices. Reprinted from *Cortex*, 48 (1), Michael Petrides, Francesco Tomaiuolo, Edward H. Yeterian, and Deepak N. Pandya, The prefrontal cortex: comparative architectonic organization in the human and the macaque monkey brains, pp. 46–57, Copyright (2012), with permission from Elsevier. Please see color plate section.

type of widespread connectivity with other brain regions that was present only in our most recent ancestors (Allman et al. 2005). When Goulas et al. (2014) constructed whole brain connectomes using diffusion-weighted magnetic resonance imaging (MRI) in humans and the CoCoMac neuroinformatics database (http://cocomac.g-node.org) in macaques, they found that the anterior cingulate cortex showed poor cross-species correspondence. Pandya and Yeterian (1996) have also noted some differences in the functional connectivity from, to, and between prefrontal regions in monkeys and humans. Despite these specific differences, however, the literature suggests that non-human primate models are a good approximation of human architecture.

Indeed, the work of Goldman-Rakic and colleagues with non-human primates was seminal in understanding the specialization of the frontal lobes in terms of working memory and online processing (e.g., Goldman-Rakic 1987, 1996), supporting the findings from lesion studies (e.g., Petrides and Milner 1982) and neuroimaging data (e.g., Owen 1997; D'Esposito et al. 1998; Petrides 2000a). Although Burgess (2011) states that data acquired using one research technique may question the conclusions of another, it is important that researchers and clinicians consider different strands of evidence to determine brain regions that are essential for specific functions.

Fractionation models of frontal lobe functions state that there are distinct frontal processes localized in different subregions within the frontal lobes (Stuss and Benson 1986; Stuss and Alexander 2000; Shallice 2002). Stuss et al. (1995, p. 206) proposed that, "… the frontal lobes (in anatomical terms) or the supervisory system (in cognitive terms) do not function as a simple (inexplicable) homunculus…. The different regions of the frontal lobes provide multiple interacting processes." Norman and Shallice (1980, 1986) propose the Supervisory Attentional System Model, which is a monitoring system that oversees and controls action and deals with novelty in conditions where the routine range of actions is inadequate. In relation to the Supervisory Attentional System Model (Norman and Shallice 1980, 1986), Shallice and Burgess (1996) proposed that there is a variety of subsystems located in the prefrontal cortex which put into operation different processes in these non-routine situations (see also Stuss and Alexander 2007; Shallice and Cooper 2011). Patients with prefrontal lesions might perform poorly due to difficulties in "energization" where they fail to initiate a non-routine task, "task-set" where patients have difficulty switching from a novel to a routine state, "monitoring" where patients are poor at monitoring their task performance and adjusting their behavior if necessary, and, more recently, "attentiveness" where patients care less about performing well on a highly demanding task (Shallice et al. 2008). Authors have argued for the fractionation of these executive processes into multiple components (Shallice and Burgess 1993, 1996; Burgess and Shallice 1994; Baddeley 1996; Burgess 1997; Collette et al. 2006) and more recently for the localization of these different processes in different frontal subregions (Shallice et al. 2008).

Only recently have lesion studies begun to differentiate patients with frontal lesions into separate groups (e.g., Stuss et al. 1995; Shallice and Burgess 1996; Stuss and Alexander 2005) rather than categorizing different frontal impairments under the umbrella of a "frontal lobe syndrome." Nearly 30 years ago, Marcel Mesulam (1986, pp. 321–322) wrote in an editorial,

These quantifiable deficits in standard tests are not always impressive. In fact, some patients with sizable frontal lobe lesions may have routine neurological and neuropsychological examinations that are quite unremarkable. This creates a problem in the assessment of these patients, especially since the behavioral derangements—which sometimes constitute the only salient features—are also too complex to test in the office.... It is not uncommon to find patients with a history of major behavioral difficulties who behave impeccably in the office.... The clinical adage that judgment and complex comportment cannot be tested in the office is particularly pertinent to the evaluation of patients with frontal lobe damage.

At that time, it was difficult to quantify frontal lobe deficits because suitable instruments to identify and quantify the various cognitive impairments associated with frontal lobe damage were not available. Since then, better instruments have been developed.

In 1995, Donald Stuss and colleagues argued that one reason why frontal tests do not typically correlate strongly with one another is because "... they evaluate anatomically and functionally separate systems within the frontal lobes" (Stuss et al. 1995, p. 192). Frontal patients with damage to one of these systems will perform poorly on tasks tapping that system but may perform well on tasks tapping the unaffected systems within the frontal lobes. Indeed, lesions in the dorsolateral prefrontal cortex have been shown to impair tests thought to tap executive processes including mental flexibility, initiation, inhibition, and problem-solving (Milner 1963; Petrides and Milner 1982; Stuss and Benson 1986; Goldman-Rakic 1987), with patients performing poorly on traditional tests assessing executive processes such as the Delayed Response task (Vérin et al. 1993), Recency Judgment (Milner et al. 1991), the Self-Ordered Pointing task (Petrides and Milner 1982), the Stroop task (Vendrell et al. 1995), and the Wisconsin Card Sorting task (Milner 1963). Damage to the orbitofrontal cortex can affect emotional processing and the regulation of social behavior whereby patients might display emotional lability, a lack of impulse and anger control, or produce inappropriate laughing, crying, and sexual behavior (Rolls 1996). Lesions in the orbitofrontal cortex of non-human primates and humans can also impair the ability to alter behavior flexibly in response to a change in stimulus–reward associations (Rudebeck et al. 2008). Patients have been reported to perform poorly on the Reversal Learning Task (Rolls et al. 1994) and the Faux Pas task (Stone et al. 1998). Finally, the anterior cingulate cortex is thought to act as a conflict-monitor when multiple possible behaviors compete for selection (Botvinick 2007) or track environmental volatility and unexpected events (Rushworth and Behrens 2008). Patients with dorsal anterior cingulate lesions have been shown to perform poorly on stimulus–response compatibility tasks such as the Stroop task (Turken and Swick 1999; Stuss et al. 2001b). In summary, recent clinical studies provide support for the existence of dissociations between the effects of damage to different frontal subregions.

1.4 **Fractionation and frontal lobe assessment**

There are several tests used in clinical practice and research worldwide that have been devised to assess the functions subsumed by the frontal lobes of the brain. Such tests have tended to focus on understanding and assessing higher-order control of goal-directed behavior rather than the more emotional and social aspects of frontal lobe functions. Even the "bibles" of neuropsychological assessment do not consider frontal tasks tapping more emotional and social frontal functions (e.g., Strauss et al. 2006; Lezak et al. 2012). A lack of standardized tests may explain why such tasks have not characteristically been included in neuropsychological assessments. Even now, many of these tests are still in an experimental form and do not have normative data, although experimental tasks can be useful in understanding and evaluating the impairments that patients might exhibit (Lezak et al. 2004). Practising clinicians tend to use standardized tests that are readily available and provide normative data. Even if experimental tests are used to further understand the specific cognitive impairment associated with the clinical diagnosis, clinicians would not typically report the results due to the lack of normative data, which might present difficulties in medico-legal cases.

Until recently, assessments of emotional and social frontal functions have relied upon naturalistic observations reported by family members which may point the clinician towards certain difficulties that the patient might have. These observations are particularly useful in the case of frontal patients who might perform well on structured standardized tests of frontal executive abilities in a clinical setting but who perform poorly on more open-ended tasks in a real-life setting (Newcombe 1987; Shallice and Burgess 1991; Capitani 1997). Another method of assessing whether frontal patients have undergone social and emotional changes caused by their brain damage has been self-report and family-report questionnaires. These provide a more structured method of identifying patient difficulties than naturalistic observations. However, frontal patients who lack insight into their condition may fail to recognize their impairments; as the face validity of these questionnaires is often evident, this may lead relatives to deny the presence of some behavioral disabilities in their family member, even when certain behaviors are evident during the testing session. Moreover, when self- and family-report questionnaires are completed, these can provide conflicting information and so care has to be taken when considering whether they are reliable or valid guides to an individual's ability. Hence, there has been a move for clinicians and researchers to devise experimental tasks assessing more social and emotional aspects of frontal lobe function, although few provide normative data as yet (e.g., Judgment of Preference task, Moral Decision-Making, Reading the Mind in the Eyes, Ultimatum Game).

It is important that clinicians be aware that different frontal tasks might tap processes associated with distinct regions of the frontal lobes. If a neuropsychological assessment only includes traditional frontal executive measures, as has typically been the case in the past, it might be concluded that a patient performing within normal limits on those tasks does not have frontal lobe dysfunction. Yet, a patient's relatives may still complain that the patient performs poorly on everyday tasks that involve emotional and social processing or multi-tasking (Burgess et al. 2009). There are several single case reports of patients as well as clinical groups, including frontotemporal dementia (Lough et al. 2001; Gregory et al. 2002) and amyotrophic lateral sclerosis (Girardi et al. 2011), showing a dissociation between impaired social processing and intact executive function (Eslinger and Damasio 1985; Shallice and Burgess 1991; Brazzelli et al. 1994; Rolls et al. 1994). There are also examples of patients in the literature showing the opposite dissociation of intact social and emotional processing but impaired executive abilities (e.g., Bechara et al. 1998). Diagnosis of the nature of the frontal lobe involvement in these patients can be achieved through the appropriate neuropsychological assessment, which includes a small number of tasks thought to tap the distinct frontal subregions. By doing so, the assessment will be more focused and less time-consuming, and provide a thorough account of the nature of the frontal deficit and its effect on an individual's daily living. Cubelli et al. (in press) maintain that the job of the neuropsychologist is to design and refine the clinical assessment, to interpret the findings, and to disentangle the patient's observed pattern of performance; in other words, examining a patient is a skilled and time-consuming task, which requires specific and interdisciplinary competence and expertise. Without diagnostic interpretation, tests results are void. Cubelli and Della Sala (2011) highlight that a clinical neuropsychological assessment should include four steps: (1) an interview to obtain a personal and clinical history; (2) a concise screening battery; (3) a full-scale neuropsychological examination to diagnose the gross clinical syndrome (e.g., dysexecutive syndrome, episodic amnesia, Wernicke's aphasia); and finally (4) experimental tests to determine the specific cognitive impairment associated with the clinical syndrome. Therefore, it is important for clinicians and researchers to be made aware of the functions assessed by individual frontal tests and to understand which frontal regions might be impaired in their patient groups.

Some extensive manuals of neuropsychological tests have been published, encompassing various cognitive domains (Strauss et al. 2006; Lezak et al. 2012). Such compendiums supply useful descriptions of how to administer neuropsychological tests and to which populations, including scoring instructions and copies of the procedure. However, whereas they clearly acknowledge that executive functions can be subdivided into different higher-order processes (e.g., planning, initiation, inhibition, flexibility), the manuals largely neglect the issue of localization within the frontal lobes and simply include a chapter discussing "executive function." Moreover, frontal tasks assessing more social and emotional processing are not discussed. It has become evident that the frontal lobes cannot simply be considered in terms of executive abilities but also in terms of other more social and emotional type tasks, goal neglect, and multi-tasking. In this book, the influence of focal frontal lesions on test performance on the wide array of tasks purporting to tap the frontal region and the regions of activation determined through neuroimaging will be discussed. The aim is to link each test to the best possible evidence of what subregions within the frontal lobe (and which cognitive processes) the tests really tackle. Clinicians or researchers wanting to use a given test will have the opportunity to examine what this test is thought to assess, and select the best instrument for their purposes.

Some of the tests reviewed here are published tests that can be purchased from publishers and include normative data. Others, however, are more experimental in nature and may be available only from the author directly. We appreciate that there are no behavioral measures that can exclusively tap the functioning of one region alone. However, a review of the current literature suggests that tasks do exist which may be more sensitive to the dysfunction of one frontal region than another, though how best to quantify the behavioral sequelae of region-specific insult within the frontal lobes is the subject of ongoing debate. Only those frontal tests with evidence from lesion and neuroimaging studies to support the involvement of particular frontal subregions have been considered. This means that only neuropsychological studies involving patients with focal frontal lesions (e.g., tumors, stroke) or studies examining structural brain changes in neurodegenerative diseases will be considered, as they allow us to conclude that the structure damaged by the lesion is necessary for performing that task.

One of the difficulties with reviewing the frontal lobe test literature is that different versions of the same task may exist. For example, the Tower tests refer to a group of tests including the Tower of London (Shallice 1982) and its several versions (e.g., Allamanno et al. 1987), Tower of Hanoi (Byrnes and Spitz 1977), the Stockings of Cambridge subtest from the Cambridge Neuropsychological Test Automated Battery (Robbins et al. 1994), and the Tower subtest from the Delis–Kaplin Executive Function System (Delis et al. 2001). While the overall processes involved in successfully performing the Tower tests are likely to overlap, different versions of the same test may vary in terms of the stimuli presented, rules the participants must follow, or indices of performance calculated. Even small differences in the administration and scoring of a test might result in differences in terms of the localization of the processes associated with performing those tests (Gilhooly et al. 1999, 2002; Phillips et al. 1999, 2003). Therefore, within each test summary, multiple versions of the same test will be described under the same heading, with the commonalties and differences between the versions of the test discussed.

Different test batteries are also available within the clinical psychology literature, allowing clinicians to create a profile of patients' strengths and weaknesses in terms of their frontal lobe abilities. For example, the Delis–Kaplan Executive Function System (Delis et al. 2001) was devised to allow clinicians to assess executive abilities such as mental flexibility, initiation, and problem-solving within the same battery of tests. Similarly, the Cambridge Neuropsychological Test Automated Battery (Robbins et al. 1994) is a computerized set of neuropsychological tests developed to examine aspects of cognition including executive abilities. The Behavioral Assessment of the Dysexecutive Syndrome (Wilson et al. 1996) was devised to assess executive dysfunction in patients with frontal lobe lesions in a way that might generalize on to performance in the real world, and the INECO Frontal Screening is a brief tool to assess executive abilities in neurodegenerative diseases (Torralva et al. 2009a). The Frontal Assessment Battery (Dubois et al. 2000) was devised to identify neurodegenerative diseases with frontal involvement and the Executive and Social Cognition Battery (Torralva et al. 2009b) was devised to identify deficits in executive abilities and social cognition in early behavioral variant frontotemporal dementia. More recently, the Rotman–Baycrest Battery to Investigate Attention (Stuss et al. 2005) was developed to probe levels of attention and cognitive control. Whereas we acknowledge that such test batteries exist, the aim of this book is to examine relationships between the processes underlying specific frontal tests and localization of these processes within frontal subregions. It is difficult to provide evidence of localization of an entire test battery. In such cases, individual components of the test battery will be discussed when they correspond with an overall test such as the Tower Tests from the Delis–Kaplin Executive Function System.

It may also be the case that some of the frontal tests reviewed could be categorized as assessing more than one frontal-related function. Therefore, a test could easily be considered under multiple headings. For example, the Hayling Sentence Completion test could be considered a test of initiation and inhibition *and* of mental flexibility (T. Shallice, personal communication). In this instance, a test is related to the heading associated with the cognitive ability that the authors/manual claim it was initially devised to assess. However, where appropriate, the test description will discuss related frontal processes associated with performing that task.

1.5 **Classification of frontal lobe subregions**

In terms of the localization of frontal processes, the frontal subregions will be described in terms of the dorsolateral prefrontal cortex (BAs 9 and 46), the orbitofrontal cortex (BAs 11, 12, 13, 14, and 47) and the anterior cingulate cortex (BAs 24, 25, 32, and 33). The term "ventromedial" prefrontal cortex is frequently used in the neuropsychology literature to refer to both orbital and medial frontal regions, although this region is often not explicitly defined in terms of Brodmann's areas. Therefore, the term ventromedial prefrontal cortex will be used to refer to the orbitofrontal cortex and ventral portions of the anterior cingulate cortex. The dorsal/ventral demarcation within the anterior cingulate is dorsal to the genu of the corpus callosum (after Bush et al. 2000; Beckmann et al. 2009; Van Overwalle 2009). In addition, whereas the frontal pole is often categorized together with the ventromedial prefrontal cortex, it has been associated with performance on a wide variety of tasks including multi-tasking and prospective memory (for reviews see Burgess et al. 2005 and Gilbert et al. 2006). Consequently, the frontal pole will be considered separately to provide a clearer overall picture of the localization of processes within the frontal lobes. See Figure 1.7 for the frontal subregions.

1.6 **Issues of frontal lobe assessment**

One difficulty with investigating fractionation of frontal lobe functions is that the terms "frontal" and "executive" are used interchangeably in the literature, and yet these terms are not synonymous (Stuss 2006). Baddeley (1996) proposed that the frontal lobes are a possible substrate for the executive control of cognitive functions, although he identifies that there are problems with using cognitive accounts to support arguments about localization. Whereas the frontal lobes are likely to be where executive abilities are best represented, executive functions do not necessarily relate to anatomical structure

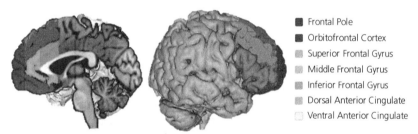

- Frontal Pole
- Orbitofrontal Cortex
- Superior Frontal Gyrus
- Middle Frontal Gyrus
- Inferior Frontal Gyrus
- Dorsal Anterior Cingulate
- Ventral Anterior Cingulate

Fig. 1.7 Subdivision of the frontal lobes. Please see color plate section.

and executive tests are somewhat unreliable diagnostic tools for determining frontal lobe damage (Phillips 1997; Rabbitt 1997). Clinicians know how often relatives complain of dramatic behavioral changes in frontal patients which off-the-shelf tests fail to identify. There are studies in the literature that have reported severely disturbed frontal patients who perform well on these tests (Eslinger and Damasio 1985; Shallice and Burgess 1991; Brazzelli et al. 1994). There are also non-frontal patients who perform poorly on executive tests (Anderson et al. 1991; Reitan and Wolfson 1994). Task purity is a particular problem for executive tests, as performance on these measures may involve cognitive functions dependent on brain regions other than the frontal lobes (Burgess 1997; Rabbitt 1997). As the frontal lobes form neural circuits with several other regions of the brain, such as the posterior association cortex, the limbic and subcortical structures (Petrides 1994; Rolls 1996, 1999), extra frontal damage may produce similar deficits to those brought about by frontal lobe lesions. In other instances, non-frontal lesions may disrupt functions distinct from frontal lobe functions but which are also responsible for successful performance on executive tasks (Mayes and Daum 1997). Burgess (1997) argues that due to the complexity of executive measures, there will always be additional non-frontal processes involved in the performance of such tasks. Given that there are many different ways of performing or indeed failing frontal tasks, poor performance on such tasks may say little about a patient's frontal abilities and more about other cognitive abilities such as their processing speed, visual acuity, sustained attention etc. Careful consideration of task purity is important when evaluating and interpreting performance on tasks thought to tap frontal lobe functions.

Lesion studies involving frontal patients also have the difficulty that there are no clinical conditions in which the damage is confined to the frontal lobes, and different etiologies result in frontal damage predominantly involving different subregions (Stuss et al. 1995; Stuss and Alexander 2009). For example, dorsolateral prefrontal lesions are typically due to unilateral infarctions or traumatic brain injury, whereas more medial lesions tend to be more mixed in their etiology and bilateral in nature. Orbitofrontal lesions are often due to the rupture of an anterior communicating artery aneurysm and are more focal. Therefore, when comparing different subgroups, patients' etiologies may differ and the cognitive deficits reported may be related to etiology rather than lesion location, although this is less likely if the patients are in the chronic rather than the acute stage (Alexander et al. 2005). It should also be pointed out that precise localization of lesions within frontal regions may be confounded in cross-study (or even cross-participant) comparison. As frequently occurs in lesion studies, the damaged site is transferred into standard coordinates[1] which are not sympathetic to the individual differences in gyrification and are therefore less likely to be an accurate indicator of underlying anatomical and functional significance (Uylings et al. 2005; Devlin and Poldrack 2007; Cox et al. 2014). In functional neuroimaging or whole-brain methods of structural analysis (e.g., voxel-based morphometry), co-registration of participants' brains is also employed to enable comparison. Among relatively small regions that share multiple boundaries, or in structures such as the anterior cingulate cortex whose trajectory is primarily posterior to anterior and whose underlying structure and connectivity alters along its course (Paus et al. 1993; Beckmann et al. 2009), even small variations in the spatial relationship between the lesion or focus of activation and the underlying morphological features can be introduced by co-registration. Thus, the noise introduced by the potentially inconsistent classification of frontal regions could well contribute to inconsistencies in the behavioral profiles reported in relation to lesion site, or loci of functional activation. Finally, the extent to which the white matter tracts beneath the frontal gyri are damaged is likely to vary between studies, but this is not always alluded to in studies themselves. This is partially due to limitations in accurately identifying which tracts may be affected, yet damage to long-range white matter connections is likely to elicit very different types of behavioral sequelae compared to cortical lesion alone (Brotis et al. 2009). Therefore, it is important to bear in mind that these factors might contribute to discrepant findings among lesion and functional imaging studies.

Another important consideration when describing frontal tests is the effect of healthy adult aging on performance on these tasks. The frontal region of the brain is particularly susceptible to the effects of age; its gross volume, cortex (volume and thickness) and white matter (volume and tract-based measure of integrity) show disproportionate age-related decreases compared with other parts of the brain (Sullivan and Pfefferbaum 2007; Driscoll et al. 2009; Fjell

---

[1] Note that the method of transfer can also differ between reports. Because the lesioned region no longer exists (and pre-lesion scans very rarely exist), assumptions must be made about the spatial characteristics of the area that has been damaged. Most commonly the lesions are traced directly onto a template brain or onto the contralateral hemisphere of the same participant. The former introduces variance due to an inevitable discord between the micro and macro topographical variance between the subject and template, whereas the latter is more likely to have far more commonality and therefore will more accurately represent the characteristics of the missing regions. However, given that results from the latter method will be registered to a template at a later stage for the purposes of inter-subject comparison (and thus introduce similar problems of concordance), it is unclear precisely how much of a benefit this method is.

et al. 2009; Burzynska et al. 2011). This deterioration of the frontal lobes and their connectivity is thought by some to be responsible for many age-related cognitive changes (Moscovitch and Winocur 1995; O'Sullivan et al. 2001; MacPherson et al. 2002). Age has been reported to affect the structure of different frontal subregions differentially, though studies do not necessarily agree on which are most and least affected (Resnick et al. 2003; Grieve et al. 2005; Raz et al. 2010). Several reports suggest that the lateral frontal lobe exhibits greater volumetric decrease with age than other frontal regions (Grieve et al. 2005; Raz et al. 2005; Driscoll et al. 2009; Fjell et al. 2009; Burzynska et al. 2011), though others identify predominantly orbital and medial frontal decline (Resnick et al. 2003).

It is logical to assume that age-related decrements in frontal subregions will also have a functional impact. Whereas the frontal regions are by no means the only brain areas to exhibit decline (which then contribute to cognitive performance), there have been several reports that functions thought to be subserved by the dorsolateral prefrontal cortex exhibit decline more rapidly than those that rely on the orbitofrontal cortex, which remain relatively unchanged, or even improve (Happé et al. 1998; MacPherson et al. 2002; Maylor et al. 2002; Keightley et al. 2006). However, others have identified age-related cognitive decline in both tasks tapping the orbitofrontal cortex and dorsolateral prefrontal cortex (Lamar and Resnick 2004; Resnick et al. 2007). A recent review suggests that there is at least some age-related decline in social cognition (an ability generally associated with the orbitofrontal cortex), but that this decline appears to be at least partially independent of a decline in general cognitive function and executive abilities (primarily thought to tap the dorsolateral prefrontal cortex; Kemp et al. 2012). Thus, it does not appear that the frontal lobes unitarily decline with age and it is important for clinicians to be aware of the frontal tasks that do show age effects. This booklet will therefore also include a discussion of the evidence that some frontal tests are sensitive to cognitive aging but not others (MacPherson et al. 2002; Phillips et al. 2002b).

It is also important to note that low socio-cultural background, including level of education, can influence performance on neuropsychological assessments (Della Sala et al. 1992, 1995; Capitani et al. 1988, 1992). Individuals with higher levels of education score higher on most neuropsychological tests (Spinnler and Tognoni 1987; Ardila et al. 1989; Rosselli et al. 1990; Ostrosky et al. 1999) and even a difference of only one or two years of education may affect how an individual performs (Ostrosky-Solis et al. 1998). In terms of assessing frontal executive dysfunction, associations between education level and performance on tests such as the Cognitive Estimation task (e.g., Della Sala et al. 2003; MacPherson et al. 2014), Stroop Test (e.g., Van der Elst et al. 2006a), verbal fluency (Phillips et al. 1996; Tombaugh et al. 1999; Meguro et al. 2001; Dursun et al. 2002; Machado et al. 2009), and the Wisconsin Card Sorting Test (e.g., Boone et al. 1993; Heaton et al. 1993; Laiacona et al. 2000; MacPherson and Della Sala 2001) have been found. Therefore, when administering the tests included in this book as part of a clinical assessment, it is important to consider an individual's level of education before concluding that they might have frontal executive impairment. In particular, populations from developing countries who are poorly educated present a challenge for assessing frontal executive dysfunction, and normative data from such populations are required.

At the end of each test section, tables summarizing the findings from the main text are provided. First, there is a table including the patient and lesion studies that have investigated localization of the processes within the frontal subregions. The list of Brodmann's areas includes all those that were damaged in the patients assessed on that test, including those that did not demonstrate impairments. Second, there is a table summarizing the findings from neuro-imaging studies. Finally, the studies that have examined whether healthy adult aging influences performance on the test are listed. These tables are created simply as a handy guide to allow clinicians and researchers to have a brief overview of the tasks, but they come with certain caveats. For example, different studies label frontal regions differently (e.g., the ventromedial prefrontal cortex) and different image registration algorithms have been used for the functional MRI data. Therefore, we recommend that theses tables be treated as a companion to the text rather than vice versa.

When reviewing the frontal lobe literature, it seems difficult to conceive of the frontal lobes as a single entity subserving a unitary function. Therefore, the tests that clinicians and researchers include in their clinical and experimental work to assess frontal lobe function should tap the various frontal subregions. Existing neuropsychological assessment textbooks do not discuss localization of frontal processes or some of the more recent tests that assess social and emotional aspects of frontal lobe function; a review of the frontal lobe test literature is timely.

Chapter 2

Abstraction

2.1 Brixton Spatial Anticipation Test

2.1.1 Task description

The Brixton Spatial Anticipation Test (Burgess and Shallice 1996a) is a rule-detection task comprising a series of 56 cards, presented to the participant in turn. Each card contains 10 circles numbered in sequence in a 2 × 5 arrangement. One of the circles is filled whereas the remaining nine circles are unfilled (see Figure 2.1). The location of the filled circle changes systematically from card to card based on a simple rule. The goal is to identify the current rule (based on the previously presented cards) in order to predict the location of the filled circle on the next card. Over the course of the test, there are nine rules governing the change in position of the filled circle. Each rule operates for three to eight consecutive cards before switching to a different rule so that rule changes cannot be easily anticipated. For example, the filled circle might begin at position 5, then move to position 6, then to 7, and so on. After several cards following this pattern, the filled circle might instead begin to alternate between two positions over several consecutive cards, or stay in the same location over several cards.

The total number of errors is usually used as the main outcome variable. The raw total number of errors can also be converted into a scaled score of between 1 and 10, where a higher scaled score represents fewer errors (e.g., those who make between zero and seven total errors will receive a scaled score of 10, whereas those who make more than 31 errors will receive a scaled score of 1). Errors arise when participants do not correctly identify the next position in the sequence. However, the initial score (which must be a guess) is not scored, and trials on which the rule changes are scored as correct if the participant correctly applies a previously contingent rule (as they have no way of knowing that the rule is about to change). The errors that participants make can also be subdivided into three types: (1) perseverative errors (e.g., continually selecting the same incorrect response); (2) following rules that were previously relevant but are now no longer so; and (3) bizarre responses or guesses (where there is no clear underlying logic or justification for a participant's response).

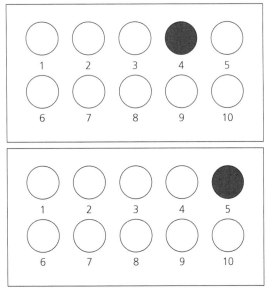

Fig. 2.1 Illustration of a sequential rule (x + 1) in the Brixton Spatial Anticipation Test. In this example, the participant sees circle 4 colored blue on the first page (upper) and then has to work out where the colored circle will appear on the next page (lower). Please see color plate section.

2.1.2 **Patient and lesion studies**

When comparing the performance of patients with frontal lesions to those with posterior lesions and healthy control participants, Burgess and Shallice (1996a) found that the frontal group made significantly more overall errors than both other groups. Additionally, those with posterior lesions did not make significantly more errors than controls. Reverberi et al. (2005a) administered the Brixton Spatial Anticipation Test to 40 patients with focal frontal lesions and 43 healthy controls. They found that those with left frontal lesions made significantly more errors than those with right frontal lesions and the control group. However, the authors also found that a significantly greater proportion of patients with right lateral lesions attained a "stay-the-same" rule (where the filled circle does not shift position for six cards) when compared to controls (reported in Reverberi et al., 2005b, Appendix 1).[1] There was also a trend

---

[1] This fits with the theory that the dorsolateral prefrontal cortex facilitates problem-solving by 'shaping the response space'. That is, it narrows down our search for possible solutions to a problem by imposing constraints on our initial representation of a problem. One such constraint—the tautology constraint—is thought initially to *exclude* possible solutions involving repetition. Though a generally useful assumption, normal individuals are consequently less able quickly to identify tautological solutions, such as the Brixton

for frontal patients with left lateral lesions to outperform controls on this specific rule, but the difference did not reach significance.

By contrast with those studies above which intimate frontal lobe involvement in the Brixton Spatial Anticipation Test, Andrés and Van der Linden (2001) reported that the performance of a group of frontal patients did not significantly differ from healthy controls in terms of total errors, or different error types. They also found no effect of lesion laterality, though their sample sizes were small (left, $n = 6$; right, $n = 4$) and both groups' lesions were not confined to a specific locus within the frontal lobes, instead appearing relatively diffuse.

Posterior lesions, on the other hand, do not appear to impair performance on the Brixton Spatial Anticipation Test. For example, patient P36 (Cubelli et al. 2011) suffered a left middle cerebral artery stroke which resulted in left brain damage in the posterior frontal lobes, the temporal and parietal lobes, insula, and part of the putamen. P36 achieved a scaled score of 4 out of a possible 10, which is classed as low–normal on the Brixton Spatial Anticipation Test. Moreover, a group of patients with temporal lobe epilepsy (and associated amygdala damage) did not show an impairment on the Brixton Spatial Anticipation Test compared to healthy controls either prior to, or following, neurosurgery for an anterior temporal lobe resection (Shaw et al. 2007).

Research concerning the effect of lesions within specific frontal subregions on Brixton Spatial Anticipation Test scores (Table 2.1) suggests that damage to the orbital aspect of the frontal lobe does not impair performance. Mitchell et al. (2006) reported two patients, DK and CL, who both suffered traumatic brain injury resulting in orbitofrontal damage, and yet they performed within normal limits on the Brixton Spatial Anticipation Test. In a different study, Kapur et al. (2009) found no impairment on the Brixton Spatial Anticipation Test for patient GS, who had a self-inflicted transoral gunshot wound to the orbitofrontal cortex. Similarly, two patients with cingulate lesions due to the resection of prefrontal gliomas showed no impairment on the Brixton Spatial Anticipation Test compared to normative data (Baird et al. 2006), though it should be noted that both patients' lesions were in no way restricted to the anterior cingulate cortex.[2] Likewise, Telling et al. (2010) report the Brixton Spatial Anticipation Test scores of a series of patients with either

circle remaining in the same position for multiple cards. Reverberi et al. (2005b) supplies a discussion and an additional example of dorsolateral prefrontal patients outperforming controls on a problem related to the tautology constraint.

[2] Patient 1 had right-sided damage to regions including the anterior cingulate cortex toward the frontal pole, anterior superior frontal gyrus, anterior corpus callosum, supplementary motor area and some frontal white matter. Patient 2 had left-sided damage including anterior cingulate cortex, left medial, superior and middle frontal gyri, orbitofrontal cortex, medial thalamus, insula and hippocampus.

Table 2.1 Brixton Spatial Anticipation Test: Patient and lesion studies

Study	n	Patient/ Control Groups	Study type	Brodmann Areas	FP	DL	OF	ACC
Critchley et al. (2003)	3	ACC	Lesion	–				X
Baird et al. (2006)	2	ACC	Lesion	8, 11, 12, 24, 25, 32			X	X
Mitchell et al. (2006)	2; 13	OF; HA	Lesion				X	
Kapur et al. (2009)	1; 5	OF; HA	Lesion	8, 24, 25, 32			X	
Telling et al. (2010)	6; 3; 9	DL; VM; HA	Lesion	8, 24, 25, 32		✓	X	

FP = frontal pole; DL = dorsolateral prefrontal cortex; OF = orbitofrontal cortex; ACC = anterior cingulate cortex; HA = healthy adults; VM = ventromedial prefrontal cortex; ✓ = frontal region damaged and impairment found; X = frontal region damaged but no impairment.

lateral ($n = 6$) or bilateral medial ($n = 3$) lesions. Patients with damage including the right lateral frontal lobe (patients JQ, AS, PW, and FK) performed either below or at the cut-off, but patients with damage mainly to the temporal lobes (SP and GA) or to the left frontolateral (DS) or focal right frontolateral region (TT: right middle frontal gyrus) showed no impairment. However, the diffuse involvement of several brain regions in each patient (many of which involve multiple lobes and all but one that involve multiple subregions) makes these data difficult to interpret with respect to regional frontal localization of function. A similar criticism may be leveled at another study in which three patients with anterior cingulate lesions were tested on the Brixton Spatial Anticipation Test (Critchley et al. 2003). Only patient 1 showed impaired task performance compared with healthy controls, but her bilateral anterior cingulate lesion also extended to the orbital and lateral frontal cortical and white matter areas.

2.1.3 Neuroimaging studies

To our knowledge, only one study has investigated the performance of healthy individuals performing the Brixton Spatial Anticipation Test using functional neuroimaging (Table 2.2). Crescentini et al. (2011) employed functional magnetic resonance imaging (fMRI) to investigate the neuroanatomy of the processes involved in inductive reasoning; specifically rule search and rule following. They administered a computerized version of the Brixton Spatial Anticipation Test to 26 healthy participants, and categorized their responses either as those pertaining to rule search or as rule following (once the rule had been acquired). These could

Table 2.2 Brixton Spatial Anticipation Test: Neuroimaging studies

Study	n	Patient/ Control Groups	Study type	Stimuli	Brodmann Areas	FP	DL	OF	ACC
Crescentini et al. (2011)	26	HA	fMRI	Letters	6, 8, 9, 45, 46	✓			

FP = frontal pole; DL = dorsolateral prefrontal cortex; OF = orbitofrontal cortex; ACC = anterior cingulate cortex; HA = healthy adults; fMRI = functional magnetic resonance imaging; ✓ = frontal region involved.

equally be interpreted as phases of incorrect and correct performance. Crescentini et al. (2011) reported significant blood oxygen level-dependent (BOLD) activity in the mid-dorsolateral prefrontal cortex during rule search, which remained until the rule had been acquired. By contrast, the rule-following phase was associated with temporal, motor, and medial/anterior prefrontal activity, though the authors also noted sustained activity in the frontal pole during both the rule-search and rule-following phases until a rule became familiar. The authors therefore concluded that the dorsolateral prefrontal cortex is implicated in inductive reasoning during the Brixton Spatial Anticipation Test, whereas a wider network of medial frontal and non-frontal areas take over as soon as the rule has been identified. The consistent frontopolar activity reported in this study during both phases concurs with associations made elsewhere between frontal pole activity and the monitoring and integration of internal subgoals while maintaining information in working memory (e.g., Braver and Bongiolatti 2002; Orr and Banich 2013).

2.1.4 **Aging studies**

Andrés and Van der Linden (2000) compared the performance of older ($n = 48$; mean age = 65 years) and younger ($n = 47$; mean age = 23 years) adults on the Brixton Spatial Anticipation Test (Table 2.3). The older group made significantly more errors than the younger group, but when the error types were considered separately, they found no age effect. The group difference in the total number of errors remained when the authors controlled for processing speed abilities (measured using a basic color-naming task). However, this finding is not surprising as the Brixton Spatial Anticipation Test is not timed. The Brixton Spatial Anticipation Test has also been administered to a larger group of 441 healthy older individuals, aged 53–90 years (Bielak et al. 2006). Older age, less education, and gender (being female) were significantly associated with higher total error rates, and these factors uniquely accounted for 11%, 2%, and 1% respectively of the error variance on the Brixton Spatial Anticipation Test. Van den Berg et al. (2009) provided a series of norms adjusted for age and education for a group of older individuals ($n = 283$ aged between 55 and 92 years) together with patient groups including stroke ($n = 106$),

Table 2.3 Brixton Spatial Anticipation Test: Aging studies

Study	n	Participant age groups (years)	Study type	Age effect
Andrés and Van der Linden (2000)	47; 48	Younger, mean = 22.8; older, mean = 65.0	Cross-sectional (behavioral)	✓
Beliak et al. (2006)	441	53–90	Cross-sectional (behavioral)	✓
Geerlings et al. (2009)	522	Mean = 57.0	Cross-sectional (behavioral)	✓
Van den Berg et al. (2009)	283	55–92	Cross-sectional (behavioral)	✓

✓ = age effect found; X = age effect not found

diabetes mellitus ($n = 376$), mild cognitive impairment/early dementia ($n = 70$), psychiatric disorders ($n = 63$), and Korsakoff's syndrome ($n = 41$). Within the healthy older group, the authors reported a significant effect of age, education, and IQ, but not gender, on the total number of task errors made. Van den Berg et al. (2009) go on to provide an equation to calculate the expected total score on the Brixton Spatial Anticipation Test based on age and education, and create a percentile distribution table for reference. All patient groups except for those with mild cognitive impairment/dementia and diabetes performed more poorly than the healthy older control group on the Brixton Spatial Anticipation Test.

Finally, Geerlings et al. (2009) investigated the relationship between white matter lesions and cognitive performance (including the Brixton Spatial Anticipation Test) in a cross-sectional analysis of 522 patients with atherosclerotic disease (mean age = 57 years; SD = 10 years). They found that greater age-related white matter lesion volume was associated with poorer performance on the Brixton Spatial Anticipation Test even when controlling for age, sex, education, and crystallized intelligence (Geerlings et al. 2009).

2.1.5 Summary

There are relatively few data regarding the neural underpinnings of the Brixton Spatial Anticipation Test. The extant lesion and fMRI data might suggest that the dorsolateral prefrontal cortex is at least involved in, if not necessary for, the ability to search for and acquire the appropriate rule, though the data supporting the role of this region to the exclusion of other frontal subregions is scarce and difficult to interpret. There has also been some interesting preliminary work examining the possible hemispheric lateralization of function in the dorsolateral prefrontal cortex, but replications and well-powered studies using diverse groups of lesion patients are lacking. In addition, the fact that lesions typically involve both cortical and white matter damage potentially confounds inferences about the frontal local-ization of Brixton Spatial Anticipation Test performance, given that age-related white matter damage is related to test score. On a practical note, it is worth men-tioning that the lesion patients evaluated by Burgess and Shallice (1996a) had a higher than average estimate of premorbid IQ. Whereas the normative data pro-vided in the Thames Valley Test Company manual of this test have been statisti-cally adjusted for, the suitability of this test for patients with a lower-than-average IQ is unclear. Age effects associated with Brixton Spatial Anticipation Test perfor-mance have been consistently reported, with older participants making fewer cor-rect responses. These deficits in performance may be partially due to age-related white matter damage (Geerlings et al. 2009), but the absence of data combining white matter and cortical data makes it impossible to know to what degree these different cerebral characteristics contribute uniquely to age-related decline in Brixton Spatial Anticipation Test performance.

2.2 Proverb Interpretation Task

2.2.1 Task description

The Proverb Interpretation Task was originally devised to assess abstract lan-guage processing (Gorham 1956) and is now one of the subtests included in the

---

Box 2.1 Adapted Proverb Interpretation Test

1. Don't cry over spilt milk
2. Rome wasn't built in a day.
3. Where there's a will there's a way.
4. Strike while the iron is hot.
5. The grass is always greener on the other side.
6. Let sleeping dogs lie.
7. All that glitters is not gold.
8. Too many cooks spoil the broth.

Reproduced from Patrick Murphy, Tim Shallice, Gail Robinson, Sarah E. MacPherson, Martha Turner, Katherine Woollett, Marco Bozzali, and Lisa Cipolotti, Impairments in proverb interpretation following focal frontal lobe lesions. *Neuropsychologia*, 51(11), pp. 2075–2086, Appendix B, http://dx.doi.org/10.1016/j. neuropsychologia.2013.06.029. Copyright © 2013 Patrick Murphy, Tim Shallice, Gail Robinson, Sarah E. MacPherson, Martha Turner, Katherine Woollett, Marco Bozzali, and Lisa Cipolotti. Creative Commons Attribution Non Commercial License.

Delis–Kaplan Executive Functions System (D-KEFS) battery (Delis et al. 2001). It includes eight familiar sayings that convey widely known facts or social rules for the country in which it is administered (see Box 2.1 for examples). The proverbs are read aloud to the participant (e.g., "Too many cooks spoil the broth") and participants should either provide an oral explanation of the proverb without help or prompts (free inquiry) or choose the best meaning of the proverb from a number of alternatives (multiple choice). In the D-KEFS version of the task, participants perform both the free inquiry followed by the multiple-choice version of the task. The Proverb Interpretation Task assesses the ability to interpret proverbs in an abstract rather than literal (concrete) way as the meaning of proverbs should be generalizable to more situations than the specific situation described in the proverb (Delis et al. 2001). In the case of, "Too many cooks spoil the broth," an abstract understanding might be that too many people (cooks) involved in performing the same task might ruin it (spoil the broth). A more literal explanation not applying to all situations might be that one person is better at making soup or cooking than several people. In the multiple-choice version of the Proverb Interpretation Task, the alternatives typically include (with examples taken from the D-KEFS): (1) the correct, abstract explanation (e.g., "A plan can go wrong when a lot of people are involved"); (2) a correct but concrete explanation (e.g., "One person can make a meal better than ten"); (3) a phonemically analogous response (e.g., "Many cooks think too many spices spoil the soup"); and (4) an unrelated metaphor (e.g., "A penny saved is a penny earned"). The tendency to produce more concrete or literal explanations of proverbs rather than abstract ones is thought to be due to impairments in higher-order executive processes, as poor performance on the Proverb Interpretation Task has been associated with poor performance on other measures of frontal executive function such as verbal fluency, the Stroop Task, and the Trail Making Task (Albert et al. 1990; Uekermann et al. 2008). The Proverb Interpretation Task from the D-KEFS is a standardized test providing clinicians with normative data to assess whether patients are impaired in terms of their verbal abstraction abilities.

2.2.2 Patient and lesion studies

Whereas the Proverb Interpretation Task is commonly used as an assessment tool in clinical practice, few studies have examined the involvement of the frontal lobes in the ability to interpret proverbs. Yet, as early as the 1920s, Zeigarnik (1927) reported that patients with frontal lobe lesions were poor at explaining the meaning of proverbs (cited in Luria 1966). Benton (1968) demonstrated that bilateral frontal lesions resulted in significantly poorer proverb interpretation scores than unilateral frontal lesions. Patients with unilateral left and right frontal lesions did not significantly differ from one another. In terms of scoring below the cut-off for normal Proverb Interpretation Task performance, Benton (1968) reported that 20% of patients with left unilateral frontal lesions, 25% of patients with right unilateral frontal lesions, and 70% of patients with bilateral frontal lesions, were impaired. Roca et al. (2010) administered the Proverb Interpretation Task to 15 frontal patients with lesions mainly due to tumor resection or cerebrovascular disease and 25 healthy controls. Their frontal group produced significantly poorer explanations on the three-item free-inquiry version of the Proverb Interpretation Task (Hodges 1994) compared to the healthy controls. Even when the authors controlled for fluid intelligence, the significant difference between the groups remained, suggesting that intellectual abilities cannot fully explain proverb interpretation in frontal patients.

Few studies have examined the localization of the processes within the frontal lobes that underlie Proverb Interpretation Task performance (Table 2.4). Roca et al. (2010) administered a battery of frontal tests to 21 frontal patients subdivided into those with superior medial ($n = 2$), inferior medial ($n = 3$), left lateral ($n = 5$), right lateral ($n = 8$), and multiple lesions ($n = 3$). Only 15 of those patients were assessed on the Proverb Interpretation Task and no significant difference between the frontal subgroups was found. However, it was not clear to which frontal subgroups these 15 patients belonged, and the authors acknowledged that their patient subgroups were small. Roca et al. (2010) then conducted further lesion overlap analysis with the six frontal patients who had performed most poorly across a group of frontal tests, which included the Proverb Interpretation Task, and found that lesion-related deficits were not entirely explained by a loss of intelligence. Lesions to the anterior frontal

Table 2.4 Proverb Interpretation Task: Patient and lesion studies

Study	n	Patient/ Control Groups	Study type	Task type	Brodmann Areas	FP	DL	OF	ACC
Keifer (2010)	14; 14; 18	VM; DL; NF	Lesion	D-KEFS	–		✓		
Roca et al. (2010)	21; 25	FL; HA	Lesion	Hodges (1994)	10	✓			
Murphy et al. (2013)	17; 16; 13; 52	M; LL; RL; HA	Lesion	D-KEFS	6, 8, 9, 10, 23, 24, 32, 33, 44, 45, 46, 47	✓	✓		✓

FP = frontal pole; DL = dorsolateral prefrontal cortex; OF = orbitofrontal cortex; ACC = anterior cingulate cortex; VM = ventromedial prefrontal cortex; NF = non-frontal cortex; D-KEFS = Delis–Kaplan executive function system; FL = frontal lobe; HA = healthy adults; M = medial frontal cortex; LL = left lateral prefrontal cortex; RL = right lateral prefrontal cortex; ✓ = frontal region damaged and impairment found; X = frontal region damaged but no impairment.

lobes (particularly the right) were associated with poor proverb interpretation. Around the same time, in an unpublished PhD dissertation, Keifer (2010) assessed 14 patients with ventromedial prefrontal cortex lesions, 14 patients with dorsolateral prefrontal cortex lesions, and 18 patients with non-frontal lesions on the Proverb Interpretation Task subtest from the D-KEFS. Whereas a significant difference between the three patient groups was not found, when Keifer (2010) examined the percentage of patients in each subgroup who had performed in the impaired range (≤5th percentile), a greater percentage of dorsolateral prefrontal patients (14%) was impaired on the Proverb Interpretation Task than ventromedial prefrontal patients (0%) or non-frontal (6%) patients. Most recently, Murphy et al. (2013) assessed a large group of patients with unselected frontal lobe lesions, mainly due to tumor resection or cerebrovascular incidents, who were subdivided into medial ($n = 17$; BAs 6, 8, 9, 10, 23, 24, 32, and 33), left lateral ($n = 16$), and right lateral ($n = 13$; BAs 6, 8, 9, 44, 45, 46, and 47) frontal subgroups. When compared on the free inquiry version of the Proverb Interpretation Task, only the medial frontal group scored significantly lower than the healthy controls. However, when the nature of the response (i.e., abstract versus concrete) was compared, only the left lateral group produced significantly more concrete responses in relation to their errors made, compared to the healthy controls. Overall, these findings suggest that both the lateral and medial prefrontal regions play a role in performance on the Proverb Interpretation Task. However, it remains difficult to reconcile the differences in terms of lateralization found by Roca et al. (2010), who recorded mainly right frontal involvement, and Murphy et al. (2013), who recorded mainly left frontal involvement.

2.2.3 Neuroimaging studies

There do not appear to be any neuroimaging studies in the literature specifically examining the neural correlates of the processes associated with the Proverb Interpretation Task. However, understanding proverbs is thought to require the ability to understand metaphors or idioms (Gibbs and Beitel 1995) and a number of fMRI studies have investigated metaphor or idiom comprehension in healthy individuals. Metaphors are phrases applied to an object or action which cannot be applied literally and which describe something by referring to it as something different (e.g., "A blanket of snow"). Idioms are thought of as constant metaphors, as they are common phrases in everyday language but mean something other than the words that create them, and thus the meaning of idioms cannot be deduced if it is unknown (e.g., "I heard it on the grapevine").

Event-related fMRI has been employed to examine metaphor comprehension (Table 2.5). For example, Rapp et al. (2004) asked 14 participants to read

Table 2.5 Proverb Interpretation Task: Neuroimaging studies

Study	n	Patient/ Control Groups	Study type	Stimuli	Brodmann Areas	FP	DL	OF	ACC
Rapp et al. (2004)	14	HA	ER-fMRI	Metaphors	45/47				
Stringaris et al. (2006)	12	HA	ER-fMRI	Metaphors	47				
Rizzo et al. (2007)	14	HA	rTMS	Idioms	9		✓		
Zempleni et al. (2007)	17	HA	fMRI	Idioms	45, 47				
Lauro et al. (2008)	22	HA	fMRI	Idioms	9, 45				
Hillert and Buračas (2009)	21	HA	ER-MRI	Idioms	8, 9, 11, 44, 45, 47			✓	

FP = frontal pole; DL = dorsolateral prefrontal cortex; OF = orbitofrontal cortex; ACC = anterior cingulate cortex; HA = healthy adults; ER-MRI = event-related magnetic resonance imaging; rTMS = repetitive transcranial magnetic stimulation; fMRI = functional magnetic resonance imaging; ✓ = frontal region involved.

metaphors or literal sentences silently and to indicate whether the sentence was positive or negative in valence, and their performance was compared with a no-sentence condition. When judging metaphor valence was compared with judging literal sentences, the left inferior frontal gyrus (BA 45/47), the left inferior temporal gyrus (BAs 19 and 20), and the left posterior middle/inferior temporal gyrus (BA 37) were activated. In a similar study by Stringaris et al. (2006), 12 participants were asked to read metaphors and literal sentences silently. The sentences were followed by a word, and participants had to judge whether it was semantically related to the sentence or not. The results demonstrated that metaphor understanding involves activation of the right ventrolateral prefrontal cortex (BA 47).

As well as metaphors, idiom processing has also been examined using neuroimaging. In an fMRI study, Lauro et al. (2008) presented 22 healthy participants with written sentences that were either idiomatic or literal in nature. A picture appeared 2000 ms after the sentence was initially presented and participants had to judge whether the picture corresponded to the meaning of the sentence (see Figure 2.2). The network of activation associated specifically with the idiomatic or non-literal sentences included the left superior medial frontal gyrus (BA 9), the left inferior frontal gyrus (BA 45), and the left inferior

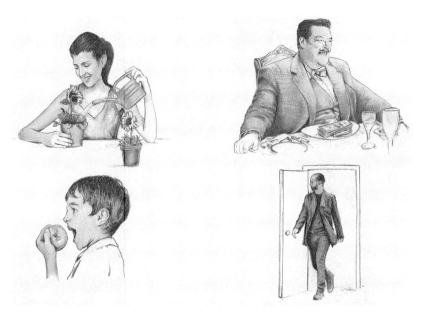

Fig. 2.2 Examples of the pictures presented in the Idiom Comprehension Task. Upper left: a correct picture for the idiom, "To have green fingers." Upper right: an incorrect picture for the idiom, "To tighten one's belt." Lower left: a correct picture for the literal sentence, "The boy is eating an apple." Lower right: an incorrect picture for the literal sentence, "The man is opening the window." Reproduced from Leonor J. Romero Lauro, Marco Tettamanti, Stefano F. Cappa, Costanza Papagno, Idiom comprehension: a prefrontal task?, *Cerebral Cortex*, 18 (1), pp. 162–170. doi:10.1093/cercor/bhm042. © 2008, Oxford Unviersity Press. http://cercor.oxfordjournals.org/content/18/1/162.full. For permission to reuse this material, please visit http://www.oup.co.uk/academic/rights/permissions.

temporal gyrus, as well as the right superior and middle temporal gyri. In another fMRI study, Zempleni et al. (2007) presented 17 Dutch participants with a series of written sentences and then asked them to decide whether the word written in red capital letters presented after the sentence was related in meaning. There were four conditions (the examples have been translated into English): (1) metaphoric sentences with an ambiguous idiom (e.g., "During the testimony of the witness, the jury smelled a rat"); (2) literal sentences with an ambiguous probable idiom (e.g., "Down in the tunnel under the barn, the terrier smelled a rat"); (3) metaphoric sentences with an unambiguous idiom (e.g., "Due to the strike of the railroad-workers, the travelers were in a blue funk"); and (4) unambiguously literal sentences (e.g., "Due to the workload of the employees, the manager hired a new caseworker"). The areas of activation associated with idiomatic compared to literal sentences included the inferior frontal gyrus (BA 47 extending into BA 45) and the middle temporal gyrus (BA 21) bilaterally. Finally, using event-related fMRI, Hillert and Buračas (2009) presented 21 participants with spoken sentences that were explicit idiomatic sentences (e.g., "He was shooting the breeze"), ambiguous idiomatic sentences (e.g., "The woman held the torch"), literal sentences (e.g., "He met her in the new mall"), or implausible phrases (e.g., "He ate the green wall"). Participants performed a rapid sentence decision task in which they had to indicate, as fast as possible, whether they believed the sentence to be meaningful or not. The findings demonstrated that the idiomatic sentences were associated with activation in the left ventral dorsolateral prefrontal cortex (BAs 11, 44, 45, and 47) and the superior and medial frontal gyrus (BAs 8 and 9).

The role of the dorsolateral prefrontal cortex in idiom comprehension has also been demonstrated using repetitive transcranial magnetic stimulation (rTMS). Rizzo et al. (2007) asked 14 participants to perform a sentence-to-picture match-ing task in which they were presented with written, unambiguous idiomatic sentences and literal sentences followed by four pictures. The participants had to choose the picture that matched the meaning of the sentence. This matching task was performed when rTMS was delivered to the left dorsolateral prefrontal cortex, the right dorsolateral prefrontal cortex, and under sham conditions in the same group of participants. Rizzo et al. (2007) found that when rTMS was applied either to the left or to the right dorsolateral prefrontal cortex, partici-pants exhibited significantly slower response times for both idioms and literal sentences, relative to the sham condition. By contrast, accuracy in the two rTMS conditions was significantly poorer than in the sham condition, but only for the idiomatic sentences. These results suggest that the dorsolateral prefrontal cortex plays a role in monitoring idiomatic responses.

In summary, whereas performance on the Proverb Interpretation Task has not been examined using neuroimaging, other forms of figurative language task performed in the fMRI scanner suggest that both the lateral and medial prefrontal cortex play an important role in conveying non-literal meanings.

2.2.4 Aging studies

One of the earlier studies examining the influence of healthy adult aging on prov-erb interpretation examined 89 men aged between 30 and 80 years (Albert et al. 1990) (Table 2.6). Participants were subdivided into their various age decades (i.e., 30–39, 40–49, 50–59, 60–69, and 70–80 years) and were administered both the free-inquiry and the multiple-choice formats of the Proverb Interpretation Task. The results showed that, although performance on both versions of the task seemed to decline from 60 years of age onwards, only the older adults in their 70s performed significantly more poorly than the participants in their 30s.

Table 2.6 Proverb Interpretation Task: Aging studies

Study	n	Participant age groups	Study type	Task	Age effect
Albert et al. (1990)	16; 8; 22; 21; 22	30–39; 40–49; 50–59; 60–69; 70–80	Cross-sectional (behavioral)	PIT	✓
Nippold et al. (1997)	52; 43; 41; 41; 49; 43; 40; 44	13–14; 16–17; 20–29; 30–39; 40–49; 50–59; 60–69; 70–79	Cross-sectional (behavioral)	PIT	✓
Uekermann et al. (2008)	35; 35; 35	20–39; 41–57; 60–79	Cross-sectional (behavioral)	PIT	✓

PIT = Proverb Interpretation Task; ✓ = age effect found; X = age effect not found.

The authors also demonstrated that although performance on the vocabulary subtest from the Wechsler Adult Intelligence Scale and verbal fluency predicted performance on the Proverb Interpretation Task, intellectual abilities were not responsible for the age-related decline in older adults. In another study, Nippold et al. (1997) administered a proverb explanation task to 353 participants aged between 13 and 79 years. Again, it was found that older adults in their 70s showed a significant age-related decline in their proverb interpretation abilities, this time compared to adolescents and individuals in their 20s. Finally, Uekermann et al. (2008) assessed the proverb interpretation abilities of 105 healthy participants who were subdivided into three age groups: a younger group of 35 participants aged 20–39 years, a middle-aged group of 35 participants aged 41–57 years, and an older age group of 35 older participants aged between 60 and 79 years. Participants performed a 32-item multiple-choice version of the Proverb Interpretation Task. Despite the proverbs being rated using a five-point scale as more familiar in the older age group, older adults correctly interpreted significantly fewer proverbs than the younger and middle-aged groups, showing a greater tendency to choose the more literal, concrete answers. These studies suggest that healthy adult aging results in an increased tendency to interpret proverbs in a more literal way.

2.2.5 **Summary**

The Proverb Interpretation Task is often used clinically to assess frontal executive dysfunction. The few lesion studies in the literature that have examined the performance on the Proverb Interpretation Task in frontal patients suggest that medial prefrontal lesions are associated with lower overall scores on the task, whereas left lateral prefrontal lesions are associated with a higher percentage of errors that are concrete in nature. Neuroimaging studies have also provided support for the notion that both the dorsolateral prefrontal cortex and medial prefrontal regions are important for performance on the Proverb Interpretation Task. In terms of the effects of healthy adult aging, studies have consistently demonstrated that older adults score more poorly on the Proverb Interpretation Task, often producing or selecting more literal responses than younger individuals. Nonetheless, as is the case for lesion studies, few studies in the literature have examined the effects of healthy adult aging on verbal abstraction abilities using the Proverb Interpretation Task.

Chapter 3

Initiation and inhibition

3.1 AX-Continuous Performance Task

3.1.1 Task description

The AX-Continuous Performance Task (Rosvold et al. 1956) refers to a variant of a classic continuous performance task, and involves participants fixating on a series of briefly presented visual stimuli, usually letters, and responding to a certain pattern of cues. Normally, participants are asked to respond only if they see an A cue followed by an X probe, not other patterns such as AY or BX (note that non-target cues are any letter other than A, and non-target probes are any letter other than X; see Figure 3.1 for an example time-course). However, more recent versions (e.g., MacDonald et al. 2005) have required participants to respond to non-target trials too, using a different response key. Successful AX-Continuous Performance Task performance requires participants to hold within working memory contextual information about the current trial. In particular, depending on the cue (target trial: A; non-target trial: non-A), participants must keep in mind the relevant response options until the probe appears and they are able to select the correct response—inhibiting or overriding any prepotent response tendencies as necessary.

The AX-Continuous Performance Task is widely used to investigate response conflict. There are three types of non-target trials (AY, BY, and BX), each created to provide a differing amount of expectancy, and thus different non-target trials can lead to different types of errors. With the least amount of expectancy, BY trials (where a non-target cue is followed by a non-target probe) are often used as a baseline condition (e.g., in neuroimaging studies) as participants are easily able to narrow down the potential responses to those that are appropriate for a non-target from the cue. Target trials (AX trials) also create little conflict, as the expectancy from the A cue helps individuals to select the appropriate response in preparation for the X probe. Errors on these trials are usually errors of omission in which an individual fails to make the target response, and participant groups with impaired context maintenance abilities—such as schizophrenics (Cohen et al. 1996; MacDonald et al. 2003)—should be able to perform well on these trials simply by using the probe to inform their response. BX trials (where a non-target cue is followed by a target probe) create a moderate amount of conflict for participant groups with context maintenance problems, as, although

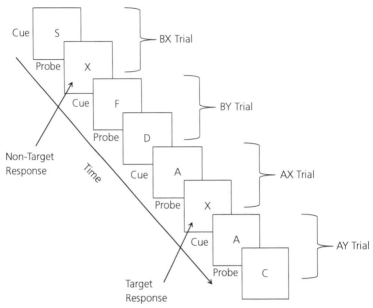

Fig. 3.1 Example time-course of the AX-Continuous Performance Task. Adapted from Braver, Todd S.; Barch, Deanna M.; Keys, Beth A.; Carter, Cameron S.; Cohen, Jonathan D.; Kaye, Jeffrey A.; Janowsky, Jeri S.; Taylor, Stephan F.; Yesavage, Jerome A.; Mumenthaler, Martin S.; Jagust, William J.; Reed, Bruce R., Context processing in older adults: Evidence for a theory relating cognitive control to neurobiology in healthy aging, *Journal of Experimental Psychology: General*, 130(4), pp. 746–763. doi: 10.1037/0096-3445.130.4.746. © 2001, American Psychological Association.

the cue should narrow down the response to that appropriate for a non-target, if the probe is relied on too heavily, then the target response is instead generated. The most interesting trial type in many studies is the AY trial (in which a target cue is followed by a non-target probe). In these trials, expectancy works against participants to encourage errors—the A cue strongly biases toward the target response, which is sometimes sufficient to override the effect of the non-target probe. In these situations, participants should show increased error rates (i.e., responding with a target response to a non-target trial) or increased reaction times (RTs), due to the additional time required to resolve the conflict when the probe appears. Many variations of the AX-Continuous Performance Task exist with changes to the sensory modality, the frequency of targets, the duration of a trial, or the type, integrity, or color of stimuli (see Riccio et al. 2002 for a review).

3.1.2 Patient and lesion studies

Although originally used to assess young adults with different types of brain damage (Rosvold et al. 1956), and more widely to assess deficits in conditions

Table 3.1 AX-Continuous Performance Task: Patient and lesion studies

Study	n	Patient/ Control Groups	Study type	Stimuli	Brodmann Areas	FP	DL	OF	ACC
Ringholz (1989)	29; 28; 25	DL; VM; HA	Lesion	Numbers	–			✓	✓
Baird et al. (2006)	1; 5	ACC, HA	Lesion (single case)	Letters	8, 24, 25, 32				✓

FP = frontal pole; DL = dorsolateral prefrontal cortex; OF = orbitofrontal cortex; ACC = anterior cingulate cortex; VM = ventromedial prefrontal cortex; HA = healthy adults; ✓ = frontal region damaged and impairment found; X = frontal region damaged but no impairment.

such as bipolar disorder and schizophrenia (e.g., McClure et al. 2005; Yoon et al. 2008), focal lesion studies have utilized the AX-CPT to investigate prefrontal involvement (Table 3.1). For example, traumatic brain injury patients with damage to the dorsolateral or orbital prefrontal regions have been noted to exhibit a deficit in AX-Continuous Performance Task performance, with both lesion groups performing more poorly than healthy controls (Ringholz 1989, unpublished doctoral dissertation, as cited in Riccio et al. 2002). However, Ringholz observed no differences between the performance of the predominantly dorsolateral and predominantly orbital patient groups. Furthermore, Baird et al. (2006) found that a patient with a unilateral anterior cingulate lesion showed no significant difference in AX-Continuous Performance Task accuracy when compared to healthy control participants. The patient did, however, perform significantly slower in terms of RTs when a long delay was presented between cue and probe (Baird et al. 2006, patient 1).

3.1.3 Neuroimaging studies

Several studies have investigated the performance of healthy individuals performing the AX-Continuous Performance Task using neuroimaging (Table 3.2). Carter et al. (1998) examined the role of the anterior cingulate cortex in error monitoring using the AX-Continuous Performance Task with event-related functional magnetic resonance imaging (fMRI). In particular, they found that greater anterior cingulate activation was related to the presentation of non-target trials that were initially similar to the target but incorrect. For example, participants showed greater anterior cingulate activation during AY trials compared to BY trials. Carter et al. (1998) concluded that the anterior cingulate cortex plays a vital role in tasks that create response competition, and that this increased activity of the anterior cingulate cortex in trials with a strong

Table 3.2 AX-Continuous Performance Task: Neuroimaging studies

Study	n	Patient/Control Groups	Study type	Stimuli	Brodmann Areas	FP	DL	OF	ACC
Barch et al. (1997)	11	HA	fMRI	Letters	6, 9, 44, 46		✓		
				Delay:					
				Difficulty:	8, 32, 44, 45, 47			✓	✓
Carter et al. (1998)	13	HA	fMRI	Letters	6, 9, 9/46, 24/32, 44/45		✓		✓
Breiter and Rosen (1999)	10	HA	fMRI	Letters	6, 9/46, 24/32, 44/45		✓		✓
Barch et al. (2001b)[a]	14; 12	schiz; HA	fMRI	Letters	6, 9, 24, 32, 44		✓		✓
Braver and Bongiolatti (2002)	21	HA	fMRI	Words			✓	✓	✓
				Semantic:	32, 44/45/47;				
				Maintenance:	9/46;				
				Subgoal:	9/46, 10	✓			
Dias et al. (2003)	11	HA	ERP	Letters	–				✓
MacDonald et al. (2005)[a]	18; 12; 18	schiz; PS; HA	fMRI	Letters	6, 8, 9/44		✓		✓
Paxton et al. (2008)[b]	20; 21	OA; YA	fMRI	Words			✓	✓	✓
				Cue:	4, 6, 24, 45, 46, 47;		✓	✓	✓
				Probe:	6, 9, 44/6;		✓	✓	✓
				Delay:	4, 6, 9, 10, 11, 32, 46, 47	✓			
Yoon et al. (2008)[a]	25; 24	Schiz; HA	fMRI	Letters	6, 8, 9, 10		✓		✓
Mayda et al. (2011)[b]	16; 15; 15	OW; OA; YA	fMRI	Letters	8, 9, 32, 46		✓		✓

FP = frontal pole; DL = dorsolateral prefrontal cortex; OF = orbitofrontal cortex; ACC = anterior cingulate cortex; HA = healthy adults; fMRI = functional magnetic resonance imaging; schiz = schizophrenia patients; PS = non-schizophrenic psychosis; ERP = event-related potential; ✓ = frontal region involved

OW = older adults with white matter impairment; OA = older adults; YA = younger adults;

[a] Only the healthy controls reported in the study.

[b] Both the healthy younger and older groups reported in the study.

prepotent response could indicate some role in performance-monitoring (see also MacDonald et al. 2005). Yoon et al. (2008) performed a functional imaging investigation where both schizophrenic and healthy individuals performed a version of the AX-Continuous Performance Task. Yoon et al. (2008) found that schizophrenic patients made significantly more errors on the AX and BX trials of the task (i.e., when participants experience a high degree of response competition), but performed as normal for other trials. More importantly, however, they found evidence of both anterior and posterior cingulate activation in healthy individuals, as well as significant activation within premotor areas such as Brodmann Area (BA) 6. This pattern of activation was not present in schizophrenic patients.

An earlier study by Barch et al. (1997) had highlighted the association between transient anterior cingulate cortex activation and the difficulty of the AX-Continuous Performance Task presented, with increasing activation noted only for the duration of trials in which the letter-stimuli were visually degraded. However, they also identified sustained dorsolateral prefrontal activation across the task, which was not associated with the difficulty of the task, but instead with the load placed upon the working memory system. In particular, this dorsolateral prefrontal activation was present when a long delay (8 s) separated the cue and probe, and lasted for the entirety of the delay period. Such a pattern of transient anterior cingulate activation within trials and sustained dorsolateral prefrontal activation across trials has been replicated in several recent studies (Barch et al. 2001b; Paxton et al. 2008; Yoon et al. 2008). This sustained, general activation of the dorsolateral prefrontal cortex likely represents the maintenance of task demands such as task rules and contextual information (Breiter and Rosen 1999; Braver and Bongiolatti 2002; MacDonald et al. 2005). A similar role has been proposed for the frontal pole in light of significantly higher activation in the AX-Continuous Performance Task versus two control tasks— semantic classification (without maintenance demands) and an AX-Continuous Performance Task with minimal maintenance and processing demands (Braver and Bongiolatti 2002). In accordance with this, increasing the maintenance demands placed on working memory appears to increase dorsolateral prefrontal activation (Cohen et al. 1996; Barch et al. 1997). For example, dorsolateral prefrontal activation changes in line with manipulations of delay—with higher activation for longer cue–probe intervals (Barch et al. 2001b; Braver and Bongiolatti 2002; MacDonald et al. 2003, 2005). Also, dorsolateral prefrontal activation increases in healthy individuals when distracters, including overlapping A cues, are placed serially between the cue and the target, thus suppressing rehearsal and impairing maintenance of the cue (Breiter and Rosen 1999, Experiment 3).

Interestingly, in healthy adults, BA 9 of the dorsolateral prefrontal cortex shows increased activation after the presentation of a B (non-target) cue, compared to an A (target) cue (MacDonald et al. 2005). By contrast, schizophrenic patients committed significantly more BX trial errors and did not show such a dissociation in activation between B and A cues (MacDonald et al. 2005). The authors suggest that task-related dorsolateral prefrontal activity reflected the initiation of the maintenance process and the application of cognitive control in preparation for a non-target response. Event-related potential (ERP) studies, using source mapping, have similarly associated the response monitoring and inhibition processes with signals originating from the anterior cingulate/dorsolateral prefrontal cortex, and parietal signals with the preparation of response (Dias et al. 2003; see also Silberstein et al. 2000).

3.1.4 **Aging studies**

Aging studies have investigated AX-Continuous Performance Task task performance both in terms of accuracy and RTs (Table 3.3). Chen et al. (1998) have compared the performance of older adults with that of adolescents on a number version of the AX-Continuous Performance Task (where target trials are 9 preceded by a 1). Older adults exhibited a significantly lower hit-rate and a higher rate of false alarms than adolescents. Braver et al. (2001c) observed that older and younger adults differed in terms of RTs and accuracy on the AX-Continuous Performance Task. In particular, older individuals committed significantly more errors and exhibited significantly longer RTs than younger individuals on BX and AY trials, which had a high degree of response conflict compared to AX or BY trials. Similarly, Mani et al. (2005) examined performance under either "clear" (i.e., a clear letter on a black background) or "noisy" (i.e., a degraded

Table 3.3 AX-Continuous Performance Task: Aging studies

Study	n	Participant age groups (years)	Study type	Stimuli	Age effect
Chen et al. (1998)	115; 53; 56; 56	Adolescents, mean = 14.0; 20–34; 35–49; 50–65	Cross-sectional (behavioral)	Digits	✓
Braver et al. (2001c)	175; 81	18–39; 65–85	Cross-sectional (behavioral)	Letters	✓
Mani et al. (2005)	32	19–82	Cross-sectional (behavioral)	Letters	✓
Mayda et al. (2011)	15; 15; 16	19-29; 66–89; 66–89	Cross-sectional (neuroimaging)	Letters	✓

letter on a background of white noise) conditions, and noted that overall accuracy decreased with age, regardless of the condition. Commission errors (e.g., making a target response to an AY or BX trial) were found to increase with age, suggesting a specific response inhibition deficit in older individuals.

Mayda et al. (2011) examined the performance and activation (using fMRI) of two groups of older adults (i.e., those with and without white matter damage; aged 66–89 years) and a group of younger adults performing the AX-Continuous Performance Task. Healthy older adults with severe white matter hyperintensity load (over the whole brain, measured by percentage of total cranial volume) exhibited both reduced dorsolateral prefrontal activation and increased rostral anterior cingulate activation following B trials (in which greater control is required to suppress the more frequently used target response) when compared to healthy older adults without white matter damage (Mayda et al. 2011). Furthermore, individuals with white matter damage performed significantly more poorly in terms of accuracy than healthy younger individuals on AX and BX trials (suggesting problems maintaining contextual information). Though there were age-related differences in RTs over AX, BX, and AY trials, there were significantly greater interference effects (BX RTs minus AX RTs) for older adults with hyperintensities—but only when compared to younger adults. In contrast to younger adults and older adults without hyperintensities, older adults with high white matter hyperintensity load exhibited reduced functional connectivity between frontal regions.

3.1.5 Summary

Anterior cingulate cortex and premotor/supplementary motor area involvement during the AX-Continuous Performance Task appears to be representative of competition resolution and error monitoring (e.g., MacDonald et al. 2005), whereas the dorsolateral prefrontal cortex and frontal pole are involved in the maintenance of contextual information necessary to select the probe-appropriate response. In summary, there is some evidence for age-related decline on particular trial types such as BX and AY trials, but the evidence for this is both limited and mixed.

3.2 Go/No-Go Task

3.2.1 Task description

The original Go/No-Go Task was developed by Luria and requires participants to raise their index finger in response to a single auditory "tap" (a Go trial) but make no movement in response to two "taps" (a No-Go trial; Luria 1973). Many of the more recent Go/No-Go Tasks involve visual paradigms, with cues ranging in stimulus dimensions such as color (e.g., "Go when you see a green cue") or identity (e.g., "Go when you see an X"). One of the most common versions of the Go/No-Go Task uses letters presented in the middle of a computer screen, and requires participants to respond with a button press to any letter other than an "X" (e.g., Casey et al. 1997, see Figure 3.2). Importantly, the Go/No-Go Task relies on participants being able to respond quickly during Go trials but inhibit responses during No-Go trials. As the No-Go trials are relatively infrequent (commonly around 25% of the total number of trials), participants are also required to maintain task-relevant information over time (i.e., the rule regarding the No-Go stimulus) and to monitor for any response conflict, especially during No-Go trials where inhibition is required to prevent irrelevant responses. The Go/No-Go Task is typically scored in terms of hits and false alarm rates.

3.2.2 **Patient and lesion studies**

The evidence from patient and lesion studies regarding frontal lobe involvement when performing the Go/No-Go Task is somewhat contradictory, particularly regarding regional specificity among frontal subregions. Several studies indicate some general frontal lobe involvement in Go/No-Go Task performance. Godefroy et al. (1996) compared the performance of patients with

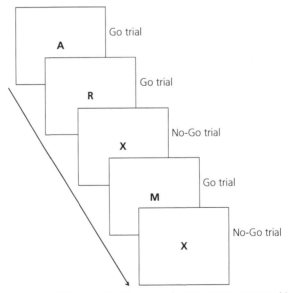

Fig. 3.2 Example of a widely used Go/No-Go Task. Letters are presented in the middle of a computer screen and participants should press the same button for all letters except for the letter "X."

prefrontal lesions, patients with more posterior lesions and healthy controls. They found that the prefrontal lesion patients committed significantly more commission errors (i.e., a Go response on a No-Go trial) and responded more slowly than the posterior lesion and healthy control groups. Poor performance was particularly associated with lesion volume in BAs 8, 9, 10, 11, 32, 44, 45, 46, and 47. Black et al. (2000) noted that schizophrenic patients who had previously undergone large resections of the prefrontal cortex as treatment for their schizophrenia were significantly impaired on the Go/No-Go Task, committing more errors than non-leukotomized schizophrenic controls, despite similar performance on more basic motor tasks without a No-Go element. In another study, 18 patients with right frontal lesions due to aneurysm, hemorrhage or meningioma exhibited slow RTs on both Go and No-Go trials when compared to 16 healthy controls (Aron et al. 2003). However, another study found no significant difference in RTs between patients with frontal or temporal lobe lesions and healthy controls performing a Go/No-Go Task (Décary and Richer 1995). A study by Rieger et al. (2003) has demonstrated that tasks relying on inhibiting ongoing responses may be less sensitive to left frontal lesions. Patients with right or bilateral frontal lesions appear to perform more poorly on the Stop Signal task[1] than patients with left frontal lesions or healthy controls (Rieger et al. 2003).

The evidence from lesion studies relating Go/No-Go deficits to specific frontal subregions is somewhat mixed (Table 3.4). The extent of damage to the inferior frontal gyrus, middle frontal gyrus, and anterior cingulate cortex region correlates positively with RTs after a No-Go stop-signal delay (Aron et al. 2003). A case report by Malloy et al. (1993) described patient JC who had significant ventromedial prefrontal damage after a head injury following a car accident. Malloy et al. administered two motor Go/No-Go Tasks to patient JC. The first required the patient to tap the desk once on hearing two taps, and to tap twice on hearing one tap. The second task required the patient to tap on hearing the word "Stop" but to withhold a response on hearing the word "Go". Patient JC exhibited profound impairments on both Go/No-Go Tasks, during which he

---

[1] The Stop Signal task is similar to the Go/No-Go task and involves two elements. The first is very similar to a Go trial in which participants perform a two-choice discrimination task. For example, Rieger et al. (2003) asked participants to discern between circles and squares. The second task, running concurrently but on only a minority of trials (e.g., 25%) prompts participants to withhold their response on a given trial (i.e., a No-Go trial). In the Stop Signal task used by Reiger et al. (2003), for example, a tone signalled a 'stop' trial. The further into the trial that the stop signal is presented, the harder it is to inhibit the 'Go' response (see Logan 1994).

Table 3.4 Go/No-Go Task: Patient and lesion studies

Study	n	Patient/ Control Groups	Study type	Task	Brodmann Areas	FP	DL	OF	ACC
Leimkuhler and Mesulam (1985)	1	Medial PFC	Lesion (single case)	Motor	–			✓	✓
Verfaellie and Heilman (1987)	2	Medial PFC	Lesion (single case)	Motor	–				✓
Malloy et al. (1993)	1	VM	Lesion (single case)	Motor	–			✓	
Fellows and Farah (2005a)	4; 12	dACC; HA	Lesion	Digits	–				X
Swick et al. (2008)	12; 5; 16	IFG; VM; HA	Lesion	Letters	6, 9, 10, 11, 13, 25, 44, 45, 46, 47	X	✓	X	X

FP = frontal pole; DL = dorsolateral prefrontal cortex; OF = orbitofrontal cortex; ACC = anterior cingulate cortex; PFC = prefrontal cortex; VM = ventromedial prefrontal cortex; dACC = dorsal anterior cingulate cortex; HA = healthy adults; IFG = inferior frontal gyrus; ✓ = frontal region damaged and impairment found; X = frontal region damaged but no impairment.

would start following the instructions but soon began to tap the same number of times as the assessor. It should be noted that these tasks differ from most Go/No-Go Tasks, which tend to use novel stimuli, as both tasks required reversal of an already learned and habitual response pattern. Therefore, the deficit shown by patient JC may simply be one relating to reversal learning (see Section 4.2) rather than inhibition per se. Indeed, while Swick et al. (2008) demonstrated that patients with lesions in the left inferior frontal gyrus (including primarily the dorsolateral prefrontal cortex and pre-supplementary motor area) committed significantly more errors than healthy controls, especially when response competition was high (i.e., in low-frequency No-Go trials), their patients with primarily ventromedial prefrontal lesions did not show a similar impairment.

An early study by Verfaellie and Heilman (1987) described impaired No-Go trial performance on Luria's (1966) version of the task in a patient with a right medial prefrontal lesion (including the supplementary motor area and anterior cingulate cortex) due to a hemorrhage but not in a patient with a left medial prefrontal lesion due to an infarction. The deficit in the right-hemisphere patient was only found when inhibiting a motor response with the left hand (i.e., contralateral to the lesion) (Verfaellie and Heilman,

1987). Interestingly, Leimkuhler and Mesulam (1985) described a patient with a large medial prefrontal meningioma who preoperatively exhibited almost complete disinhibition on the Go/No-Go Task, committing >75% commission errors on No-Go trials. After removal of the meningioma, the patient's performance improved over a seven-week recovery period to near-perfect levels (with only one commission error), suggesting not only that the medial prefrontal regions are key to No-Go performance but also that intervening in the putative cause of the impairments can have a significant effect on performance (Leimkuhler and Mesulam 1985). This being said, patients with focal lesions only in the dorsal portion of the anterior cingulate cortex, compared to the more diffuse anterior cingulate cortex lesions investigated in previous studies, do not appear to perform differently from healthy controls in terms of error rates and are not differentially impaired by high conflict (i.e., 25 No-Go trials in a block of 200 trials; Fellows and Farah 2005a). However, care must be taken in interpreting this finding, as the conclusion is based on the data from only three patients, and the baseline condition (125 No-Go trials in a block of 200 trials) still involves some degree of conflict between Go and No-Go responses.

3.2.3 **Neuroimaging studies**

One of the main contributions of neuroimaging studies to the Go/No-Go literature has been the association of distinct recruitment patterns specific to the functions required to perform the task (Table 3.5). Response competition has been associated with activation in the dorsolateral prefrontal cortex, ventrolateral prefrontal cortex, and anterior cingulate cortex, and response execution with motor and premotor regions (Menon et al. 2001). Both Go and No-Go trials activate the dorsolateral prefrontal cortex and anterior cingulate region, but the extent of this recruitment appears more dorsolateral (with some extra ventrolateral activation) in No-Go trials specifically (Konishi et al. 1998b; 1999b; Watanabe et al. 2002). Liddle et al. (2001) presented healthy participants, while undergoing event-related fMRI, with an equal number of Go and No-Go trials rather than a frequent number of Go trials and an infrequent number of No-Go trials. This was to ensure that the No-Go trials were not considered novel "oddball" stimuli. When Liddle et al. (2001) contrasted Go and No-Go trial activation directly, Go trials showed more recruitment of motor and premotor regions whereas No-Go trials showed more recruitment of the dorsolateral and ventrolateral prefrontal cortex; the authors suggested that this indicated the involvement of inhibitory processes during the No-Go trials. Similarly, in an electroencephalography (EEG) study, Alegre et al. (2004)

Table 3.5 Go/No-Go Task: Neuroimaging studies

Study	n	Patient/Control Groups	Study type	Stimuli	Brodmann Areas	FP	DL	OF	ACC
Sasaki et al. (1993)	5	HA	MEG	Color No-Go:	—				
Roberts et al. (1994)	21	HA	EEG	Letters No-Go:	—		✓		✓
Kawashima et al. (1996)	9	HA	PET	Color	4, 6, 8, 9, 24, 32, 47	✓		✓	✓
Casey et al. (1997)	9	HA	fMRI	Letters No-Go:	6, 8, 9, 10, 11, 24, 32, 45, 46, 47		✓	✓	✓
Shibata et al. (1997)	10	HA	EEG	Shapes No-Go:	—	✓	✓	✓	✓
Kiefer et al. (1998)	16	HA	ERP	Auditory No-Go:	—	✓	✓	✓	✓
Konishi et al. (1998)	5	HA	fMRI	Color Go: No-Go:	9, 10, 24, 32, 45; 9, 32, 44, 45, 46	✓	✓		✓ ✓
Garavan et al. (1999)	14	HA	ER-fMRI	Letters No-Go:	9, 10, 32	✓	✓		✓
Konishi et al. (1999b)	6	HA	ER-fMRI	Color No-Go:	45/44				
De Zubicaray et al. (2000)	8	HA	fMRI	Shapes	6, 8/9, 10	✓	✓		✓

Study	N	Group	Method	Task	Areas			
Kiehl et al. (2000)	14	HA	ER-fMRI	Letters Commission errors: Correct No-Go: Correct Go:	6, 10, 32; 6, 32; 4, 6, 13, 32	✓		✓ ✓ ✓
Bokura et al. (2001)	13	HA	ERP	Digits No-Go:	–			✓
Braver et al. (2001a)	14	HA	ER-fMRI	Letters	6, 32, 44/45, 46/9		✓	✓
Liddle et al. (2001)	16	HA	ER-fMRI	Letters Go: No-Go:	–		✓	✓ ✓
Menon et al. (2001)	14	HA	fMRI	Letters Error: Inhibition: Go:	24/32, 47; 6, 9/46, 24, 45/47; 4/6, 6		✓	✓ ✓
Rubia et al. (2001)	15	HA	fMRI	Objects Go/No-Go: Stop-Signal:	6, 8, 9, 24, 44/45; 6, 32, 44/45		✓	✓ ✓
Durston et al. (2002)	10	HA	ER-fMRI	Characters Frequency: Go: No-Go:	9/44, 32, 44/46; 4; 6, 8		✓	✓
Garavan et al. (2002)	14	HA	ER-fMRI	Letters Correct No-Go: Commission Errors:	6, 9, 13, 24/6, 32, 44; 6, 9/6, 32/24/6		✓ ✓	✓ ✓

(continued)

Table 3.5 Continued

Study	n	Patient/Control Groups	Study type	Stimuli	Brodmann Areas	FP	DL	OF	ACC
Watanabe et al. (2002)	11	HA	ER-fMRI	Color					
				Response Preparation:	6, 32;				✓
				Go:	4, 24;				✓
				No-Go:	9, 10	✓	✓		
Booth et al. (2003)	12	HA	fMRI	Color/shape					
				No-Go:	6, 10, 13, 32/8, 45	✓			✓
Mostofsky et al. (2003)	48	HA	ER-fMRI	Color/					
				Counting					
				Go:	6;				
				No-Go:	6				
Nieuwenhuis et al. (2003)	12	HA	ERP	Letters					✓
Alegre et al. (2004)	9	HA	EEG	Motor					
				Inhibition:			✓		✓
				Decision-making:				✓	
				Response preparation:					✓
Asahi et al. (2004)	17	HA	fMRI	Letters	6, 9, 46		✓		✓
Bellgrove et al. (2004)	42	HA	ER-fMRI	Letters					
				Correct No-Go:	6, 9, 13, 32/24, 44/6, 46		✓		✓
Hester et al. (2004b)	15	HA	ER-fMRI	Letters					
				Correct No-Go:	6, 9/6, 10/46, 46/9;	✓	✓	✓	✓
				Commission Errors:	10, 13, 32, 44, 47	✓	✓	✓	✓

Study	N	Group	Method	Task / Brodmann areas
Kelly et al. (2004)	15	HA	ER-fMRI	Letters Fast presentation, Correct No-Go: 9, 9/46, 13; Slow presentation, Correct No-Go: 9, 10
Wager et al. (2005)	14	HA	fMRI	Letters 9/46, 10, 13, 32
McNab et al. (2008)	14	HA	fMRI	Color Go/No-Go Task: 9, 9/46, 13/47, 47; No-Go: 10/46, 47/13; Stop Task: 6, 8, 9, 14, 32, 47/13; Stops: 6, 47, 47/13, 47/32
Simmonds et al. (2008)	11 studies	HA	Meta-analysis (fMRI)	Simple Go/No-Go: 6/32; Complex Go/No-Go: 6/32, 9/44, 46
Chikazoe et al. (2009)	25	HA	fMRI	Color Inhibition: 6, 6/9/44, 10, 10/46, 24/23, 32, 44/45, 47/12; Frequency: 6, 6/9/44, 10

FP = frontal pole; DL = dorsolateral prefrontal cortex; OF = orbitofrontal cortex; ACC = anterior cingulate cortex; HA = healthy adults; MEG = magnetoencephalography; EEG = electroencephalography; PET = positron emission tomography; fMRI = related functional magnetic resonance imaging; ERP = event-related potentials; ER-fMRI = event-related functional magnetic resonance imaging; ✓ = frontal region involved associated changes in central signals with motor preparation and response, increases in medial frontal activity with decision-making, and increases in frontocentral activity with inhibition processes (see also Roberts et al. 1994; Shibata et al. 1997).

Indeed, the Go/No-Go Task can be divided into temporally distinct phases—preparation and inhibition—each of which recruits different brain regions. For example, Hester et al. (2004b) administered a Go/No-Go Task in which responses were withheld for No-Go trials (inhibition), and contrasted this activation with activation during a preparatory cue period. Hester et al. (2004b) demonstrated a pattern of preparatory activation and deactivation within the anterior cingulate, parietal, and insula regions during the phase prior to No-Go responses, which predicted a successful withholding of response. It has also been shown that activation associated with both the preparation phase and Go trials is primarily motor-oriented (BAs 4, 6, 24 and 32; Watanabe et al. 2002). In the preparatory phase, participants are readying both the Go response and the task-relevant information necessary to interpret quickly and process a No-Go response. This allows the preparation of a Go response to be inhibited before the response is made. These phases require different component functions—inhibition of inappropriate responses, storing cues or keeping No-Go rules within working memory, and processing of conflict during infrequent No-Go trials—and these functions have been associated with different frontal lobe regions.

3.2.3.1 Inhibition

Various frontal and non-frontal regions have been implicated in Go/No-Go Task performance, with No-Go (i.e., inhibitory) activation observed within the frontal pole (BA 10), posterior cingulate cortex (BA 23) and anterior cingulate cortex (BAs 6 and 32) (Booth et al. 2003; see also Kawashima et al. 1996; de Zubicaray et al. 2000). Significant dorsolateral prefrontal cortex and pre-supplementary motor area activity has been noted during No-Go trials using both magnetoencephalography (MEG; Sasaki et al. 1993) and fMRI (Wager et al. 2005). Asahi et al. (2004) noted that the dorsolateral prefrontal cortex (BAs 9 and 46) and temporal lobe (BAs 22 and 37) were significantly activated after subtracting Go activation from No-Go activation. Furthermore, activation within the dorsolateral prefrontal cortex (BA 9) was negatively correlated with performance on a motor impulsiveness questionnaire, with greater activation associated with less-impulsive tendencies (Asahi et al. 2004). Individual differences in the variability of Go-trial RTs have been associated with frontal activation, with those participants showing greater RT variability also showing increased recruitment of the dorsolateral prefrontal cortex (BAs

9 and 46) and anterior cingulate cortex (BAs 6, 24 and 32) during No-Go trials (Bellgrove et al. 2004).

In terms of the involvement of the ventrolateral and ventromedial prefrontal cortex in Go/No-Go performance, the findings here are less consistent, despite these regions being associated with performance on other inhibition tasks. In line with previous fMRI studies, Garavan et al. (1999) reported activation in the frontal pole, dorsolateral prefrontal cortex, and anterior cingulate cortex, but not the ventrolateral or ventromedial prefrontal cortex (see also Hester et al. 2004b). In a later study, Garavan et al. (2002) combined event-related fMRI with EEG techniques, and found distinguishable activation within different components of task performance. In particular, successful inhibition was associated with activation in the right dorsolateral prefrontal cortex, parietal lobe and cingulate, whereas inhibition failure was associated with the anterior cingulate and pre-supplementary motor area activation, which potentially represents conflict and response monitoring. The actual modulation of responses after an error was associated with anterior cingulate and left dorsolateral prefrontal activation. However, again, the ventromedial and ventrolateral prefrontal regions were not associated with any part of the task.

Yet, McNab et al. (2008) reported activation in the ventrolateral prefrontal cortex, as well as the dorsolateral prefrontal cortex and the frontal pole when Go trial activation was subtracted from No-Go activation. The authors also noted common activation between No-Go trials and the Stop-Signal task in the dorsolateral and ventrolateral prefrontal cortex (BAs 46 and 47; McNab et al. 2008). In the Stop-Signal task, a "Go" signal is sometimes (e.g., in 25% of trials) closely followed by a "Stop" signal which indicates that the participant is to quickly withhold their response. Though both tasks measure inhibition, the main difference between this task and the Go/No-Go Task is that the "Stop" signal is not cued and appears once participants have already begun preparing their response. Whereas inhibition tasks appear to share common recruitment of the ventrolateral prefrontal cortex and anterior cingulate regions, the Go/No-Go Task (when compared to other inhibition tasks) appears to differentially recruit the dorsolateral prefrontal cortex and parietal regions (BAs 7, 9, 40, and 46; Rubia et al. 2001; Wager et al. 2005). Furthermore, source-analysis in ERP studies has implicated both the ventrolateral prefrontal cortex and anterior cingulate cortex in inhibitory processes during the Go/No-Go Task (Kiefer et al. 1998; Bokura et al. 2001). In a review of Go/No-Go Tasks, including the Stop Signal task, Chikazoe (2010) noted the importance of the ventrolateral prefrontal cortex and pre-supplementary motor area in the inhibition of responses.

It should be noted that whereas most neuroimaging studies contrast activation during frequently presented Go trials with infrequent No-Go trials, contrasting infrequent No-Go activation with infrequent Go activation gives a more accurate measurement of response inhibition (Chikazoe et al. 2009). In any case, this too shows extensive recruitment both within (BAs 9, 10, 12, 44, 45, 46, and 47) and beyond (BAs 6, 19, 21, 24, and 32) the prefrontal cortex (Chikazoe et al. 2009). Furthermore, a more circumscribed pattern of dorsolateral, ventrolateral and anterior cingulate activation has been associated with the processing of infrequently presented Go and No-Go trials (Chikazoe et al. 2009).

3.2.3.2 Working memory

There has been some suggestion that inhibition tasks, such as the Go/No-Go Task, and working memory tasks, such as the N-Back and dot-location tasks, share common neural components and recruit similar regions (especially BA 47; McNab et al. 2008). Furthermore, Mostofsky et al. (2003) suggest that dorsolateral prefrontal involvement is only required when working memory is required to successfully perform the Go/No-Go Task. In order to manipulate the working memory demands on the Go/No-Go Task, Mostofsky et al. asked participants to respond to all green spaceships, but also to red spaceships that were preceded by an even number of green spaceships. Thus, participants were required to count green spaceships and store this count in an accessible manner. Mostofsky et al. (2003) compared activation associated with this working memory version of the Go/No-Go Task with a basic version of the task in which the "Go" rule was defined only by the color of the stimulus, and thus minimizing the working memory demands. The authors noted significantly greater dorsolateral prefrontal activity during performance of the high-load task, but only activation in the primary motor, pre-supplementary motor and cerebellar areas during performance of the low-load task (Mostofsky et al. 2003). Similarly, a meta-analysis of neuroimaging studies has suggested that low working memory load (in which there is only one type of No-Go stimulus) and high working memory load (in which there are several types of No-Go stimuli) versions of the Go/No-Go Task share some activation patterns (particularly the dorsolateral prefrontal cortex, parietal lobe, frontal pole, pre-supplementary motor area and anterior cingulate cortex), but that high working memory load versions rely more heavily on the dorsolateral prefrontal cortex and parietal regions (Simmonds et al. 2008). Furthermore, when demand on the response-selection process is maximized (e.g., by shortening the decision time), activation patterns change to recruit the dorsolateral prefrontal cortex and frontal pole more during successful No-Go performance

(Kelly et al. 2004). Durston et al. (2002) noted that the dorsolateral prefrontal cortex (BA 9), ventrolateral prefrontal cortex (BA 44) and anterior cingulate cortex (BA 32) activation modulated with the number of Go trials presented before a No-Go trial. Importantly, for No-Go trials, BAs 6 and 8 showed differential activation when the No-Go trial was preceded by five Go trials compared to when one or three Go trials preceded the No-Go trial.

3.2.3.3 Conflict-monitoring

Donkers and van Boxtel (2004) implicated specific EEG signal changes with conflict-monitoring when they examined the Go/No-Go Task and a Go/GO task. In the Go/No-Go Task, participants had to respond to white (Go) stimuli and withhold responses to red (No-Go) stimuli. In the Go/GO task, participants also had to generate a speeded response to white (Go) stimuli but respond with maximum force to green (GO) stimuli. The Go/No-Go Task involved both response inhibition and conflict-monitoring whereas the Go/GO task involved conflict-monitoring only. Donkers and van Boxtel (2004) found changes in the N2 component localized within the anterior cingulate region, which had the largest amplitude for both GO and No-Go trials when presented in among frequent Go trials. These findings suggest that the N2 component reflects conflict-monitoring rather than response inhibition. In support of this, when Nieuwenhuis et al. (2003) recorded EEG signal changes while participants performed the Go/No-Go Task with 20%, 50%, and 80% No-Go conditions (and 80%, 50%, and 20% Go conditions respectively), an N2 signal change was even apparent when participants made less frequent Go responses among more frequent No-Go trials. Similarly, Braver et al. (2001a) identified the importance of the role of the anterior cingulate cortex in monitoring response conflict in Go/No-Go Tasks (see also Bush et al. 2000). Indeed, the anterior cingulate cortex modulates its activation in response to the frequency with which No-Go trials are presented—with greater blood oxygen level-dependent (BOLD) activation in low-frequency No-Go conditions than when No-Go and Go trials are presented in equal proportions (Braver et al. 2001a).

3.2.3.4 Error processing

Using fMRI, Kiehl et al. (2000) noted that when subtracting correct-inhibition activation from commission error activation—designed to specify error-related processing—the rostral anterior cingulate and dorsolateral prefrontal cortex remained significantly activated. Specific correlations between commission errors and anterior cingulate activation have previously been reported by Casey et al. (1997). In a large-scale fMRI study in which 102 participants performed the Go/No task (Steele et al. 2014), contrasting false alarms with correct inhibitions revealed significant activation in the dorsal and rostral anterior cingulate cortex (BA 24), which extended caudally into the posterior cingulate cortex and superiorly to the supplementary motor area (BA 6). There was also bilateral activation in the superior frontal gyrus (BAs 8 and 10) and left medial frontal gyrus (BAs 9 and 10). Furthermore, the rostral anterior cingulate cortex, posterior cingulate cortex, and insular regions appear to be differentially activated in error processing when compared to other functions such as response inhibition and competition (Menon et al. 2001). In a review of tasks requiring action-selection and decision-making, Rushworth et al. (2004) suggest that the pre-supplementary motor area is primarily concerned with selecting appropriate actions, whereas the anterior cingulate cortex and posterior cingulate cortex regions are involved in associating such actions with their outcomes (e.g., error monitoring) and feeding this into the decision-making process.

When considering the evidence above, it is clear that the Go/No-Go Task is complex and that, during the task, diverse recruitment of brain regions—both frontal and non-frontal—takes place. Breaking the task into components can go some way to understanding this diversity—for example, recruitment during Go trials is particularly centered around motor and premotor regions, whereas recruitment during No-Go trials relies on regions of the prefrontal cortex and temporal lobes. Furthermore, these patterns of activity are highly dependent on aspects of the Go/No-Go Task, such as the frequency of each trial type and the complexity of the No-Go rule.

3.2.4 Aging studies

Studies have examined the effects of healthy adult aging on Go/No-Go Task performance both in terms of accuracy and RTs (see Table 3.6). Villardita et al. (1985) found no age-related differences in accuracy on the classic auditory Go/No-Go Task, with younger (*n* = 10, aged 15–24 years), middle-aged (*n* = 10, aged 45–54 years), younger-old (*n* = 10, aged 55–64 years), and older-old (*n* = 10, aged 65–74 years) participants performing similarly. However, this lack of an age-related impairment may be the result of the small sample size. In a more recent visual Go/No-Go Task, Rush et al. (2006) observed that older adults (*n* = 56, mean age = 74.8 years) exhibited no age-related impairment in terms of errors on either Go or No-Go trials when compared to younger individuals (*n* = 51, mean age = 19.8 years), despite age-related deficits in the Stop-Signal task. However, in a large cross-sectional study of 1265 participants ranging in age from 17 to 96 years, Fozard et al. (1994) found that error rates on an auditory Go/No-Go Task (including total errors, omission errors, and commission errors) exhibited a linear increase over the lifespan. This trend also existed longitudinally, with increasing age

Table 3.6 Go/No-Go Task: Aging studies

Study	n	Participant age groups (years)	Study type	Stimuli	Age effect
Villardita et al. (1985)	10; 10; 10; 10	15–24; 45–54; 55–64; 65–74	Cross-sectional (behavioral)	Motor	X
Pfefferbaum and Ford (1988)	8; 12; 12; 6; 10; 16; 2	20–25; 26–35; 36–45; 46–55; 56–65; 66–75; 76–85	Cross-sectional (neuroimaging)	Motor	✓
Fozard et al. (1994)	1265	16–24; 25–34; 35–44; 45–54; 55–64; 65–74; 75–84; ≥85	Cross-sectional (behavioral)	Tones	✓
Reuter-Lorenz et al. (1999)	24; 24	18–25; 65–75	Cross-sectional (neuroimaging)	Letters	✓
Langenecker and Nielson (2003)	11; 11	Younger, mean = 28.1 Older, mean = 72.8	Cross-sectional (neuroimaging)	Letters	✓
Rush et al. (2006)	51; 56	Younger, mean = 19.8 Older, mean = 74.8	Cross-sectional (behavioral)	Letters	X
Langenecker et al. (2007)	11; 11	25–32; 67–77	Cross-sectional (neuroimaging)	Letters	✓

✓ = age effect found; X = age effect not found

associated with increasing RTs and omission error rates, but decreasing commission error rates.

Go/No-Go studies examining RTs tend to concur that performance slows with age. Pfefferbaum and Ford (1988) administered a visual Go/No-Go Task to 66 adults aged 20–85 years. The authors found that as age increased, RTs increased and the ERPs associated with inhibition peaked later after the Go/No-Go stimuli had been presented. These effects were more pronounced on Go trials. Furthermore, the amplitude of the inhibitory ERPs decreased with age, but only in central and parietal sites, not frontal sites. This age-related increase in RTs was also found using an auditory version of the Go/No-Go Task, where the slowing was much greater for Go/No-Go performance than for performance on a simple RT task (Fozard et al. 1994). Interestingly, this slowing process appears to begin around 20 years of age with a relatively linear increase in RTs across the lifespan. However, Falkenstein et al. (2002) noted that the slowing of response, and a delay in the appearance of ERPs associated with decision-making, was present across both Go and No-Go trials and across modalities, suggesting an age-related slowing in decision-making.

In a replication of a previous neuroimaging study, Langenecker and Nielson (2003) observed that older individuals exhibited more bilateral activation in the dorsolateral prefrontal cortex and anterior cingulate cortex than younger individuals, despite somewhat similar performance. Crucially, similar dorsolateral prefrontal and anterior cingulate involvement in older individuals was observed both at first-test (Nielson et al. 2002) and at re-test (Langenecker and Nielson 2003); suggesting that such bilateral activation recruited during Go/No-Go performance is reliable and may be compensatory. A later fMRI study by Langenecker et al. (2007) attempted to assess activation and volumetric correlates of age-related change specifically on Go trial performance. Behaviorally, the authors noted that older adults ($n = 11$, aged 67–77 years) performed as well as younger adults ($n = 11$, aged 25–32 years) in terms of accuracy on No-Go trials and RTs on Go trials, but older adults committed significantly more errors on Go trials. During Go trials, older adults exhibited greater activation in the putamen/globus pallidus and lower activation in the caudate than younger adults. Furthermore, poor performance across the age groups was associated with greater activation of these regions. By contrast, age-related changes in the volume of these two regions did not predict Go trial performance. It has also been shown that older individuals ($n = 24$, aged 65–75 years) show a pattern of more bilateral activation during the Go/No-Go Task, which supports the Hemispheric Asymmetry Reduction in Older Adults hypothesis (see Cabeza 2002), in which older adults perform better when stimuli are presented bilaterally compared to unilaterally (Reuter-Lorenz et al. 1999). Interestingly, younger individuals ($n = 24$, aged 18–25 years) do not show poorer performance with unilateral stimuli unless the complexity of the task is very high (Reuter-Lorenz et al. 1999).

3.2.5 Summary

Lesion evidence clearly points to the importance of the dorsolateral prefrontal cortex, anterior cingulate cortex, and supplementary motor area in successful performance on the Go/No-Go Task. However, it is less clear whether ventromedial or ventrolateral prefrontal lesions impair Go/No-Go Task performance. By contrast, neuroimaging has helped to clarify that, although the Go/No-Go Task recruits both frontal and non-frontal regions, the role of each of these regions is associated with different cognitive processes required to perform the task. Specifically, the anterior cingulate cortex, insula, and parietal regions may be recruited to help prepare for upcoming trials and responses. The pre-supplementary motor area may be particularly important for selecting an appropriate response, whereas the dorsolateral prefrontal cortex and anterior cingulate cortex (and perhaps the ventrolateral and ventromedial prefrontal cortex) play key roles in inhibiting inappropriate responses. Furthermore, the cingulate (particularly the anterior cingulate) monitors for errors and tracks the outcomes of decisions. Finally, the evidence of an age-related impairment in terms of errors is mixed (at least for visual Go/No-Go Tasks), with little agreement on which type of error (omission or commission), if any, increases in frequency with age. There is some evidence that increased errors on Go trials may due to age-related changes in basal ganglia functioning. Several studies, involving both visual and auditory versions of the Go/No-Go Task, suggest that older individuals are slower to make decisions and to inhibit responses than younger individuals. This impaired inhibitory functioning may be due to the need to recruit both hemispheres of the brain when performing the Go/No-Go Task in older individuals.

3.3. **Hayling Sentence Completion Task**

3.3.1 **Task description**

The Hayling Sentence Completion Task (Burgess and Shallice 1996b) contains two conditions: one developed to measure response initiation, another to assess response suppression.[2] In Part A (response initiation), the researcher reads aloud a series of sentences, one at a time. In each one, the final word is omitted (e.g., "He posted a letter without a…."). After hearing each sentence, participants are required to supply a word that could plausibly complete the sentence (e.g., stamp). In Part B (response suppression), participants are required to provide a word that makes no sense in the context of the sentence to be completed (e.g., "London is a very busy… tripod."). The test comprises 30 different incomplete sentences in total (15 for each condition), which are taken from completion norms for 329 sentences (Bloom and Fischler 1980). The sentences selected for the Hayling Sentence Completion task were chosen because they have a particularly high probability of being completed with a particular response. In both conditions, participants are given two practice sentences (also taken from Bloom and Fischler 1980) and instructed that they must provide their response as quickly as possible when the researcher has finished reading. The time taken to respond is recorded for each trial, and a maximum time of 60 s is allowed per sentence. If participants fail to provide an unrelated word on a trial in Part B, participants are reminded of the task instructions. The total times for completing the sentences in Parts A and B are

---

[2] Technically, Part B measures both response initiation and response suppression. However, since Part A measures inhibition only, controlling scores on Part B for those on Part A results in a measure of response suppression.

recorded separately, and the time for Part B minus Part A can be calculated in order to quantify response inhibition, taking into account individual differences in response initiation. In the Burgess and Shallice (1996b) version of the test, response times for Parts A and B are converted into scaled scores. The number of errors made on Part B is recorded separately for category A errors (words that are connected to the meaning of the sentence) and category B errors (words that are somewhat connected). These can also be converted to scaled scores and a total scaled score can be derived by summing the scaled scores for Part A completion time, Part B completion time, and Part B errors.

3.3.2 Patient and lesion studies

Burgess and Shallice (1996b) assessed groups of patients with frontal and non-frontal lesions (total $n = 91$) on the Hayling Sentence Completion Task. They found that frontal lobe patients took longer to respond to Part A and Part B, and made more Part B errors than those with non-frontal lesions, suggesting some specific involvement of the frontal lobes on task performance. Burgess and Shallice (1996b) also investigated group differences on B–A latencies (thought to represent the additional thinking time and remove the potential confounding effect of initiation), and found that frontal patients' latencies were significantly longer than those of healthy controls. Yet, using smaller groups, Channon and Crawford (2000) did not find a significant effect of anterior ($n = 19$) versus posterior ($n = 12$) lesion location on Part A and B completion times or error scores (similarly reported in Channon and Crawford 1999 with a lower number of the same participants), although left lateral lesion patients ($n = 6$) were significantly slower than healthy controls on Part A. Moreover, Andrés and Van der Linden (2001) found that a group with frontal lesions had longer response latencies than healthy controls on Part B (but not Part A). Yet, there was no difference in the number of Part B errors. Using an abbreviated form of the Hayling Sentence Completion Task,[3] a frontal lesion group ($n = 21$) achieved a significantly poorer score than healthy controls (Roca et al. 2010). The possible specificity of the Hayling Sentence Completion Task to frontal lesions was investigated by Robinson et al. (2012), who found that a group of 47 frontal patients had significantly lower total Hayling Sentence Completion Task scores but that patients with posterior lesions ($n = 20$) were unimpaired relative to healthy controls.

---

[3] Parts A and B contained only three sentences each. Only Part B was scored: 2 for an unrelated word, 1 for a related word, and 0 for the expected word itself. The maximum score was 6.

In terms of localization of the processes associated with Hayling Sentence Completion Task performance, three studies have examined the contribution of medial prefrontal lesions predominantly involving the anterior cingulate cortex to performance, though each is limited by its small sample size (Table 3.7). Patients' total scaled scores on the Hayling Sentence Completion Task were poorer when compared to healthy controls (Critcheley et al. 2003, $n = 2$; Bird et al. 2004, $n = 1$; Baird et al. 2006, $n = 2$). However, the lesion loci were not well circumscribed, extending in all cases to more dorso- and ventromedial prefrontal areas, and in some cases including the insula, corpus callosum, and other frontal white matter. These data alone therefore cannot clarify the role of the anterior cingulate cortex in Hayling Sentence Completion Task performance.

One recent approach for examining localization within frontal subregions combined voxel-based morphometry and diffusion tensor imaging (Hornberger et al. 2011). In this study, the authors investigated the neural correlates of Hayling Sentence Completion Task performance in patients with the behavioral (frontal) variant of frontotemporal dementia ($n = 14$), Alzheimer's disease ($n = 15$), and healthy controls ($n = 18$). Both patient groups performed more poorly than controls, and MRI analysis implicated poorer integrity

Table 3.7 Hayling Sentence Completion Task: Patient and lesion studies

Study	n	Patient/ Control Groups	Study type	Brodmann Areas	FP	DL	OF	ACC
Critchley et al. (2003)	2	ACC	Lesion (single case)	–				✓
Bird et al. (2004)	1	ACC	Lesion (single case)	–				✓
Baird et al. (2006)	2	ACC	Lesion (single case)	8, 11, 12, 24, 25, 32				✓
Hornberger et al. (2011)	14; 15; 18	fvFTD, AD, HA	Lesion (VBM)	–			✓	✓
Robinson et al. (2012)	10; 8; 12; 20; 35	LL, RL, SM, post, HA	Lesion	–		✓		✓
Volle et al. (2012)	45; 110	Lesions; HA	Lesion (VBM)	–		✓	✓	

FP = frontal pole; DL = dorsolateral prefrontal cortex; OF = orbitofrontal cortex; ACC = anterior cingulate cortex; fvFTD = frontotemporal dementia (frontal variant); AD = Alzheimer's disease; HA = healthy adults; VBM = voxel-based morphometry; LL = left lateral frontal; RL = right lateral frontal; SM = superior medial frontal; post = posterior (non-frontal); ✓ = frontal region damaged and impairment found; X = frontal region damaged but no impairment.

in a network including the orbital and medial frontal areas as well as their connective tracts (uncinate fasciculus, genu of the corpus callosum and forceps minor). Conversely, Robinson et al. (2012) reported that lateral frontal lesion groups showed the lowest Hayling Sentence Completion Task total score, although those with superior medial lesions ($n = 18$) were still impaired relative to posterior lesion patients ($n = 20$) and healthy controls. However, Robinson et al. (2012) did not compare any group with orbital and ventral cingulate lesions due to low numbers, precluding comparison of this study with that of Hornberger et al. (2011). Finally, Volle et al. (2012) used a large sample of patients with frontal ($n = 26$), non-frontal ($n = 19$) and controls, using both *a priori* groupings of patients and two voxel-based lesion methods. They identified a role for the medial rostral prefrontal cortex in initiation (Part A), the right lateral frontal prefrontal cortex including the inferior, medial, and superior frontal gyri in slowness during both initiation (part A) and inhibition (part B), and the orbital areas in the number of Part B errors.

3.3.3 Neuroimaging studies

Attempts to examine the neural correlates of the Hayling Sentence Completion Task using fMRI or positron emission tomography (PET) are relatively scarce (Table 3.8). Using PET, Nathaniel-James et al. (1997) contrasted performance on Parts A and B of the Hayling Sentence Completion Task with a condition in

Table 3.8 Hayling Sentence Completion Task: Neuroimaging studies

Study	n	Patient/ Control Groups	Study type	Brodmann Areas	FP	DL	OF	ACC
Nathaniel-James et al. (1997)	6	HA	PET	45, 32			✓	✓
Collette et al. (2001)	12	HA	PET	9, 10, 45	✓	✓		
Lawrie et al. (2002)	8; 10[a]	schiz; HA	fMRI	6, 8, 9, 46,47		✓		✓
Whalley et al. (2004)	69; 21[a]	schizR; HA	fMRI	–		✓		✓
Royer et al. (2009)[a]	19; 12	schiz; HA	fMRI	9, 10, 24, 32, 45, 46	✓	✓		✓

FP = frontal pole; DL = dorsolateral prefrontal cortex; OF = orbitofrontal cortex; ACC = anterior cingulate cortex; HA = healthy adults; PET = positron emission tomography; schiz = schizophrenia patients; fMRI = functional magnetic resonance imaging; schizR = younger participants at high genetic risk of developing schizophrenia; ✓ = frontal region involved.

[a]Both groups reported in the study.

which participants had simply to read the final word of the sentence. Activation for Parts A and B was reported in the left operculum (BA 45) and right anterior cingulate cortex (BA 32), but there were no supplementary foci of activation when Parts A and B were directly contrasted. However, as the sentences were presented every 6 s, participants who responded more quickly than this had to await the next presentation, and thus were not consistently cognitively engaged in the task during scan acquisition (Collette et al. 2001). Consequently, Collette et al. adapted the task to present the next sentence as soon as participants had responded. Consistent with Nathaniel-James et al. (1997), they reported that initiation was related to left inferior frontal gyrus activation (BA 45/47), also finding that response inhibition led to left lateral activation (BAs 9, 10, and 45) using PET.

The processes associated with performance on the Hayling Sentence Completion Task have been further examined in three fMRI studies involving healthy controls and individuals with schizophrenia (Lawrie et al. 2002; Whalley et al. 2004; Royer et al. 2009). In each case, there were no group differences in the loci of the BOLD response (only Royer et al. reported significant group differences in task performance in the form of more errors and longer RTs). However, pooling the patient and control groups consistently showed activation in the left lateral prefrontal cortex (inferior and dorsolateral) and medial superior frontal cortex including the anterior cingulate cortex. Nonetheless, Royer et al. (2009) reported bilateral activation of dorsolateral, ventrolateral, and cingulate regions.

3.3.4 **Aging studies**

The extant literature suggests a significantly negative relationship between age and performance on various indices of the Hayling Sentence Completion Task (Table 3.9). When 48 older adults aged 60–70 years were compared with 47

Table 3.9 Hayling Sentence Completion Task: Aging studies

Study	n	Participant age groups (years)	Study type	Age effect
Andrés and Van der Linden (2000)	47; 48	Younger, mean = 23 Older, mean age = 65	Cross-sectional (behavioral)	✓
Crawford and Channon (2002)	30; 30	Younger, mean age = 25 Older, mean age = 68	Cross-sectional (behavioral)	✓
Bielak et al. (2006)	441	53–90 years	Cross-sectional (behavioral)	✓

✓ = age effect found; X = age effect not found

younger adults aged 20–30 years, the older group made significantly more over-all errors in Part B and also a significantly larger number of category A-type errors (i.e., words that are connected to the meaning of the sentence; Andrés and Van der Linden 2000). The age-related differences were only partially explained by group differences in processing speed. When performance on a speeded color-naming task was introduced into a partial correlation between Hayling Sentence Completion Task score and age, the effect of age on Part B latency was attenuated to non-significance, but age effects on Part B score remained. In another study, older participants were also slower on both Parts A and B, but there was more pronounced slowing for Part B (30 in each group; Crawford and Channon 2002). Finally, in a study of 457 participants aged between 53 and 90 years, advancing age was associated with general slowing (but more so for part B) as well as increasing category A and B errors, and these were partially independent of the effects of age on intelligence (Beliak et al. 2006).

3.3.5 Summary

Frontal lesions appear to result in increased slowing in response to items on the Hayling Sentence Completion Task, and this is more pronounced for Part B. Whereas there is relatively sparse evidence to implicate specific frontal subre-gions in Hayling Sentence Completion Task performance, there does appear to be a small degree of consistency between functional imaging and lesion studies regarding the significance of the lateral frontal cortex, possibly on the left side. However, there is also evidence that the ventral frontal and cingulate regions may be involved, although definite conclusions are limited by small sample sizes and the absence of well-characterized lesion groups. Increasing age leads to poorer scores on all principal Hayling Sentence Completion Task indi-ces: response latency to Parts A and B, and increased number of Part B errors.

3.4 Stimulus–response compatibility tasks

3.4.1 Task description

The Stroop Task (Stroop 1935), Flanker Task (Eriksen and Eriksen 1974), Simon Task (Simon 1969), and Motor Stroop (Lu and Proctor 1995) are all types of stimulus–response compatibility task, thought to create conditions of response competition (see Figure 3.3), even though the source of the compat-ibility effects differs between tasks (Egner 2008). These tasks require partici-pants to make a response (e.g., left or right key press in the case of the Simon Task) based on one dimension of a stimulus (e.g., color, in the Simon Task) while ignoring another equally salient dimension (e.g., stimulus location—left or right in the Simon Task). Congruent trials are those on which both stimulus

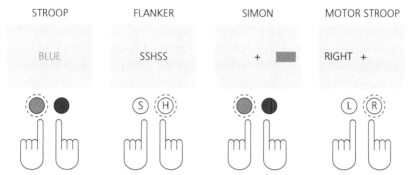

Fig. 3.3 Stimulus–response compatibility tasks showing sources of conflict. For each task, the depicted stimulus presented to participants (inside grey boxes) is for the incongruent condition. Circles indicate response options, and the broken outline indicates the correct response. Note that different stimuli (e.g., arrows) and response dimensions (e.g., verbal or motor) can be used. Adapted from *Trends in Cognitive Sciences*, 12 (10), Tobias Egner, Multiple conflict-driven control mechanisms in the human brain, pp. 374–80, Copyright (2008), with permission from Elsevier.

features (e.g., position and color) require the same response, and incongruent trials are those in which two conflicting responses are elicited by stimulus features. These tasks are thought to elicit enhanced performance-monitoring by co-activating two possible responses to task stimuli. One is an automatic response tendency and the other is appropriate in the context of the task instructions (Jonides and Nee 2004). Where the two are conflicting (i.e., incongruent), participants must suppress their automatic tendency to respond to the task-irrelevant dimension and use the task-relevant dimension in order to guide their behavior to respond to the other.

In the Stroop task, participants are required to respond based on the color of the ink in which a word is printed, ignoring the actual color word. Thus, congruent trials are those in which both the word and the ink color indicate the same response (e.g., "BLUE" printed in blue ink), and incongruent trials are those in which two possible responses are co-activated (e.g., "BLUE" printed in red ink). In the Flanker Task, respondents must identify a central letter or object, ignoring the conflicting stimuli to either side which relate to the alternative response route. In the Simon Task, the color of the object rather than its conflicting location is the cue for the response; in the Motor Stroop, it is the word itself that should determine action selection, rather than its location on the screen. It is worth noting that the Motor Stroop differs from the Word-color Stroop in both stimulus- and response-dimensions. For example, whereas the Word-color Stroop requires participants to ignore the semantics of the presented word, the Motor Stroop generally requires them not to ignore it.

It has been noted that significantly greater RTs are taken to respond on incongruent trials compared to congruent trials (i.e., the incongruency effect) or on the subsequent trial following an incorrect response compared to correct responses (i.e., post-error slowing; Rabbit 1966). This response-slowing is thought to represent a triggered behavioral adaptation to conflict between stimulus and response or the presence of errors,[4] and a large body of evidence suggests a central role for the anterior cingulate cortex in this type of behavior. Once detected, subsequent cognitive control processes are facilitated (subserved by the dorsolateral prefrontal cortex) in order to minimize future errors (Miller and Cohen 2001).

On a practical note, it is worth observing that administration of tests such as the Stroop in a clinical setting may tend to rely more on the number of errors made, rather than on precise timing of time taken to complete congruent and incongruent trials. In addition to the general floor effect for total errors (which means that error scores on this test are not informative for higher-functioning individuals), the experimental evidence is primarily derived from the calculation of the incongruency effect from response times, rather than from errors, and so the diagnostic utility of this variable is less clear.

3.4.2 Patient and lesion studies

It is clear from lesion studies that the dorsolateral prefrontal cortex is involved at some stage of stimulus–response compatibility task performance (Perret 1974; Vendrell et al. 1995; Stuss et al. 2001b) (Table 3.10). The fact that lesions in the dorsolateral prefrontal cortex also impair patients' ability to name colors in a control condition of the Stroop, however, suggests that the dorsolateral prefrontal cortex may not be directly sensitive to incongruency and error (Floden et al. 2011). Moreover, post-error slowing appears to be unaffected following ventromedial prefrontal lesions (Turken and Swick 2008).[5] Rather, early lesion studies report

---

[4] It is a matter of debate whether post-error slowing reflects the engagement of cognitive control mechanisms to improve subsequent performance (Schroder and Infantolino 2013) or simply that low frequency of error orients attention away from the task (Noteabaert et al. 2009).

[5] Szatowska et al. (2007) report that resection of the right, but not left, gyrus rectus to patients following anterior communicating artery rupture resulted in significantly larger difference in RTs between incongruent and neutral Stroop conditions, although it is not clear whether general slowing could be a factor, as proportionate data were not used, nor was a control for speeded RT. Also, those patients with anterior communicating artery ruptures who did not undergo resection did not show this effect, suggesting that the surgical resection may be causally related.

Table 3.10 Stimulus–response compatibility tasks: Patient and lesion studies

Study	n	Patient/ Control Groups	Study type	Test	Brodmann Areas	FP	DL	OF	ACC
Richer et al. (1993)	7; 10	DM + DL; HA	Lesion	Stroop	–		✓		✓
Vendrell et al. (1995)	32; 32	FL; HA	Lesion	Stroop	–		✓		X
Cohen et al. (1999)	12; 20	CP + C; CP	Lesion	Stroop	–				✓
Turken and Swick (1999)	1; 6	Posterior dorsal ACC; HA	Lesion	Stroop Motor Stroop	–				X ✓
Pujol et al. (2001)	45; 30	MS; HA	Patient	Stroop	–				✓
Ochsner et al. (2001)	1; 8	ACC; HA	Lesion	Stroop	–				✓
Stuss et al. (2001b)	51; 13; 19	FL; non-FL; HA	Lesion	Stroop	–		✓		
Swick and Turken (2002)	1; 8	ACC; HA	Lesion	Stroop Motor Stroop	32				✓
Fellows and Farah (2005a)	4; 12	ACC; HA	Lesion	Stroop	–				X
Yen et al. (2009)	10	CP + C	Lesion	Stroop	–				✓
di Pellegrino et al. (2007)	8; 6; 11	ACC; non-FL; HA	Lesion	Simon	10, 12, 24, 32				✓[a]
Cohen et al. (2008)	1(2)	Epilepsy	Lesion (+ EEG)	Flanker	–				✓

FP = frontal pole; DL = dorsolateral prefrontal cortex; OF = orbitofrontal cortex; ACC = anterior cingulate cortex; DM = dorsomedial prefrontal cortex; HA = healthy adults; FL = frontal lesions; CP = patients with chronic intractable pain; CP + C = CP who underwent cingulotomy; MS = multiple sclerosis; EEG = electroencephalography; ✓ = frontal region damaged and impairment found; X = frontal region damaged but no impairment.

[a] Effect of lesion was only for the *directional* Simon effect.

that dorsomedial lesions in humans result in slowed responses on incongruent trials when compared to controls on stimulus–response compatibility tasks (Richer et al. 1993). A study of 51 patients with focal lesions reported that dorsomedial but not ventral cingulate or orbital lesions were associated with incongruent response-slowing *and* increased error rates

(Stuss et al. 2001b).[6] Dorsomedial lesions associated with demyelination in multiple sclerosis have been shown to account for a significant amount of variance in Stroop interference (Pujol et al. 2001). Eight patients with lesions involving the dorsal anterior cingulate cortex and adjacent medial prefrontal cortex showed slowed responses to incongruent stimuli (65 ms) compared to control participants (31 ms), but these dorsal anterior cingulate patients were not significantly slower than a comparison group with non-frontal lesions ($n = 6$, 47 ms; di Pellegrino et al. 2007). However, the dorsal anterior cingulate lesion group did show a significantly slower 'Simon effect' compared to the non-frontal patients, but only when an incongruent trial was preceded by a congruent trial. The authors interpreted this condition as eliciting the greatest level of conflict and consequently identified a key role for the anterior cingulate cortex in Simon Task performance. Nevertheless, this directional Simon effect is not a widely used variable, and, combined with the small group sizes, it is difficult to make strong claims on the basis of these data alone.

Cingulotomy patients, who had the dorsal part of their anterior cingulate cortex surgically destroyed for chronic intractable pain, showed a greater Stroop incongruency effect when compared to non-surgical controls who also had a history of intractable chronic pain (Cohen et al. 1999), though there were no pre-surgical differences in performance between the groups. When comparing the pre- and post-surgery performance of patient MT—a dorsal cingulotomy patient, on the Stroop—with that of eight healthy controls, there was a significant increase in incongruent trial response times (Ochsner et al. 2001). Similarly, removal of epileptogenic tissue[7] from a patient's anterior cingulate cortex improved performance on the Flanker task from near-chance levels (prior to surgery) to almost perfect performance following surgery (Cohen et al. 2008). Surgery also resulted in the appearance of conflict-related activity in the medial prefrontal cortex as measured by EEG; this activity was absent prior to the surgical intervention. Another study reported an individual whose

---

[6] Whereas a relatively large amount of data suggests that stimulus–response compatibility tasks involve the anterior cingulate cortex, primate studies do not replicate this finding. Although this has been used to suggest a misinterpretation of the human literature, closer examination of the data suggests that there are crucial anatomical and evolutionary differences that make human and primate cingulate cortices incommensurable (Cole et al. 2009).

[7] Removal of this tissue is a surgical intervention for some pharmaco-resistant epilepsy patients. Epileptogenic tissue is considered to be dysfunctional by the authors, and therefore likely to contribute to cognitive impairment.

rare selective lesion to the dorsal anterior cingulate cortex due to a blockage of the peri-callosal branch of the anterior cerebral artery resulted in poorer error-correction and significantly slower responses on incongruent trials when compared to healthy control participants (Swick and Turken 2002). Yen et al. (2009) recently undertook an evaluative follow-up of cingulotomy patients, in which they observed an initial increase in Stroop interference one week post-operatively, compared to baseline performance, although one month after excision the difference had fallen to a trend level of significance.

While the above work suggests that damage to the anterior cingulate cortex affects performance on stimulus–responses compatibility tasks, Vendrell et al. (1995) reported that response-slowing in patients with anterior cingulate lesions was confined not only to the interference condition, but also to the control color-naming condition despite an increase in the number of errors compared to controls. This indicated general slowing rather than a specific deficit in incongruent responding. There are also reports of cases with cingulate lesions who exhibit no congruency or error-related effects on RTs, compared to controls. Fellows and Farah (2005a) reported that four patients with extensive cingulate lesions showed no significant differences in response-slowing either on incongruent trials or post-error, when compared to controls. The authors also noted that a previous single case who showed general slowing on the Stroop would actually fall into the normal range when compared to the performance of their control group (patient RN who had a left rostral to mid-dorsal anterior cingulate lesion; Swick and Jovanovic 2002). It is also possible that lesion location within the cingulate may have different effects on performance across different modalities. For example, a patient with a unilateral lesion limited to the posterior portion of the dorsal anterior cingulate cortex showed increased errors and larger interference effects in response to colored words when motor, but not verbal, responses were required (Turken and Swick 1999).

3.4.3 Neuroimaging studies

Neuroimaging studies suggest a role for both the dorsal anterior cingulate cortex and dorsolateral prefrontal cortex in stimulus–response compatibility tasks (Table 3.11). A review of early functional imaging studies suggests that the dorsal anterior cingulate cortex is consistently activated during tasks that involve the inhibition of prepotent responses or the commission of errors (Barch et al. 2001a). Unlike the lesion data, this anterior cingulate involvement is irrespective of the response modality (verbal versus motor) or processing domain (spatial versus verbal; Barch et al. 2001a). Direct comparison of BOLD activation patterns elicited during Stroop and Simon tasks (incongruent > congruent) show considerable overlap (Peterson et al. 2002).

Table 3.11 Stimulus–response compatibility tasks: Neuroimaging studies

Study	n	Patient/Control Groups	Study type	Task	Brodmann Areas	FP	DL	OF	ACC
Barch et al. (2001a)	Review	HA	Review	Various	24, 32				✓
	13	HA	fMRI	Stroop + MStr					✓
Van Veen and Carter (2002)	Review	HA	fMRI + EEG	Various	–				✓
Ullsperger and von Cramon (2004)	Review	HA	fMRI	Various	6, 8, 9, 24/32		✓		✓
Nee et al. (2007)	Review	HA	fMRI	Various	6, 8, 9, 10, 24, 32		✓		✓
Roberts and Hall (2008)	Review	HA	fMRI	Various	6, 8, 32, 44/45		✓		✓
Zysset et al. (2001)	9	HA	fMRI	Stroop	–		✓		
Peterson et al. (2002)	10	HA	fMRI	Stroop + Simon	6, 24, 32, 46		✓		✓
Hajcak et al. (2003)	22	HA	EEG	MStr	–				✓
Kerns et al. (2004)	23	HA	fMRI	Stroop	8, 9, 10, 24/32		✓		✓
Kerns (2006)	26	HA	fMRI	Simon	9/46, 32		✓		✓
Wittfoth et al. (2008)	20	HA	fMRI	Simon variant	6, 8, 9, 24, 32, 45, 46, 47		✓		✓
Yeung et al. (2004)	16	HA	EEG	Flanker	–				✓

FP = frontal pole; DL = dorsolateral prefrontal cortex; OF = orbitofrontal cortex; ACC = anterior cingulate cortex; HA = healthy adults; fMRI = functional magnetic resonance imaging; MStr = motor Stroop; EEG = electroencephalography; ✓ = frontal region involved

It has also been reported that RTs following incongruent and post-error trials are predicted by increased anterior cingulate BOLD responses (e.g., the Stroop Task, Kerns et al. 2004; the Simon Task, Kerns 2006). Thus, whereas the precise cognitive processes underlying anterior cingulate involvement during stimulus–response compatibility tasks remain a matter of some debate, both post-error slowing and incongruent trials seem to activate this brain region.

Many functional neuroimaging studies have reported increased activation in the dorsal anterior cingulate cortex and dorsolateral prefrontal cortex when incongruent and congruent trials are compared in healthy adults (summarized in Nee et al. 2007; and in Roberts and Hall 2008). Likewise, functional imaging indicates activation in the anterior cingulate cortex associated with post-error trials (Carter et al. 2000; Braver et al. 2001a; Ullsperger and Von Cramon 2001; Garavan et al. 2003; Mathalon et al. 2003; Rubia et al. 2003; Carter and van Veen 2007; Danielmeier et al. 2011). An analysis of 14 neuroimaging studies found that activity associated with conflict shared considerable overlap with activity associated with erroneous responses; both clusters originated in the dorsal anterior cingulate cortex (Ullsperger and von Cramon 2004). This finding was subsequently corroborated using the Simon task (Wittfoth et al. 2008). Further evidence that conflict- and post-error-related activation loci are common in the anterior cingulate cortex can be found using electrophysiological recordings (Van Veen and Carter 2002; Hajcak et al. 2003; Yeung et al. 2004). In an EEG study, Mathalon et al. (2003) showed that task-related activity correlates with the BOLD response in the anterior cingulate cortex. Another study found no anterior cingulate activation when contrasting incongruent and neutral conditions in an fMRI study involving the Stroop Task (Zysset et al. 2001).

The precise nature of the processing contributions made by the anterior cingulate and dorsolateral prefrontal cortex to stimulus–response compatibility tasks has also been investigated. Using a modified Stroop Task, MacDonald et al. (2000) contrasted color-naming with word-reading. During the pre-trial instruction phase (i.e., name the color versus read the word), greater dorsolateral prefrontal activation was reported, suggesting the role of this frontal subregion in the implementation of control. When performing the actual Stroop Task, MacDonald et al. (2000) found anterior cingulate activation associated with incongruent trials, suggesting that this frontal subregion plays a role in performance monitoring. In another fMRI study using the Stroop Task, Liu et al. (2008) manipulated the ratio of congruent and incongruent trials, and found that dorsolateral prefrontal activity was primarily associated with high-ratio trials (i.e., was not sensitive to congruency), whereas anterior cingulate activation was associated with RTs for incongruent trials when there was a higher ratio of incongruent to congruent trials. The authors concluded that the dorsolateral prefrontal cortex was involved in the executive modification of behavior, whereas the anterior cingulate cortex plays a more specific role in conflict-monitoring.

To further understand the interaction between the anterior cingulate and dorsolateral prefrontal cortex when performing stimulus–response compatibility tasks, West and Travers (2008) examined the temporal dynamics of error processing using EEG. They used a Stroop variant in which participants mapped the numbers 1 to 4 on to response keys. Participants were then presented with a variable number of digits, and had to respond to the number of digits rather than the actual digits presented. Thus, a congruent trial would be "333" (because both the number of digits and the actual digits are 3) whereas an incongruent trial would be "44" (because the number of digits is 2 but the actual digits are 4). West and Travers (2008) reported that error detection is associated with concomitant activity in both the anterior cingulate cortex and lateral prefrontal cortex, with more extended subsequent frontolateral activity indicative of updating cognitive control. Further to this, King et al. (2010) employed an fMRI stimulus–response compatibility paradigm using conflicting face location (interference) and face gender (response-relevant) cues. When they contrasted erroneous and correct trials, the authors reported dorsomedial BOLD activity in response to error, which was temporally linked to *increased* activity in the left lateral prefrontal cortex and fusiform face areas, and with *decreased* sensorimotor cortex activation. King et al. (2010) interpret these data as evidence for the dorsomedial prefrontal cortex in error detection and the lateral prefrontal cortex in subsequent behavioral adjustment.

3.4.4 Aging studies

Studies generally report longer responses to incongruency in healthy older adults compared to younger adults (Table 3.12). For example, interference effects have been reported to be greater in older than younger participants in the Stroop Task (Comali et al. 1962; West and Bell 1997; Mutter et al. 2005; Van der Elst et al. 2006a; Juncos-Rabadan et al. 2008; Ludwig et al. 2010), Flanker Task (Zeef et al. 1996, but see Wild-Wall et al. 2008[8]) and Simon Task (Bialystok et al. 2004; Salvatierra and Rosselli 2011), and on greater post-error slowing on the Flanker Task (Falkenstein et al. 2001) and Stroop Task (West and Moore 2005). In addition to reporting greater age-related Stroop interference, Davidson et al. (2003) found that the age-related deficit did not diminish even with practice.

---

[8] Wild-Wall et al. (2008) did not find group differences in the Flanker interference effect between a group of young ($n = 15$, mean age = 23.7 years) and 'middle-aged' ($n = 15$, mean age = 60.9 years) adults.

Table 3.12 Stimulus–response compatibility tasks: Aging studies

Study	n	Participant age groups (years)	Test	Study type	Age effect
Comali et al. (1962)	24; 20; 20; 25; 29; 25; 29; 18; 14; 16; 15	7; 8; 9; 10; 11; 12; 13; 17–19; 25–34; 65–80	Stroop	Cross-sectional (behavioral)	✓
West and Bell (1997)	20; 19	18–28; 62–78	Stroop	Cross-sectional (EEG)	✓
Verhaegen and De Meersman (1998)	Various	Various	Stroop	Meta-analysis	X[a]
West and Alain (2000)	12; 12	Younger, mean = 27 Older, mean = 70	Stroop	Cross-sectional (EEG)	✓[b]
Milham et al. (2002)	12; 10	Younger, mean = 23 Older, mean = 68	Stroop	Cross-sectional (neuroimaging)	✓
Davidson et al. (2003)	24; 24	Younger, mean = 20 Older, mean = 75	Stroop	Cross-sectional (behavioral)	✓
Mutter et al. (2005)	12; 12	Younger, mean = 21 Older, mean = 71	Stroop	Cross-sectional (behavioral)	✓
West and Moore (2005)	12; 12	Younger, mean = 27 Older, mean = 70	Stroop PES	Cross-sectional (EEG)	✓
Van der Elst et al. (2006)	1856	24–81	Stroop	Cross-sectional	✓
Bugg et al. (2007)	281	20–89	Stroop	Cross-sectional	✓[b]
Zysset et al. (2007)	23; 24	Younger, mean = 27 Older, mean = 57	Stroop	Cross-sectional (neuroimaging)	X[a]
Juncos-Rabadan et al. (2008)	41; 31; 30; 29	19–26; 50–59; 60–69; 70–82	Stroop	Cross-sectional (behavioral)	✓

(continued)

Table 3.12 Continued

Study	n	Participant age groups (years)	Test	Study type	Age effect
Ludwig et al. (2010)	39; 75	Younger, mean = 23; Older, mean = 71	Stroop	Cross-sectional (behavioral)	✓[c]
Kousaie and Phillips (2012)	118	18–84	Stroop	Cross-sectional (behavioral)	✓
Zeef et al. (1996)	12; 12	Younger, mean = 21 Older, mean = 70	Flanker	Cross-sectional (EEG)	✓
Falkenstein et al. (2001)	12; 12	Younger, mean = 23 Older, mean = 58	Flanker PES	Cross-sectional (EEG)	✓
Wild-Wall et al. (2008)	15; 15	Younger, mean = 24 Older, mean = 61	Flanker	Cross-sectional (behavioral)	X
van der Lubbe and Verleger (2002)	11; 11	Younger, mean = 25 Older, mean = 61	Simon	Cross-sectional (EEG)	✓[b]
Bialystok et al. (2004)	20; 20	Younger, mean = 43 Older, mean = 72	Simon	Cross-sectional (behavioral)	✓
Salvatierra and Rosselli (2011)	133; 100	Younger, mean = 26 Older, mean = 64	Simon	Cross-sectional (behavioral)	✓

EEG = electroencephalography; PES = post-error slowing; ✓ = age effect found; X = age effect not found.

[a] No age effect on the interference effect above general slowing.

[b] Age effect on interference after accounting for general slowing.

[c] Age effect for computerized item-by-item task, but not for paper and pencil version.

Some studies have further aimed to identify the neural underpinnings of these reported age-related differences in stimulus–response compatibility task performance. Falkenstein et al. (2001) found that in tasks that induce errors of which the participant is aware, the error negativity (an ERP component that is a correlate of error detection) was delayed in older compared to younger participants. West and Bell (1997) found that Stroop word–color interference and task-related EEG activation was greater for older than younger participants in the medial and lateral frontoparietal areas, which they interpreted as evidence for the differential aging of frontoparietal areas. Investigating the neural correlates of age-related differences in the Stroop effect, Milham et al. (2002) found that differences between younger and older adults were related to decreased activity in the dorsolateral prefrontal cortex and parietal cortex, which they suggest relates to possible impairments in attentional control with age. There was also increased anterior cingulate activity in older (compared to younger) participants during incongruent trials. However, Zysset et al. (2007) found that there were no age-related differences in the Stroop effect (above general slowing), but they did report increased magnitude in the bilateral dorsolateral prefrontal BOLD activity in middle-aged versus young participants when contrasting incongruent versus neutral trials.

Finally, a group of studies has attempted to address potential factors that confound or modulate the reported effects of age on the interference conditions of these stimulus–response compatibility tasks. Bugg et al. (2007) attempted to identify the degree to which age differences in Stroop interference can be accounted for by general age-related slowing ($n = 281$, aged 20–89 years). They found that measures of processing speed (simple and choice RT) accounted for significant variance in the age effect on the Stroop incongruent latency, but it did not entirely attenuate the relationship between age and the Stroop effect, suggesting that the age-related differences in Stroop performance are also partially attributable to decline in task-specific processes. However, in a meta-analysis of 20 studies, Verhaeghen and De Meersman (1998) used linear regression to fit the response latencies from the baseline Stroop condition. The residuals were then used to estimate the latencies in the interference condition to test how much the interference condition latencies deviated from what could be predicted from baseline speed. The authors found that the initial regression line computed from baseline latencies was sufficient to describe the Stroop interference effect, suggesting that this effect may be an artifact of general slowing. Moreover, Salthouse (2005) reported that the significant effects of age on various measures of Stroop task performance (i.e., congruent, neutral,[9] incongruent, and incongruent minus neutral difference) in a large sample ($n = 681$) were significantly attenuated by processing speed or by fluid ability, leaving no unique contribution of age to these effects beyond the general cognitive domains.

---

[9] Neutral trials are those in which the presented text string is "XX" and the participant has to name the colour of the ink in which the text string is printed.

An alternative perspective comes from an EEG study in which the authors tested the competing hypotheses that age effects on Stroop interference are attributable either to general slowing or to a specific inhibitory deficit (West and Alain 2000). After controlling for speed on neutral trials, increased latencies on incongruent trials were found. The authors had predicted that general slowing would be instantiated by finding that the amplitude of specific modulations was comparable between groups, but that their latency would increase with age. Instead, they found an age-related reduction in the amplitude of modulations that differentiated congruent and neutral from incongruent trials in frontal and parietal regions. West and Alain (2000) propose that these data support the view that age-related inhibitory deficits underlie the reported interference effect on the Stroop Task, rather than one of general slowing. A similar finding has been reported for the Simon Task (van der Lubbe and Verleger 2002).

Addressing potential modulators of age effects on stimulus–response compatibility task performance, Bialystok et al. (2004) and Salvatierra and Rosselli (2011) found that older participants exhibited a greater Simon effect than younger participants, but that being bilingual was associated with a significantly reduced Simon effect in old age. By contrast, although an effect of age on incongruent trials in the Stroop Task was reported by Kousaie and Phillips (2012), their older participants did not appear to benefit from being bilingual. Ven der Elst et al. (2006) administered the Stroop color word test to 1856 participants (aged 24–81 years). As well as a significant effect of age (particularly on the interference effect, rather than on errors made), their findings suggested that individuals with a lower level of education experience a greater degree of decline on Stroop performance with age.

3.4.5 Summary

There are clearly inconsistencies in the literature regarding both the regional specificity of functional activations within the anterior cingulate, lesion location, and the behavioral profile in relation to stimulus–response compatibility tasks, though the implication of dorsolateral prefrontal and dorsal anterior cingulate involvement has considerable theoretical support (e.g., Botvinick et al. 2004; Dutilh et al. 2012). There also exists persuasive evidence for age-related decline in performance. Inconsistencies surrounding the involvement of the anterior cingulate cortex may be partially affected by the methods employed for the precise localization of lesions or BOLD response in this small region, confounding cross-study comparison (see Chapter 1 for a discussion of this issue). Moreover, the extent to which the white matter tract beneath the cingulate (cingulum bundle) is damaged is likely to vary between studies, but this is not always alluded to in studies of cingulate cortex lesions. Damage to this area is likely to elicit very different types of behavioral sequelae compared to a cortical lesion alone (Brotis et al. 2009), and inter-patient variance in the extent of white matter damage could also contribute to discrepant findings between lesion studies by comparison with the consistency of the functional imaging literature.

Nevertheless, some convergent evidence from lesion and imaging studies implicates the dorsal anterior cingulate cortex and dorsolateral prefrontal cortex in unimpaired performance on stimulus–response compatibility-type tasks. Healthy young control participants tend to make fewer errors and exhibit a smaller incongruency effect compared to lesioned patients and older adults; though it remains unclear to what extent the effects of age on stimulus–response compatibility conflict conditions are independent from age-related changes in processing speed and more general indices of cognitive ability.

3.5 **Verbal fluency tasks**

3.5.1 **Task description**

The verbal fluency task is often included in test batteries developed to assess frontal executive abilities (e.g., the Frontal Assessment Battery, Dubois et al. 2000; the Delis–Kaplan Executive Function Scale, Delis et al. 2001) and language abilities (e.g., Multilingual Aphasia Examination, Benton et al. 1994), as well as for dementia screening (e.g., Addenbrooke's Cognitive Examination—Revised, Mioshi et al. 2006). The task instructs participants to generate as many words as possible in a predefined time (usually one minute). Typically, participants are instructed not to produce the same word more than once, a related alternative (e.g., eat and eating), or any proper nouns such as the names of people or places. Two main versions of the task exist: (1) a phonemic version; (2) a semantic version. In the phonemic version of the task, participants are required to generate as many words as possible beginning with a particular letter. Although the letters F, A, S are the most widely used, other letters have also been included (e.g., C, L, P, B). The ability to generate words in response to letters may depend on the specific letters employed where some letters in the English language (e.g., S, C, P, T, F, B, A) are considered easier than others (R, L, G, E, N, O, I; Borkowski et al. 1967). Indeed, a recent meta-analysis showed that a version of the verbal fluency task which included only easy letters (FAS) was performed significantly better than a version of the task which included both easy and difficult letters (CFL; Barry et al. 2008). The semantic version of the task requires participants to generate as many words as possible belonging to a given category (e.g., animals, vegetables, occupations). Performance on both versions of the verbal fluency task includes measures such as the total number of words produced, the number of perseverative errors (repeated words) produced, the cluster length of words from the same phonemic (e.g., cat, car, cap) or semantic (e.g., farm animals, zoo animals) subgrouping, and the number of category switches made (i.e., switching from one phonemic or semantic category to another). Both versions of the verbal fluency task are thought to involve self-monitoring, cognitive set-shifting, inhibition of responses and working memory (Rosen and Engle 1997; Troyer et al. 1998; Schwartz et al. 2003; Henry and Crawford 2004). However, phonemic fluency is additionally thought to involve strategic search through lexical memory, whereas semantic fluency is thought to involve search through semantic memory. Therefore, individuals may fail semantic fluency due to impairments in language or semantic memory rather than executive dysfunction (e.g., see Henry and Crawford 2004) and caution should be taken when interpreting poor semantic fluency performance without the administration of additional neuropsychological tests (Phillips et al. 1996).

3.5.2 Patient and lesion studies

3.5.2.1 Localization of the processes associated with phonemic verbal fluency performance

Lesion studies have examined the frontal subregions involved in performing phonemic verbal fluency (Table 3.13). Some studies support the view that the dorsolateral prefrontal cortex is crucially involved, as reduced performance has been associated with damage to the dorsolateral prefrontal cortex (Stuss et al. 1998; Troyer et al. 1998) but not the ventromedial prefrontal cortex (Cicerone and Tanenbaum 1997; Dimitrov et al. 1999; Bird et al. 2004). In a large group study of 74 patients with focal frontal or non-frontal lesions and 37 healthy control participants, Stuss et al. (1998) demonstrated that damage to the left but not the right dorsolateral prefrontal cortex resulted in impaired performance on the phonemic verbal fluency task compared to healthy controls. In an early PET investigation with 13 patients with frontal lobe damage, Sarazin et al. (1998) found that poor performance on tests of executive abilities, including the phonemic verbal fluency task, correlated with changes in the cerebral glucose metabolism in BAs 8 and 9 bilaterally (both lateral and medial) and left BAs 45 and 46. Poor performance on the verbal fluency task in patient studies has been associated with switching deficits (i.e., the transition between subcategories of words). Support for this view comes from a lesion study in which patients with lesions involving the left dorsolateral prefrontal cortex or the superior medial frontal gyrus generated fewer words and showed fewer switches between clusters on the phonemic verbal fluency task compared to healthy controls (Troyer et al. 1998).

Table 3.13 Phonemic Verbal Fluency: Patient and lesion studies

Study	n	Patient/ Control Groups	Study type	Brodmann Areas	FP	DL	OF	ACC
Cicerone and Tanenbaum (1997)	1	TBI	Lesion (single case)	–			X	
de Zubicaray et al. (1997)	1	HFI	Lesion (single case)	–		X		
Stuss et al. (1998)	54; 20; 37	FL; non-FL; HA	Lesion	–		✓		
Troyer et al. (1998)	53; 23; 55	FL; TL; HA	Lesion	–		✓		
Dimitrov et al. (1999)	1	Penetrating injury	Lesion (single case)	8, 9, 10, 11, 24, 32	X		X	X
Szatkowska et al. (2000)	12; 12; 10	Tumor; ACoA; HA	Lesion	–		✓	X	
Bird et al. (2004)	1	ACA	Lesion (single case)	–			X	X
Ptak and Schnider (2004)	1	TBI	Lesion (single case)	9/46		X		
Baird et al. (2006)	2	ACC; ACC + OF	Lesion	8, 11, 12, 24, 25, 32			✓	✓
Baldo et al. (2006)	48	CVA	VLSM	4, 6, 44				
Davidson et al. (2008)	20; 32	Tumor; HA	Lesion	4, 6, 8, 9, 10, 11, 24, 25, 32, 44, 45, 46, 47		X		

FP = frontal pole; DL = dorsolateral prefrontal cortex; OF = orbitofrontal cortex; ACC = anterior cingulate cortex; TBI = traumatic brain injury; HFI = hyperostosis frontalis interna; FL = frontal lobes; HA = healthy adults; TL = temporal lobes; ACoA = anterior communicating aneurysm; ACA = anterior cerebral artery; CVA = cerebral vascular accident; ✓ = frontal region damaged and impairment found; X = frontal region damaged but no impairment.

Although the above evidence indicates that the dorsolateral prefrontal cortex supports phonemic verbal fluency task performance, there are also studies which suggest that the dorsolateral prefrontal cortex is not critical to perform the task (Goldstein et al. 1993; de Zubicaray et al. 1997; Dimitrov et al. 1999; Ptak and Schnider 2004; Baldo et al. 2006; McDonald et al. 2006; Davidson et al. 2008). For example, Ptak and Schnider (2004) reported normal verbal fluency performance in a patient with damage to the right dorsolateral prefrontal cortex (BA 9/46) due to a traumatic brain injury 13 years prior; although this is in line with Stuss et al. (1998) who suggest a role for the left but not right dorsolateral prefrontal cortex in phonemic fluency. Dimitrov et al. (1999) described patient MGS with a right hemisphere penetrative Vietnam war wound involving BA 8, 9, 24, and 32 as well as BAs 10 and 11 who performed well on the phonemic verbal fluency task. Whereas these cases had right hemisphere frontal damage, De Zubicaray et al. (1997) described the case of patient EW who had predominantly left dorsolateral prefrontal compression due to hyperostosis frontalis interna. The result of her neuropsychological examination showed variable performance on executive tests traditionally associated with the dorsolateral prefrontal cortex. Patient EW was significantly impaired on the Self-Ordered Pointing Task (see Section 7.4, Petrides and Milner 1982; Petrides et al. 1993a; 1993b) and borderline in terms of performance on the Modified Card Sorting Test (see Section 4.4; Nelson 1976). Yet, she performed within normal limits on the Tower of London (see Section 6.3; Shallice 1982; Owen et al. 1990) and phonemic verbal fluency, suggesting that the dorsolateral prefrontal cortex is not preferentially involved in task performance. In another patient study where performance on phonemic and semantic fluency was compared in a small group of right dorsolateral prefrontal lesion patients ($n = 12$) and right non-dorsolateral prefrontal lesion patients ($n = 8$), no significant differences in terms of words generated, clustering or switching were found (Davidson et al. 2008). In a fluorodeoxyglucose positron emission tomography (FDG-PET) study, McDonald et al. (2006) investigated the relationship between brain metabolism and phonemic verbal fluency in patients with frontal lobe epilepsy or juvenile myoclonic epilepsy and healthy controls. Verbal fluency outside the scanner was only predicted by the frontal metabolism of the frontal lobe epilepsy group in BAs 45, 46, and 47, but not in the other two groups.

The involvement of the ventromedial prefrontal cortex in performing phonemic fluency remains a matter of debate. Some studies have reported intact verbal fluency performance in patients with ventromedial prefrontal lesions. For example, in 1997, Cicerone et al. described patient SAL who suffered a traumatic brain injury affecting the orbitofrontal cortex after a car accident. She was assessed on a series of neuropsychological measures, including phonemic verbal fluency. Whereas performance on the phonemic verbal fluency task was slightly impaired six months post injury relative to normative data, it had completely remitted 14 months later. As the patient sustained a traumatic brain injury, her initial impairment may have been due to damage to brain areas outside the orbitofrontal prefrontal cortex. Similarly, Bird et al. (2004) found intact performance on the phonemic verbal fluency task in a patient with damage to the medial prefrontal cortex due to a bilateral anterior cerebral artery infarction, which included the orbitofrontal cortex, the cingulate, and medial frontal sulcus. However, there are also studies where damage to the ventromedial prefrontal cortex has impaired phonemic fluency performance. For example, Baird et al. (2006) investigated the performance of two patients who underwent surgical debulking of medial prefrontal tumors on a series of tests that measured executive abilities and attention. Patient 1 had damage involving the right anterior cingulate cortex, as well as medial BA 8, whereas Patient 2 had damage involving medial BA 8, the bilateral anterior cingulate cortex, the insular cortex (BA 44), the orbitofrontal cortex (BAs 11 and 12) as well as temporal regions. The results of the neuropsychological assessment revealed that both patients performed well on tests measuring intellectual abilities, memory, and language functions. However, Patient 2, with the more extensive medial lesion, performed poorly on phonemic verbal fluency, suggesting that damage to the ventromedial prefrontal cortex affects performance (although this could equally be attributed to his temporal lobe damage). These results must be interpreted with caution. First, the two patients were assessed at different stages: Patient 1 was tested in the acute stage post surgery whereas Patient 2 was assessed in the chronic phase. Furthermore, whereas the right anterior cingulate cortex was damaged in Patient 1, the damage was bilateral in Patient 2. As the anterior cingulate cortex has been implicated in verbal fluency performance (e.g., Barch et al. 2000; Fu et al. 2002), the poor performance of Patient 2 may also have been due to more extensive anterior cingulate cortex damage rather than ventromedial prefrontal damage.

Clinical studies investigating phonemic verbal fluency performance have often revealed that poor performance is accompanied by anomalies in the brain activation in both the dorsolateral prefrontal cortex as well as other prefrontal regions such as the frontal pole (BA 10) and the ventrolateral prefrontal cortex (BA 47). For example, using PET, Abrahams et al. (1996) compared six amyotrophic lateral sclerosis patients who were impaired on a written version[10] of the phonemic verbal fluency task and six amyotrophic lateral sclerosis patients who performed normally. Participants performed two tasks: a paced version of a word generation task and a word repetition task. The behavioral results showed that the performance of both the impaired and unimpaired amyotrophic lateral

---

[10] The written phonemic verbal fluency task includes a copy condition to account for writing speed deficits associated with amyotrophic lateral sclerosis. The patients are timed as they copy the previously generated written words. A verbal fluency index is then computed: (total time allowed for test – time to copy all words generated)/total number of words generated.

sclerosis patients matched that of healthy controls. In terms of PET, the healthy controls showed increased activation of the dorsolateral prefrontal cortex (BAs 9 and 46), the frontal pole (BA 10) and the anterior cingulate cortex (BAs 24 and 32) during the verbal fluency task compared to the control condition. The results of the impaired amyotrophic lateral sclerosis group showed reduced activation in BAs 9, 10, 24, and 46 compared to healthy controls whereas the unimpaired amyotrophic lateral sclerosis group revealed only a minor reduction in activation of the right BA 9. In a second study, Abrahams et al. (2004) compared the fMRI activation of amyotrophic lateral sclerosis patients and healthy controls during word generation and confrontation naming tasks, in which participants were instructed to say the name of visually presented line drawings. Preliminary neuropsychological investigation revealed that the amyotrophic lateral sclerosis patients performed significantly more poorly on both the spoken and the written phonemic verbal fluency tasks. The fMRI results showed reduced activation in the left middle (BA 10/46) and inferior (BA 44) frontal gyrus, as well as the right middle frontal gyrus (BA 9/46) and the anterior cingulate cortex (BA 32) as well as reduced activation in the temporal and parietal areas in amyotrophic lateral sclerosis patients compared to controls. However, the deficits in verbal fluency may be due to language dysfunction rather than to deficits in executive abilities, since the amyotrophic lateral sclerosis patients were also significantly impaired on the Graded Naming Test compared to the healthy controls, and this impairment was accompanied by reduced activation in the same regions reported for phonemic verbal fluency.

It has also been shown that metabolic values in the left middle and inferior frontal gyri (BAs 45, 46, and 47) predict phonemic verbal fluency task performance in patients with frontal lobe epilepsy but not healthy controls (McDonald et al. 2006). Patients with functional psychoses show reduced fMRI activation in BAs 9/8, rostral 24/32, and 47 compared to healthy controls while performing the phonemic verbal fluency task, despite there being no difference in their behavioral performance (Schaufelberger et al. 2005). Conversely, the patient group showed greater activation of the right prefrontal cortex (BA 10/46) and the anterior cingulate cortex, which has been associated with greater cognitive processes being required to maintain normal performance. More recently, Okada et al. (2009) investigated fMRI activity in remitted patients with major depression and healthy individuals. Although no difference was reported in task performance, the fMRI results showed reduced prefrontal activation in the remitting patients in the anterior cingulate cortex and middle frontal gyrus (BA 10).

Factors such as depression, apathy, and anxiety have also been shown to influence verbal fluency performance (Okada et al. 2003; Woodward et al.

2003; Grossman et al. 2007; Bogdanova and Cronin-Golomb 2011; Grossi et al. 2013). For example, Grossman et al. (2007) found that scores on verbal fluency were predicted by apathy levels in a group of amyotrophic lateral sclerosis patients. Negative symptoms including apathy in schizophrenia have also been linked with poor performance on phonemic verbal fluency (O'Leary et al. 2000). In another study, Bogdanova et al. (2011) investigated the relationship between (i) apathy and anxiety and (ii) performance on a series of cognitive tests, including phonemic verbal fluency, in a group of patients with Parkinson's disease. Anxiety correlated significantly with phonemic fluency performance. Other research has shown that poor clustering in phonemic fluency has been associated with psychomotor slowing (e.g., poverty of speech, reduced spontaneous movement) whereas poor switching has been associated with disorganization syndrome (e.g., thought disorder) in schizophrenia (Woodward et al. 2003). This may make it more difficult to tease apart whether the fluency deficits found in clinical patients are due to a decline in the processes associated with dorsolateral prefrontal damage or these neuropsychiatric symptoms.

Overall, the results of the studies discussed above indicate that the dorsolateral prefrontal cortex is important when performing the phonemic verbal fluency task. However, other regions of the prefrontal cortex including the frontal pole, the anterior cingulate cortex, and the ventrolateral prefrontal cortex may also be involved in task performance.

3.5.2.2 Localization of the processes associated with semantic verbal fluency performance

Neuropsychological evidence for the localization of semantic verbal fluency within the frontal lobes can also be found in the literature (Table 3.14). Contrasting evidence exists on the role of the dorsolateral prefrontal cortex. Some studies indicate that the dorsolateral prefrontal cortex is important for task performance (Stuss et al. 1998; Troyer et al. 1998; Szatkowska et al. 2000; Cilia et al. 2007). For example, Stuss et al. (1998) and Troyer et al. (1998) reported deficits in semantic verbal fluency following damage to the dorsolateral prefrontal cortex. Whereas both studies indicated that phonemic verbal fluency deficits were associated with damage to the left dorsolateral prefrontal cortex, semantic verbal fluency deficits were associated with bilateral dorsolateral prefrontal damage. Similarly, Szatkowska et al. (2000) found poorer performance on the semantic verbal fluency task in patients with either left or right dorsolateral prefrontal damage compared to healthy controls.

However, other research has not demonstrated that damage to the dorsolateral prefrontal cortex impairs performance on the semantic verbal fluency task

Table 3.14 Semantic Verbal Fluency: Patient and lesion studies

Study	n	Patient/ Control Groups	Study type	Brodmann Areas	FP	DL	OF	ACC
Cicerone and Tanenbaum (1997)	1	TBI	Lesion (single-case)	–			X	
Stuss et al. (1998)	54; 20; 37	FL; non-FL; HA	Lesion	–		✓		
Troyer et al. (1998)	53; 23; 55	FL; TL; HA	Lesion	–		✓		
Dimitrov et al. (1999)	1	Penetrating injury	Lesion (single-case)	8, 9, 10, 11, 24, 32	X	X	X	X
Szatkowska et al. (2000)	12; 12; 10	Tumor; ACoA; HA	Lesion	–		✓	✓	
Ptak and Schnider (2004)	1	TBI	Lesion (single-case)	9/46		X		
Baird et al. (2006)	2	ACC; ACC + OF	Lesion	8, 11, 12, 24, 25, 32			✓	✓
Baldo et al. (2006)	48	CVA	VLSM	4, 6, 44				
Davidson et al. (2008)	20; 32	Tumor; HA	Lesion	4, 6, 8, 9, 10, 11, 24, 25, 32, 44, 45, 46, 47		X		

FP = frontal pole; DL = dorsolateral prefrontal cortex; OF = orbitofrontal cortex; ACC = anterior cingulate cortex; TBI = traumatic brain injury; FL = frontal lobes; HA = healthy adults; TL = temporal lobes; ACoA = anterior communicating aneurysm; ACA = anterior cerebral artery; CVA = cerebral vascular accident; ✓ = frontal region damaged and impairment found; X = frontal region damaged but no impairment.

(Ptak et al. 2004; Davidson et al. 2008). For example, in the earlier-mentioned Davidson et al. (2008) study, the authors investigated associations between verbal fluency performance and the extent of brain damage in the dorsolateral prefrontal cortex (BAs 8, 9, and 46), the cingulate cortex (BAs 24, 25, 32, and 33), the anterior frontal lobe (BA 10), the inferior frontal regions (BAs 11 and 47) as well as BAs 44 and 45. The researchers administered both the phonemic and semantic verbal fluency tasks to a group of 20 patients who had undergone resection of the right frontal lobe (16 patients had frontal damage and four had frontal damage with additional non-frontal damage) and a group of healthy controls. The results showed that the patient group performed significantly more poorly than healthy controls on both versions of the verbal fluency task. Yet, when the authors mapped the patients' frontal damage, the study reported no significant association between task performance (i.e., total words produced, clustering, and switching) and dorsolateral prefrontal damage.

There is evidence to suggest that the medial regions of the prefrontal cortex are involved in semantic verbal fluency. Although some early studies did not demonstrate deficits in semantic fluency after lesions in the ventromedial prefrontal cortex (Cicerone and Tanenbaum 1997; Dimitrov et al. 1999), more recent studies have found that extensive damage to the ventromedial prefrontal cortex and the anterior cingulate cortex (Troyer et al. 1998; Szatkowska et al. 2000; Baird et al. 2006; Cilia et al. 2007) as well as damage to more posterior brain areas (e.g., the temporal and parietal regions; Troyer et al. 1998; Baldo et al. 2006, 2010) impairs task performance. Troyer et al. (1998) investigated verbal fluency performance in patients with either frontal or temporal lobe damage. The frontal patients were further grouped into those with either left or right dorsolateral prefrontal damage and those with damage involving either the superior or inferior medial prefrontal cortex. In addition to a decline in semantic fluency performance following left and right dorsolateral prefrontal damage, the researchers found that both superior and inferior medial patients produced significantly fewer words compared to healthy controls. Furthermore, damage to the left temporal lobe was associated with reduced word generation. The previously discussed Baird et al. (2006) study showed that their patient with a lesion involving the entire left anterior cingulate cortex and right dorsal anterior cingulate cortex (BAs 24 and 32) and the orbitofrontal cortex (BAs 11 and 12) performed poorly on semantic verbal fluency (as well as phonemic fluency), whereas the patient whose lesion affected the right anterior cingulate cortex performed within normal limits.

There is also some evidence that more posterior brain regions are involved in performance on the semantic verbal fluency task (e.g., Abrahams et al. 2004; Baldo et al. 2006, 2010; see Henry and Crawford 2004 for a review). In particular, the temporal lobes have been found to play a critical role in performing the semantic version of the verbal fluency task. In a study by Baldo et al. (2006), both semantic and phonemic fluency tasks were administered to 48 left-hemisphere stroke patients. The results of voxel-based lesion symptom mapping showed that phonemic verbal fluency was mainly associated with frontal damage involving BAs 4, 6, and 44 whereas performance on semantic verbal fluency was mainly associated with posterior lesions in the temporal and parietal lobes. In their later study, Baldo et al. (2010) compared the performance of a patient with large frontal lesion and a patient with a large temporal lesion on both phonemic and semantic verbal fluency. The behavioral results showed that the patient with the temporal lobe lesion generated more words than the patient with the frontal lesion on the phonemic task, but performed more poorly on the semantic task.

In summary, the majority of patient and lesion studies indicate that performance on the semantic verbal fluency task relies on a distributed brain network that includes both lateral and medial regions of the prefrontal cortex as well as more posterior regions, including the temporal and parietal lobes.

3.5.3 Neuroimaging studies

3.5.3.1 Neural correlates of phonemic verbal fluency performance

Neuroimaging studies have also examined the neural correlates of phonemic verbal fluency (see Table 3.15). The verbal fluency task is characterized by the intrinsic generation of responses in the absence of external cues, and neuroimaging evidence suggests that lateral areas of the prefrontal cortex are recruited during fluency performance. In an early PET study, Frith et al. (1991) compared brain activation during the phonemic and semantic verbal fluency tasks with a rest baseline condition, as well as counting and lexical-decision task conditions. By comparing activation associated with the verbal fluency tasks and the active baseline tasks, the researchers found that the intrinsic generation of words mainly recruited the left dorsolateral prefrontal cortex (BAs 9 and 46) with smaller foci of brain activity associated with the anterior cingulate cortex (BA 24) and the parietal region. There was also deactivation of the superior temporal gyrus.

Verbal fluency performance has been investigated using either the aloud or silent production of words (i.e., overt versus covert word production). Neuroimaging studies have investigated brain activation associated with overt verbal fluency compared either with a resting baseline (Warkentin et al. 1991; Cantor-Graae et al. 1993; Audenaert et al. 2000; Perani et al. 2003; Dan et al. 2013) or with tasks that control for speech production and for automatic generation processes (e.g., word repetition, counting; Frith et al. 1991; Cardebat et al. 1996; Phelps et al. 1997; Elfgren and Risberg 1998). The results of these neuroimaging studies suggest that phonemic verbal fluency is associated with activation of a brain network including the lateral prefrontal cortex (i.e., dorsolateral and ventrolateral prefrontal cortex), the anterior cingulate cortex, and the orbitofrontal cortex. For example, Warkentin et al. (1991) measured regional cerebral blood flow (rCBF) using PET while 39 healthy participants performed a phonemic verbal fluency task, finding increased left dorsolateral prefrontal activation compared to a rest baseline. The recruitment of the dorsolateral prefrontal cortex during phonemic verbal fluency has been associated

Table 3.15 Phonemic Verbal Fluency: Neuroimaging studies

Study	n	Patient/Control Groups	Study type	Brodmann Areas	FP	DL	OF	ACC
Frith et al. (1991)	4	HA	PET	9, 24, 46		✓		✓
Warkentin et al. (1991)	39	HA	PET	–		✓		
Cantor-Graae et al. (1993)	22	HA	PET	–		✓		
Cuenod et al. (1995)	8	HA	fMRI	6, 9, 44, 47		✓		
Abrahams et al. (1996)[a]	6; 12	ALS, HA	PET	6, 8, 9, 10, 24, 32, 44, 45, 46	✓	✓		✓
Cardebat et al. (1996)	19	HA	SPECT	–		X		
Mummery et al. (1996)	6	HA	PET	44/6				
Brammer et al. (1997)	6	HA	fMRI	9, 32, 44/9, 44/46		✓		✓
Paulesu et al. (1997)	5	HA	fMRI	45, 44/6				
Phelps et al. (1997)	11	HA	fMRI	6, 8, 24, 32, 45		✓		✓
Elfgren and Risberg (1998)	20	HA	PET	9, 10, 11, 44, 45, 46, 47	✓	✓	✓	
Friedman et al. (1998)	11	HA	fMRI	44, 45				
Sarazin et al. (1998)	13	FL	PET	8, 9, 45, 46		✓		
Hutchinson et al. (1999)	12	HA	fMRI	9, 32, 46		✓		✓
Audenaert et al. (2000)	20	HA	SPECT	24, 32, 45, 47				✓
Gaillard et al. (2000)	10; 10	Children; HA	fMRI	9, 44, 45, 46		✓		✓
Fu et al. (2002)	11	HA	fMRI	8, 9, 10, 24, 32, 45, 46, 47	✓	✓		✓
Ravnkilde et al. (2002)	46	HA	PET	6, 9, 11, 24, 25, 32, 44, 45, 47	✓	✓	✓	

(continued)

Table 3.15 Continued

Study	n	Patient/ Control Groups	Study type	Brodmann Areas	FP	DL	OF	ACC
Abrahams et al. (2003)	18	HA	fMRI	6, 9, 24, 32, 44, 45, 46, 47		✓		✓
Perani et al. (2003)[a]	5; 10	Aphasics; HA	fMRI	6, 9, 10, 44, 45, 46, 47	✓	✓		
Weiss et al. (2003)	10; 10	M; F	fMRI	32, 46, 47		✓		✓
Abrahams et al. (2004)[a]	28; 18	ALS; HA	fMRI	9/46, 10/46, 32, 44		✓		✓
Schaufelberger et al. (2005)[a]	7; 9	Psych; HA	fMRI	9/8, 24/32, 47		✓		✓
McDonald et al. (2006)[a]	18; 10; 14	FLE; JME; HA	FDG-PET	–				
Okada et al. (2009)[a]	10; 8	Rem dep; HA	fMRI	10	✓			✓
Birn et al. (2010)	14	HA	fMRI	–				
Kircher et al. (2011)	15	HA	fMRI	44, 45				
Senhorini et al. (2011)	21	HA	fMRI	6, 9, 24, 32, 44, 45		✓		✓
Vannorsdal et al. (2012)	24	HA	tDCS	–		X		
Dan et al. (2013)	28	HA	fNIRS	6, 9, 44, 45		✓		
Pereira et al. (2013)	16	PD	tDCS	–		✓		

FP = frontal pole; DL = dorsolateral prefrontal cortex; OF = orbitofrontal cortex; ACC = anterior cingulate cortex; HA = healthy adults; PET = positron emission tomography; fMRI = functional magnetic resonance imaging; ALS = amyotrophic lateral sclerosis; SPECT = single-photon emission computed tomography; FL = frontal lobes; M = males; F = females; psych = psychosis; FLE = frontal lobe epilepsy; JME = juvenile myoclonic epilepsy; FDG = fludeoxyglucose; rem dep = remitted major depression; tDCS = transcranial direct current stimulation; fNIRS = near-infrared spectroscopy; PD = Parkinson's disease; ✓ = frontal region involved.

[a]Only the healthy controls reported in the study.

with the executive and working memory demands of the task (i.e., the storage of the produced words to avoid repetition and the inhibition of irrelevant responses) as well as for strategy implementation (e.g., Brammer et al. 1997; Fu et al. 2002; Abrahams et al. 2003). For example, when Phelps et al. (1997)

investigated fMRI activation associated with phonemic verbal fluency compared to word repetition and a antonym-generating task (e.g., short-TALL), they found activation in the dorsolateral prefrontal cortex as well as the anterior cingulate cortex.

Other studies have reported activation in the inferior frontal gyrus and the anterior cingulate cortex associated with phonemic verbal fluency performance (Audenaert et al. 2000; Perani et al. 2003; Senhorini et al. 2011; see Wagner et al. 2014 for a review). For example, using single-photon emission tomography (SPET), Audenaert et al. (2000) reported increased blood flow in the left inferior frontal gyrus (BAs 45 and 47) as well as in the anterior cingulate cortex (BAs 24 and 32) when participants had to say aloud as many words beginning with a certain letter as they could, compared to alternating between counting from 1 to 100 and saying the letters of the alphabet. The involvement of the anterior cingulate cortex during verbal fluency has been explained in terms of selective attention, monitoring of conflicting responses and response selection (Barch et al. 2000; Fu et al. 2002; Ravnkilde et al. 2002).

There is also some evidence for the involvement of the orbitofrontal cortex in phonemic fluency (Abrahams et al. 1996; Elfgren and Risberg 1998; Gourovitch et al. 2000; Ravnkilde et al. 2002). For example, Ravnkilde et al. (2002) investigated PET activation during phonemic verbal fluency compared to a reading control task. In line with previous neuroimaging results, the researchers found significant activation of the left dorsolateral prefrontal cortex, including BAs 9 and 45 and the anterior cingulate cortex (BAs 24 and 32). However, the PET results revealed further activation of the inferior frontal gyrus (BA 47) and the orbitofrontal cortex (BA 11). In another PET study, Elfgren and Risberg (1998) reported increased rCBF during phonemic verbal fluency compared to a control counting condition in the left prefrontal cortex (BAs 44, 45, 46 and 47), extending into the superior frontal areas (BA 9) and the anterior orbital region (BA 10). In a subsequent analysis, participants were subdivided on the basis of the strategy they used to perform the task, as indicated by post-scan interview: 12 used a verbal strategy (e.g., try different combinations of syllables) and eight used a mixed strategy which included both verbal and visual search processes (e.g., visualizing objects whose names start with the required letter). Those employing a verbal strategy produced significantly more words than those employing a mixed strategy. These behavioral results were accompanied by increased activation in both the lateral (BAs 45, 46, and 47) and orbital (BA 11) regions associated with the verbal strategy compared to an automatic speech condition, whereas no difference emerged compared to baseline in those participants employing a mixed strategy. Therefore, the strategy used to perform verbal fluency may affect both performance as well as the recruitment of distinct brain areas.

Although the studies discussed above mainly report some degree of dorso-lateral prefrontal involvement, there are also studies that have not found any dorsolateral prefrontal activation during phonemic verbal fluency task perfor-mance (Cardebat et al. 1996; Paulesu et al. 1997; Vannorsdall et al. 2012). For example, Paulesu et al. (1997) reported fMRI activation during phonemic ver-bal fluency in the left inferior frontal gyrus (BAs 44/6 and 45) which did not extend into the dorsolateral prefrontal cortex. However, as Paulesu et al. (1997) employed a self-paced design in which participants generated words for 30 s rather than a more cognitively demanding paced design in which participants were instructed to respond on letter presentation (i.e., a cue presented every few seconds), this might explain the lack of dorsolateral prefrontal activation in their study.

Phonemic fluency tasks which employ covert word production have reported activation in both the dorsolateral and ventrolateral prefrontal cortex (Cuenod et al. 1995; Audenart et al. 2000; Gourovitch et al. 2000) as well as BAs 44 and 45 and the anterior cingulate cortex (Brammer et al. 1997; Friedman et al. 1998; Hutchinson et al. 1999; Gaillard et al. 2000). Cuenod et al. (1995) instructed their participants to generate words covertly in response to 10 different let-ters; fMRI showed activation in the left dorsolateral prefrontal cortex (BA 46/9) and the inferior frontal gyrus (BAs 44 and 47). Hutchinson et al. (1999) compared silent phonemic verbal fluency performance with silent counting and found increased activation of the dorsolateral prefrontal cortex (BAs 9 and 46) as well as the anterior cingulate cortex (BA 32) associated with verbal flu-ency performance. Other studies, however, have reported additional activa-tion of the ventrolateral prefrontal cortex and orbitofrontal cortex (Schlösser et al. 1998; Weiss et al. 2003). For example, Schlösser et al. (1998) investigated fMRI activation in men and women during phonemic verbal fluency, finding that females showed areas of activation in the orbitofrontal cortex and medial frontal cortex not shown in men. In another fMRI study, Weiss et al. (2003) reported gender differences associated with the activation in the hippocampus but not in the prefrontal cortex during the phonemic verbal fluency task. In fact, the researchers found that both males and females activated the dorsolat-eral prefrontal cortex (BA 46), ventrolateral prefrontal cortex (BA 47) as well as the anterior cingulate cortex (BA 32), although women showed greater activity in the hippocampus compared to men.

The disadvantage of using a covert phonemic fluency paradigm in the scanner is that it does not allow for performance monitoring. Fu et al. (2002) employed a compressed sequence design to overcome this limitation: participants were presented with a target letter, to which they silently produced a word in response while being scanned. After a few seconds, scanning stopped and participants overtly produced the words. Using this paradigm, Fu et al. (2002) found bilateral activation in the middle frontal gyrus (BAs 9 and 46) as well as the inferior frontal gyrus (BA 47) and the anterior cingulate cortex (BA 32) relative to the baseline condition (i.e., word repetition). Using a similar paradigm, Abrahams et al. (2003) also found activation of the left middle frontal gyrus (BAs 9 and 46), the inferior frontal gyrus (BAs 44, 45, and 47) and the anterior cingulate cortex (BAs 24 and 32). In another study, Halari et al. (2006) administered the compressed sequence design to compare the neural correlates associated with phonemic verbal fluency in men and women. The behavioral results showed that women produced significantly more words than did men. These results were accompanied by activation of the left inferior frontal gyrus as well as the superior and medial prefrontal gyri in men, whereas women showed bilateral activity of the inferior frontal gyrus but not these additional frontal subregions. These results suggest that men either recruit more frontal areas than women or that they employ a different strategy in order to perform the phonemic verbal fluency task.

Overall, these neuroimaging studies indicate that phonemic verbal fluency recruits mainly the left dorsolateral prefrontal cortex and the anterior cingulate cortex. Some studies have also reported activation associated with the ventrolateral prefrontal cortex (Audenaert et al. 2000; Gourovitch et al. 2000; Fu et al. 2002; Ravnkilde et al. 2002; Abrahams et al. 2003; Weiss et al. 2003) and the orbitofrontal cortex (Schlösser et al. 1998; Gourovitch et al. 2000; Fu et al. 2002; Ravnkilde et al. 2002). Activation in the left inferior frontal gyrus has been linked to language production, semantic processing, and switching between categories (Petersen et al. 1988; McCarthy et al. 1993; Hirshorn and Thompson-Schill 2006).

3.5.3.2 Neural correlates of semantic verbal fluency performance

Neuroimaging studies investigating the neural correlates associated with performing semantic verbal fluency have shown that this version of the task activates brain areas similar to those activated by phonemic fluency (Frith et al. 1991; Cardebat et al. 1996; Warburton et al. 1996; Paulesu et al. 1997; Audenart et al. 2000; Gourovitch et al. 2000; Crosson et al. 2001; Gurd et al. 2002; Gaillard et al. 2003; Vannorsdal et al. 2012) (Table 3.16). For example, Warburton et al. (1996) investigated brain activation associated with noun generation in response to semantic categories (e.g., furniture) using PET and reported a consistent pattern of left prefrontal activation, which included the superior and inferior frontal sulcus (BAs 9 and 44/46), as well as the anterior cingulate cortex and the supplementary motor areas (BA 6/32). Other neuroimaging investigations support the central role played by the left inferior prefrontal cortex (BAs 44 and 45) in the performance of both verbal fluency

Table 3.16 Semantic Verbal Fluency: Neuroimaging studies

Study	n	Patient/ Control Groups	Study type	Brodmann Areas	FP	DL	OF	ACC
Frith et al. (1991)	4	HA	PET	9, 46		✓		
Cardebat et al. (1996)	19	HA	SPECT	–		✓		
Mummery et al. (1996)	6	HA	PET	–		✓		
Warburton et al. (1996)	6	HA	PET	6/32, 9, 44/46		✓		✓
Paulesu et al. (1997)	5	HA	fMRI	45				
Audenaert et al. (2000)	20	HA	SPECT	10, 10/46, 24, 32, 44/45	✓			✓
Crosson et al. (2001)	15	HA	fMRI	6, 8, 9, 32, 45, 47				✓
Gurd et al. (2002)	11	HA	fMRI	–				✓
Gaillard et al. (2003)[a]	29; 16	Children; HA	fMRI	6, 6/8, 9, 11, 44/9, 46, 47	✓	✓		
Perani et al. (2003)[a]	5; 10	Aphasics; HA	fMRI	6, 9, 10, 45, 46, 47	✓	✓		
Basho et al. (2007)	12	HA	fMRI	6, 32, 44, 45				✓
Cilia et al. (2007)	20; 12	PD/STN-BDS; PD	SPECT	6, 9, 33		✓		✓
Heim et al. (2008)	28	HA	fMRI	44, 45				
Meinzer et al. (2009)[b]	16; 16	YA; OA	fMRI	11, 32			✓	✓
Whitney et al. (2009)	18	HA	fMRI	6/9, 32, 44, 45, 47				✓
Birn et al. (2010)	14	HA	fMRI	–				

(continued)

Table 3.16 Continued

Study	n	Patient/ Control Groups	Study type	Brodmann Areas	FP	DL	OF	ACC
Kircher et al. (2011)	15	HA	fMRI	44, 45				
Vannorsdal et al. (2012)	24	HA	tDCS	–		✓		
Dan et al. (2013)	28	HA	fNIRS	6, 9, 44, 45				
Pereira et al. (2013)	16	PD	tDCS	–		✓		

FP = frontal pole; DL = dorsolateral prefrontal cortex; OF = orbitofrontal cortex; ACC = anterior cingulate cortex; HA = healthy adults; PET = positron emission tomography; SPECT = single-photon emission computed tomography; fMRI = functional magnetic resonance imaging; PD = Parkinson's disease; STN-BDS = deep brain stimulation of subthalamic nucleus; YA = younger adults; OA = older adults; tDCS = transcranial direct current stimulation; fNIRS = near-infrared spectroscopy; ✓ = frontal region involved.

[a]Only the healthy controls reported in the study.

[b]Only the younger adults reported in the study.

tasks (Audenaert et al. 2000; Perani et al. 2003; Amunts et al. 2004; Basho et al. 2007; Heim et al. 2008; Whitney et al. 2009; Kircher et al. 2011; Dan et al. 2013). Whitney et al. (2009) compared fMRI activation associated with both phonemic and semantic verbal fluency paradigms, finding common brain activation in the inferior frontal gyrus (BAs 44, 45, and 47) as well as the anterior cingulate cortex (BA 32) and the premotor frontal areas (BA 6/9). Nonetheless, neuroimaging studies have also shown additional brain activation associated with semantic fluency. In their SPET study, Audenaert et al. (2000) demonstrated that whereas both phonological and semantic verbal fluency activated the left inferior prefrontal cortex (BA 44/45) and the anterior cingulate cortex (BAs 24 and 32), semantic verbal fluency additionally activated the right medial frontal gyrus (BA 10). In a SPECT study, Cardebat et al. (1996) found significant right dorsolateral (rather than the typically reported left) and medial prefrontal activation associated with semantic verbal fluency performance. However, no specific additional activation was found for the phonemic fluency task compared to the baseline. Cardebat et al. (1996) argued that, as their baseline condition might be considered a self-generation task (i.e., participants repeat aloud dysyllabic high frequency words at their convenience rather than as soon as they hear them), left dorsolateral prefrontal activation might be common to both the phonemic fluency and baseline tasks, and therefore not found when phonemic fluency is contrasted with baseline performance.

Brain stimulation and inhibition using transcranial direct current stimulation (tDCS) has also been used to investigate the brain regions important for performing phonemic and semantic verbal fluency tasks, as tDCS can result in either excitatory (i.e., anodal) or inhibitory (i.e., cathodal) stimulation. Vannorsdal et al. (2012) investigated the effect of brain stimulation and inhibition on both the phonemic and semantic fluency tasks. In this study, the authors applied anodal or cathodal tDCS on the left dorsolateral prefrontal cortex during performance of phonemic and semantic verbal fluency. The results of this study showed that the application of anodal tDCS over left dorsolateral prefrontal cortex was associated with improved semantic verbal fluency performance, whereas no effect emerged on the phonemic task, suggesting that the left dorsolateral prefrontal cortex may not be critically involved during performance on the phonemic verbal fluency task. However, anodal tDCS application over the dorsolateral prefrontal cortex appears to improve the performance on both tasks in patients with Parkinson's disease compared to stimulation of posterior brain areas (Pereira et al. 2013).

Activation of the medial prefrontal cortex and the middle frontal gyrus has also been associated with performing semantic fluency (Audenart et al. 2000; Gaillard et al. 2003; Hirshorn and Thompson-Schill 2006; Heim et al. 2008). In an fMRI study, Meinzer et al. (2009) examined the activity pattern elicited during semantic and phonemic fluency. When semantic fluency was directly compared with phonemic fluency, phonemic fluency was associated with stronger activation of the left inferior frontal gyrus (BAs 45 and 9/44), whereas semantic fluency was associated with stronger activation of the right medial prefrontal gyrus (BA 11) and left rostral anterior cingulate (BA 32). In an fMRI study, Birn et al. (2010) found that phonemic fluency activated the left inferior frontal gyrus to a greater extent than did the semantic task, whereas the semantic task resulted in greater activity in the left middle frontal gyrus. Finally, a meta-analysis by Wagner et al. (2014) including 28 neuroimaging studies showed that the regions of activation associated with semantic fluency were the left anterior cingulate gyrus (BA 32), the left superior (BAs 6 and 8) and medial frontal gyrus (BA 6), the left inferior frontal gyrus (BAs 9, 45, and 47) as well as the left claustrum, the left thalamus, and precuneus (BA 7). Phonemic fluency was associated with similar regions of activation including the left inferior and middle frontal gyri (BAs 6, 9, 44, 45, and 47), the left and right anterior cingulate gyrus (BAs 24 and 32), the left and right insula (BA 13), the left thalamus, the left precuneus (BA 7) and putamen, as well as in the right claustrum and caudate head.

Semantic fluency performance has also been associated with activation of more posterior brain regions. For example, when Billingsley et al. (2004)

compared brain activity associated with the phonemic and semantic fluency tasks using magnetic source imaging (which combines magnetoencephalography and MRI data to obtain a comprehensive understanding of the association between behavior, brain structure and function), semantic fluency was associated with greater temporal lobe activation. In a PET study by Mummery et al. (1996), semantic fluency recruited left temporal regions whereas phonemic fluency was associated with left frontal activation in BA 44/6. Notably, the left dorsolateral prefrontal activation typically associated with intrinsic word generation was not found (Frith et al. 1991) and yet both fluency tasks are thought to involve intrinsic word generation (Mummery et al. 1996). The authors argue that contrasting the brain activation associated with performing the two verbal fluency tasks had removed brain regions common to both tasks. Gourovitch et al. (2000) used PET to compare patterns of brain activation associated with phonemic and semantic verbal fluency. In particular, the phonemic fluency task revealed greater activation of the left inferior prefrontal cortex (BAs 44 and 47), the right prefrontal cortex (BAs 9 and 44), and the temporo-parietal cortex. The semantic task, instead, showed greater activation of the left temporal cortex and the medial prefrontal cortex (BA 10).

3.5.4 **Aging studies**

3.5.4.1 Aging and phonemic verbal fluency performance

Research investigating age effects on phonemic verbal fluency performance has produced conflicting results (Table 3.17). Some studies have reported age effects (Spinnler and Tognoni 1987; Zappalà et al. 1995; Isingrini and Vazou 1997; Bolla et al. 1998; Tombaugh et al. 1999; Bryan and Luszcz 2000; Dursun et al. 2002; Auriacombe et al. 2001; Brickman et al. 2005; Van der Elst et al. 2006b; McDowd et al. 2011). An early review of 32 studies published between 1992 and 1999 concluded that there is a progressive decline in phonemic fluency abilities as people age (Loonstra et al. 2001). In a large-scale study of 478 adults aged between 55 and 94 years, Bolla et al. (1998) examined phonemic and semantic fluency using the Controlled Oral Word Association. Performance on both versions of the verbal fluency task declined with age. Similarly, a meta-analysis of 26 studies examining phonemic fluency and aging demonstrated age effects from 40 years onwards and especially after 60 years of age (Rodriguez-Aranda and Martinussen 2006). A recent meta-analysis also showed that phonemic fluency declines with age, and this age effect is attributed to the executive demands of the task (Barry et al. 2008).

Despite these findings, a considerable number of studies have not revealed age-related effects on the phonemic verbal fluency task (Bolla et al. 1990;

Table 3.17 Phonemic Verbal Fluency: Aging studies

Study	n	Participant age groups (years)	Study type	Age effect
Bolla et al. (1990)	65; 64; 70	≤53; 54–60; ≥61	Cross-sectional (behavioral)	X
Tomer et al. (1993)	26; 39; 19	50–64; 65–74; 75–91	Cross-sectional (behavioral)	X
Parkin et al. (1995)	30; 29	18–25; 74–95	Cross-sectional (behavioral)	X
Zappalà et al. (1995)	160; 142; 122; 124; 98; 55	20–29; 30–39; 40–49; 50–59; 60–69; 70–79	Cross-sectional (behavioral)	✓
Bryan et al. (1997)	683	Mean = 77.18	Cross-sectional (behavioral)	✓
Crossley et al. (1997)	252; 673; 384	65–74; 75–84; ≥85	Cross-sectional (behavioral)	X
Fabiani and Friedman (1997)	14; 14	22–28; 65–88	Cross-sectional (behavioral)	X
Isingrini et al. (1997)	107	25–46; 70–99	Cross-sectional (behavioral)	✓
Troyer et al. (1997)	41; 54	18–35; 60–89	Cross-sectional (behavioral)	X
Bolla et al. (1998)	196; 195; 87	55–69; 70–79; 80–94	Cross-sectional (behavioral)	✓
Capitani et al. (1998)	102; 83; 99; 95; 97; 27	18–29; 30–39; 40–49; 50–59; 60–69; 70–81	Cross-sectional (behavioral)	X
Parkin and Java (1999)	20; 20; 20	22–31; 63–72; 75–88	Cross-sectional (behavioral)	X
Tombaugh et al. (1999)	19; 106; 132; 121; 144; 220; 334; 200; 24	16–19; 20–29; 30–39; 40–49; 50–59; 60–69; 70–79; 80–89; 90–95	Cross-sectional (behavioral)	✓
Bryan and Luszcz (2000)	565	72–95	Cross-sectional (behavioral)	✓
Crawford et al. (2000)	39; 50; 23; 11	18–30; 31–45; 46–60; 61–75	Cross-sectional (behavioral)	X
Auriacombe et al. (2001)	1133	≥65	Cross-sectional (behavioral)	✓
Kemper and Sumner (2001)	100; 100	18–28; 63–88	Cross-sectional (behavioral)	X
Meguro et al. (2001)	34; 32; 25; 8	65–69; 70–74; 75–79; ≥80	Cross-sectional (behavioral)	X

(continued)

Table 3.17 Continued

Study	n	Participant age groups (years)	Study type	Age effect
Dursun et al. (2002)	75	13–67	Cross-sectional (behavioral)	✓
Hughes and Bryan (2002)	60; 60	17–48; 65–88	Cross-sectional (behavioral)	X
Mathuranath et al. (2003)	50; 85; 18	55–64; 65–74; 75–84	Cross-sectional (behavioral)	X
Ravdin et al. (2003)	149	60–69; 70–79; ≥80	Cross-sectional (behavioral)	X
Lamar and Resnick (2004)	23; 20	20–40; 60–80	Cross-sectional (behavioral)	X
Brickman et al. (2005)	196; 87; 72; 61; 35; 20	21–30; 31–40; 41–50; 51–60; 61–70; 71–82	Cross-sectional (behavioral)	✓
Mell et al. (2005)	20; 20	Younger, mean = 23.15 Older, mean = 67.63	Cross-sectional (behavioral)	X
Henry and Phillips (2006)	69; 64	18–40; 60–88	Cross-sectional (behavioral)	✓
Van der Elst et al. (2006b)	1825	24–81	Cross-sectional (behavioral)	✓
Steiner et al. (2008)	48	30–80	Cross-sectional (behavioral)	X
Meinzer et al. (2009)	16; 16	20–33; 64–88	Cross-sectional (neuroimaging)	X
Machado et al. (2009)	135, 160; 50	60–69; 70–79; ≥80	Cross-sectional (behavioral)	X
Elgamal et al. (2011)	62; 30; 38	17–40; 41–59; 60–78	Cross-sectional (behavioral)	✓
McDowd et al. (2011)	36; 30	18–30; 65–90	Cross-sectional (behavioral)	✓
Kahlaoui et al. (2012)	16; 16	Younger, mean = 23.06 Older, mean = 70.19	Cross-sectional (neuroimaging)	X
Meinzer et al. (2012)	14; 14	19–32; 61–80	Cross-sectional (neuroimaging)	X
Heinzel et al. (2013)	325	51–82	Cross-sectional (neuroimaging)	X

✓ = age effect found; X = age effect not found

Tomer and Levin 1993; Meinzer et al. 1995; Parkin et al. 1995; Fabiani and Friedman 1997; Troyer et al. 1997; Capitani et al. 1998; Parkin and Java 1999; Ardila et al. 2000; Crawford et al. 2000; Kemper and Sumner 2001; Meguro et al. 2001; Hughes and Bryan 2002; Mathuranath et al. 2003; Ravdin et al. 2003; Rodríguez-Aranda 2003; Lamar and Resnick 2004; Mell et al. 2005; Steiner et al. 2008; Meinzer et al. 2009; Kahlaoui et al. 2012; Heinzel et al. 2013). Some studies have found that word generation performance improves with age (Henry and Phillips 2006; Elgamal et al. 2011). Small sample sizes, variation in the age ranges, and the number of age comparisons performed may explain why some studies have failed to find a statistically significant effect of age on phonemic fluency performance, given that the meta-analyses have reported age effects.

The aging studies that have not demonstrated age declines in phonemic verbal fluency performance have at the same time reported age differences on other measures of frontal executive function (Parkin et al. 1995; Fabiani and Friedman 1997; Lamar and Resnick 2004; Mell et al. 2005). For example, Mell et al. (2005) administered the phonemic verbal fluency to 20 younger (mean age = 23 years) and 20 older (mean age = 67 years) adults. They found that their older participants performed significantly more poorly than younger adults on tests such as the Stroop Task and the Self-Ordered Pointing Task. Yet, no age difference emerged on the phonemic verbal fluency task or on the Tower of London. Fabiani and Friedman (1997) reported intact phonemic fluency in a group of older adults who performed significantly more poorly than younger participants on the Wisconsin Card Sorting Test. Lamar and Resnick (2004) found age-related declines in performance on the Self-Ordered Pointing Task but not the phonemic verbal fluency task. Correlational research has also found that age is negatively associated with performance on the Wisconsin Card Sorting Task, the Stroop Task, and the Tower of London, but not with the phonemic verbal fluency task (Crawford et al. 2000).

Intact performance on the phonemic verbal fluency task in older adults has been explained in terms of verbal skills (Bryan et al. 1997; Isingrini et al. 1997; Troyer et al. 1997; Bolla et al. 1998; Phillips 1999; Crawford et al. 2000; Henry and Phillips 2006; Loonstra et al. 2001 for a review of normative data), which tend not to decline with age (Salthouse 1991). For example, in the Crawford et al. (2000) study, they explain their lack of correlation between verbal fluency performance and age in relation to the intact verbal knowledge of their older participants, which was measured using the vocabulary subtest of the Wechsler Adult Intelligence Scale—Revised (WAIS-R; Wechsler 1981). Other aging studies have also shown that verbal skills predict phonemic verbal fluency performance. For example, Bryan et al. (1997) administered phonemic verbal fluency and the National Adult Reading test (NART; Nelson 1982) to a large sample of 683 participants and found that NART error scores significantly predicted verbal fluency performance. In another study, Hughes and Bryan (2002) administered the phonemic verbal fluency task, the NART and the Extended Range Vocabulary Test (Ekstrom et al. 1976) to 60 younger participants aged 17–48 years and 60 older participants aged 65–88 years. The older adults performed significantly better than younger adults on both measures of verbal skills, and no age effect emerged on the standard phonemic verbal fluency task. Articulation speed was associated with phonemic verbal fluency performance in terms of the number of words produced and clusters in older participants.

A small number of aging studies have reported age-related decline on more demanding verbal fluency tasks (Parkin et al. 1995; Bryan and Luszcz 2000; Henry and Phillips 2006; Elgamal et al. 2011). For example, Henry and Phillips (2006) investigated the performance of younger (age range = 18–40 years) and older (age range = 60-88 years) adults on a series of verbal fluency tasks, which varied in terms of their cognitive demands: the traditional phonemic and semantic verbal fluency tasks and three alternating versions of verbal fluency: the intra-dimension alternating phonemic fluency task (i.e., alternating between letters C and P), the intra-dimension alternating semantic fluency task (i.e., alternating between the categories "color" and "occupation") and the extra-dimension alternating fluency task (i.e., alternating between the letter R and category "things to wear"). The neuropsychological battery included tests of crystallized intelligence (i.e., Mill Hill Vocabulary Test), measures of fluid intelligence (i.e., Raven's Progressive Matrices) and a measure of speed of processing. The results of the neuropsychological background revealed that older adults performed better than younger participants on the vocabulary test but more poorly on measures of fluid intelligence and speed of processing. In terms of the fluency tasks, older participants outperformed younger adults on the phonemic verbal fluency and no age effect emerged on the semantic fluency task. However, some age differences emerged on the more demanding alternating semantic task, with older adults performing more poorly than younger participants and producing more perseverative errors than younger adults. These results suggest that verbal skills might compensate for decline with age on traditional verbal fluency measures, but deficits emerge in older participants when more demanding versions of the task are administered which rely more on cognitive set-shifting. In a correlational study, Bryan and Luszcz (2000) administered three verbal fluency tasks, which differ in terms of their executive demands, to a large group of 565 older participants aged between 72 and 95 years. The participants were instructed to perform the standard version of the phonemic verbal fluency task, the Excluded Letter Task, in which participants were instructed to produce words that did not contain a specified letter, and the Uses for Object Task, in which participants produced as many uses for objects as possible (e.g., a paper clip). The Excluded Letter Task and the Uses for Object Task are thought to rely more strongly on strategic retrieval and monitoring processes. The results showed that age negatively correlated with performance on all three fluency tasks. However, age correlated more strongly with the Excluded Letter and the Uses of Objects Task than with the standard fluency paradigm. More recently, Elgamal et al. (2011) investigated the effect of processing speed on phonemic verbal fluency performance in young (age range = 17-40 years), middle-aged (age range = 41-59 years), and older (age range = 60-78 years) adults. Processing speed was measured with Parts A and B of the Trail Making Test and the Digit-Symbol Substitution Test. Performance on phonemic verbal fluency did not decline with age. By contrast, the younger group performed significantly better the middle-aged and older age groups on processing speed measures. However, when the age decline on processing speed abilities was controlled for, an age effect on the verbal fluency task emerged, with older adults performing better than younger adults, suggesting that slow word generation may mask an older-age advantage for phonemic verbal fluency performance.

Other factors such as gender and education are thought to affect verbal fluency task performance. Some evidence suggests that gender affects performance on the phonemic fluency task (Zappalà et al. 1995; Crossley et al. 1997; Capitani et al. 1998; Loonstra et al. 2001; Rodriguez-Aranda and Martinussen 2006). A meta-analysis conducted by Rodriguez-Aranda et al. (2006) reported better performance in women compared to men. Other studies have found that better task performance was associated with higher levels of education (Capitani et al. 1998; Tombaugh et al. 1999; Meguro et al. 2001; Dursun et al. 2002; Mathuranath et al. 2003; Machado et al. 2009). Mathuranath et al. (2003) administered the phonemic and semantic fluency tasks to 153 participants aged between 55 and 84 years divided into three age groups: 55–64, 65–74 and 75–84 years. No age effect was found on the phonemic verbal fluency task, whereas the oldest age group performed significantly more poorly than the youngest age group and the intermediate age group on the semantic fluency task. The results also revealed that education influenced performance on both fluency tasks.

3.5.4.2 Aging and semantic verbal fluency performance

Performance on the semantic version of the verbal fluency task appears to decline consistently with age (Spinnler and Tognoni 1987; Tomer and Levin

1993; Parkin et al. 1995; Crossley et al. 1997; Troyer et al. 1997; Bolla et al. 1998; Kempler et al. 1998, 2001; Parkin and Java 1999; Sakatani et al. 1999; Ardila et al. 2000; Mathuranath et al. 2003; Ravdin et al. 2003; Rodríguez-Aranda 2003; Brickman et al. 2005; Van der Elst et al. 2006b; Fichman et al. 2009; Meinzer et al. 2009; Elgamal et al. 2011; Meinzer et al. 2012), although a few studies have not reported age-related decline on the task (e.g., Maki et al. 1999; Henry and Phillips 2006) (Table 3.18). This age effect on semantic verbal fluency performance has been associated with reduced switching abilities (i.e., shifting between clusters of semantically related words). For example, Troyer et al. (1997) found that younger adults (age range = 18–35 years) produced more words and switched more often than older participants (age range = 60–89 years) when performing the semantic verbal fluency task.

Other factors have also been shown to influence performance on semantic verbal fluency tasks. Rodríguez-Aranda (2003) investigated the role of psychomotor slowness in terms of oral articulation and handwriting on vocal and written versions of the phonemic and semantic verbal fluency tasks in younger and older participants (age groups: 20–39, 40–59, 60–69, 70–79, >80 years). The results showed a significant decline with age from 60 years onwards in terms of both oral and written versions of the semantic fluency task, but only on the written, not the oral, version of the phonemic task. Furthermore, verbal knowledge, as measured using the vocabulary subtest of the WAIS-R, predicted performance on all versions of the verbal fluency task, except the oral semantic condition. Writing speed and verbal knowledge predicted performance on both written fluency tasks, whereas reading speed and verbal knowledge predicted performance on the oral fluency tasks. Thus, deficits on verbal fluency task might be affected by both verbal and psychomotor skills. Bolla et al. (1998) have also reported that verbal abilities significantly predict semantic verbal fluency performance.

Level of education also influences semantic fluency task performance. Crossley et al. (1997) administered the semantic and the phonemic verbal fluency tasks to 635 older participants divided into three age groups: 65–74 years, 75–84 years, and >85 years. The results showed that higher levels of education (≥13 years) resulted in significantly better performance on both versions of the verbal fluency task. However, there was no significant interaction between age and level of education. In another study, Brickman et al. (2005) found that years of education significantly correlated with performance on both fluency tasks. However, as education did not interact with age, the age decline on the task was not moderated by years of education. Fichman et al. (2009) found a significant negative correlation between age and semantic fluency performance in two groups of older participants: young-old (i.e., aged <75 years) and

Table 3.18 Semantic Verbal Fluency: Aging studies

Study	n	Participant age groups (years)	Study type	Age effect
Tomer and Levin (1993)	26; 39; 19	50–64; 65–74; 75–91	Cross-sectional (behavioral)	✓
Parkin et al. (1995)	30; 29	18–25; 74–95	Cross-sectional (behavioral)	✓
Crossley et al. (1997)	252; 673; 384	65–74; 75–84; ≥85	Cross-sectional (behavioral)	✓
Troyer et al. (1997)	41; 54	18–35; 60–89	Cross-sectional (behavioral)	✓
Bolla et al. (1998)	196; 195; 87	55–69; 70–79; 80–94	Cross-sectional (behavioral)	✓
Kempler et al. (1998)	195; 122	55–74; 75–99	Cross-sectional (behavioral)	✓
Maki et al. (1999)	33; 19; 15; 20; 22; 52; 25	<40; 40–49; 50–59; 60–69; 70–79; ≥80	Cross-sectional (behavioral)	X
Parkin et al. (1999)	20; 20; 20	22–31; 63–72; 75–88	Cross-sectional (behavioral)	✓
Tombaugh et al. (1999)	19; 106; 132; 121; 144; 220; 334; 200; 24	16–19; 20–29; 30–39; 40–49; 50–59; 60–69; 70–79; 80–89; 90–95	Cross-sectional (behavioral)	✓
Auriacombe et al. (2001)	1133	≥65	Cross-sectional (behavioral)	✓
Kemper and Sumner (2001)	100; 100	18–28; 63–88	Cross-sectional (behavioral)	✓
Mathuranath et al. (2003)	50; 85; 18	55–64; 65–74; 75–84	Cross-sectional (behavioral)	✓
Ravdin et al. (2003)	149	60–69; 70–79; ≥80	Cross-sectional (behavioral)	✓
Brickman et al. (2005)	196; 87; 72; 61; 35; 20	21–30; 31–40; 41–50; 51–60; 61–70; 71–82	Cross-sectional (behavioral)	✓
Henry and Phillips (2006)	69; 64	18–40; 60–88	Cross-sectional (behavioral)	X
Van der Elst et al. (2006)	1825	24–81	Cross-sectional (behavioral)	✓
Fichman et al. (2009)	203; 116	<75; >75	Cross-sectional (behavioral)	✓

(continued)

Table 3.18 Continued

Study	n	Participant age groups (years)	Study type	Age effect
Meinzer et al. (2009)	16; 16	20–33; 64–88	Cross-sectional (neuroimaging)	✓
Elgamal et al. (2011)	62; 30; 38	17–40; 41–59; 60–78	Cross-sectional (behavioral)	✓
Kahlaouoi et al. (2012)	16; 16	Younger, mean = 23.06 Older, mean = 70.19	Cross-sectional (neuroimaging)	X
Meinzer et al. (2012)	14; 14	19–32; 61–80	Cross-sectional (neuroimaging)	✓
Heinzel et al. (2013)	325	51–82	Cross-sectional (neuroimaging)	✓

✓ = age effect found; X = age effect not found

old-old (i.e., aged >75 years). Further analyses, however, revealed that the age effect disappeared when education level was controlled for. One main difference between the Brickman et al. (2005) and Fichman et al. (2009) studies is that many of the participants in the latter study are considered illiterate as ~50% of them have fewer than five years of education. Studies have shown that individuals with low levels of education are at a much higher risk of being cognitively impaired, even without dementia (Leibovici et al. 1996; Barnes et al. 2004; Nitrini et al. 2004).

Fluid intelligence abilities have also been found to contribute to the age effects on semantic verbal fluency (Parkin and Java 1999; Henry and Phillips 2006; Elgamal et al. 2011). For example, Henry and Phillips (2006) administered semantic verbal fluency to 69 younger (aged 18–40 years) and 64 older (aged 60–88 years) adults, as well as Raven's Progressive Matrices to assess fluid abilities, the Mill Hill Vocabulary Test to assess verbal abilities, and the Digit–Symbol Substitution Test to assess processing speed. Fluid intelligence abilities accounted for 12.5% of the variance on semantic fluency, with processing speed only contributing to another 0.4% of the variance, verbal abilities contributing zero, and age contributing a further 1.3% variance. In another study, Parkin and Java (1999) reported age effects on the semantic verbal fluency task with performance on speed of processing (i.e., Digit–Symbol Substitution Test) and fluid intelligence (i.e., AH4) measures accounting for the variance on this fluency task. Finally, Isingrini and Vazou (1997) found that older adults performed significantly more poorly than younger adults on the Wisconsin Card Sorting Task, and the phonemic and semantic versions of the verbal fluency task. Further analysis revealed that performance on tests involving fluid intelligence (i.e., Cattell's Matrices and Similarities from the WAIS-R) correlated with performance on both the semantic and phonemic verbal fluency tasks in older but not younger participants.

Neuroimaging studies have investigated the neural correlates of semantic verbal fluency in younger and older adults. In an fMRI study, Meinzer et al. (2009) found that the age decline on the semantic task performance was accompanied by additional brain activation involving the inferior and middle frontal cortex (BAs 44 and 47), the cingulate gyrus (BA 23) and the superior temporal gyrus (BA 42) in older participants. Further analysis showed that brain activation in the inferior and middle frontal cortex negatively correlated with task performance. A second fMRI investigation by Meinzer et al. (2012) found that the age decline in semantic fluency performance was accompanied by greater right hemisphere activation including the medial, middle, and inferior frontal areas in older adults. This right lateralized activity negatively correlated with performance (e.g., number of words produced) in older participants.

3.5.5 Summary

Overall, patient and lesion studies suggest that the dorsolateral prefrontal cortex is important when performing verbal fluency tasks, although other frontal regions including the frontal pole, the anterior cingulate cortex, and the ventrolateral prefrontal cortex may also be involved in phonemic fluency performance, and the ventrolateral and medial prefrontal regions, the temporal cortex, and parietal cortex have been associated with semantic fluency. Neuroimaging studies also suggest dorsolateral prefrontal cortex and anterior cingulate cortex involvement as well as additional activation of the orbitofrontal cortex and inferior frontal gyrus. In addition, semantic verbal fluency appears to rely to a greater extent on temporal lobe activation. In terms of aging, whereas semantic fluency performance is consistently reported to decline with age, age-related decline in phonemic fluency is less consistently reported. This may be because phonemic word generation is thought to rely on verbal knowledge and crystallized intelligence abilities, which show little decline with age.

Chapter 4

Mental flexibility

4.1 **Goal Neglect Task**

4.1.1 **Task description**

The Goal Neglect Task was designed to measure deficits in the ability to maintain task rules online (i.e., the instructions) so that the rules can be used during the task. Importantly, these deficits arise despite intact understanding and recall of the task rules at the end of the task (Duncan et al. 1996). The task consists of a mixture of letter-only and number-only pairs sequentially presented on a computer screen so that one character appears on the left of the screen and the other character appears on the right of the screen. Participants are given three rules they should follow while monitoring the presented letter and number pairs. First, participants are instructed to attend only to letters, and to ignore numbers, reading the letters aloud as they occur. Second, participants are told to pay attention only to characters presented on the side of the screen determined by a written instruction presented at the start of each trial ("WATCH LEFT" or "WATCH RIGHT"). Third, after ten pairs have been presented, participants are given a second side-instruction that they must follow. A symbol (e.g., + or –; > or <) is shown that instructs participants either to continue to watch the same side or to change side for the final three pairs in the trial (e.g., + indicates to watch right and—indicates to watch left). An example of the sequence of stimuli presented is shown in Figure 4.1. The task requires participants to report only letters and only from the cued side (ignoring numbers and letters from the non-cued side) and to switch side accurately for the final three pairs if indicated by the cue. Performance is measured in terms of errors, and the phenomenon of goal neglect usually manifests as the tendency to report letters from the non-cued side. In particular, Duncan et al. (1996) propose that the weakest task rule (i.e., the rule most likely to be neglected) is the one presented to the participant last during the instruction phase of the task. This means that the second side-instruction is most usually neglected, especially when it is in direct competition with the first side-instruction (i.e., when the second side-instruction requires participants to switch sides; Duncan et al. 1996, 2008). Task performance closely relates to performance on measures of general intelligence (Spearman's g-factor; e.g., Cattell's Culture Fair

WATCH RIGHT

6	9
E	J
R	U
4	8
2	3
G	P
Q	S
1	5
7	6
B	F
+	
9	4
N	W
Z	H

Fig. 4.1 Example of the stimulus sequence from the Goal Neglect Task. The task requires participants to follow the first side-instruction (e.g., WATCH RIGHT), report only letters (not numbers), and to follow the second side-instruction when it appears. Correct responses in this trial would be "J, U, P, S, F, W, H." The typical neglect-like response, where the second side-instruction is not followed, may take the form of "J, U, P, S, F, N, Z."

Test; Duncan et al. 1996) and tests assessing executive functions (e.g., verbal fluency, Wisconsin Card Sorting Test, WCST; Duncan et al. 1997).

4.1.2 Patient and lesion studies

Deficits in maintaining task demands, despite intact understanding of the task instructions, were described by Luria (1966). In one example, patients with frontal lobe damage were asked to squeeze a rubber ball when a light was switched on. Such patients often failed to follow the instruction despite reporting that they "must squeeze" (Luria 1966). Since then, the effect of brain damage on the ability to maintain task demands has not been extensively investigated, although some evidence suggests that task performance declines following damage to the frontal lobes. Duncan et al. (1996, Experiment 4) administered the Goal Neglect Task to a group of 10 patients with frontal lesions, eight patients with posterior lesions not involving the frontal lobes, and 18 healthy controls who closely matched each patient in terms of age, sex, socio-economic status, and performance on the National Adult Reading Test (Nelson 1982). The brain damage of three frontal patients involved the inferior and medial regions of the frontal lobes. In the remaining seven frontal patients, the brain damage involved both frontal and posterior brain areas (i.e., temporal and parietal). As these latter frontal patients sustained lesions from closed head injuries, the damage was relatively diffuse and substantial, and no reference to specific frontal subregions was made. The ability to attend initially to the stimuli before the second side-instruction was presented was comparable across groups. However, after the second side-instruction (i.e., the "+" or "–" symbols), the task performance of the frontal patients declined compared to the performance of the patients with posterior damage and the healthy control group. The majority of frontal patients (i.e., seven out of 10) showed complete neglect of the task requirement to switch sides, and instead attended to the side cued by the first side-instruction for the entire trial. By contrast with the frontal patient group, the performance of the posterior patients did not differ from that of healthy matched controls.

In a correlational study, Duncan et al. (1997) investigated the relationship between the ability to maintain task rules and the locus of brain damage. Duncan et al. administered the Goal Neglect Task to 24 head-injury patients, with damage involving both frontal and non-frontal regions. Though no control group was recruited, performance of the patient group was poor in comparison to normative data taken from previous work (see Duncan et al. 1996). Furthermore, performance on the Goal Neglect Task significantly correlated with performance on executive tasks (e.g., verbal fluency, Self-Ordered Pointing Task), which are thought to tap dorsolateral prefrontal functions (e.g., Petrides and Milner 1982; Stuss et al. 1998; Troyer et al. 1998). Duncan et al. examined the relationship between performance on these executive tasks, the Goal Neglect Task, lesion volume for the frontal, parietal, and temporal areas, and global brain atrophy (i.e., ventricular enlargement). In this group of head-injured individuals, performance on the Goal Neglect Task and a composite measure of executive abilities were both shown to correlate with global brain atrophy. Although correlations were also noted between performance and focal brain damage (i.e., frontal, parietal, and temporal regions), these were not as strong. However, the severity and location of damage was not described in these patients, and so it is unclear which frontal subregions (and to what degree) are involved. The study does not rule out the necessity of the dorsolateral prefrontal cortex or other frontal subregions during the performance of the Goal Neglect Task.

4.1.3 **Neuroimaging studies**

Neuroimaging techniques have not been used extensively to investigate the neural mechanisms associated with Goal Neglect Task performance. However, goal neglect appears to relate closely to measures of general intelligence and executive abilities (Duncan et al. 1996). As the lateral prefrontal regions are recruited during tests of general intelligence (see Duncan et al. 2000 for a review) and tests of executive abilities, such as the AX-Continuous Performance Test, verbal fluency, WCST, anti-saccade and Stroop Tasks (Frith et al. 1991; Marenco et al. 1993; Rezai et al. 1993; Barch et al. 1997; Phelps et al. 1997; Peterson et al. 1999; Nieuwenhuis et al. 2004), the dorsolateral prefrontal cortex may also be involved in performing the Goal Neglect Task.

Recent investigations suggest that one component of the task (i.e., learning new rules) involves the frontoparietal brain network (see Duncan 2013 for a review). Duncan et al. (2008) showed that the phenomenon of goal neglect is affected by the complexity of the rules given in the instruction phase before performing the actual task. Duncan et al. proposed that a task model (i.e., the mental representation of relevant facts and rules required for the execution of the task) is built during the learning phase of a new task. As rule complexity increases, relevant information and facts may be neglected. Thus, the task representation is simplified and its role in shaping the appropriate task execution is weakened. Support for the involvement of the frontoparietal network associated with task model formation comes from a series of fMRI studies (Hampshire et al. 2008; Dumontheil et al. 2011; Woolgar et al. 2011). For example, Woolgar et al. (2011) employed fMRI to investigate brain activation associated with the processing of task-relevant information (e.g., cue processing and response formation) during the performance of a stimulus–response mapping task. In the task, participants were required to respond to a blue square presented in one of four horizontal locations with the designated button on a keypad. Importantly, the mapping of the keys was either simple (e.g., the left index finger responded to outermost right-sided stimuli) or complex (e.g., the left middle finger responded to outermost right-sided stimuli), resulting in different amounts of spatial incongruity. The results revealed the activation of a frontoparietal network during the processing of task-relevant information. In the main, four areas were recruited: the inferior frontal sulcus, the anterior insular/frontal operculum, the anterior cingulate cortex/pre-supplementary motor area, and the inferior parietal sulcus. These brain areas coded different components of the task: the anterior insular/frontal operculum coded both the stimulus–response mapping rules and the cue indicating what rules to apply. The inferior frontal sulcus coded the mapping rules, the target position, and response. The inferior parietal sulcus was involved in coding the rules, the cue and the target position, and a trend emerged for the anterior cingulate cortex/pre-supplementary motor area to be involved in rules and response coding.

There is evidence to suggest that brain activation is modulated by rule complexity (Dumontheil et al. 2011; Hampshire et al. 2011). For example, using fMRI, Hampshire et al. (2008) investigated brain activation associated with the performance of a non-verbal reasoning task and found that activation of the middle frontal gyrus (including BAs 10 and 46), the superior parietal cortex, and the precuneus increased as the complexity of the rules increased. Dumontheil et al. (2011) administered several complex tasks during fMRI in which participants had to perform tasks designed to measure the ability to maintain task rules, similar to the Goal Neglect Task. By contrast with the Goal Neglect Task, these tasks involved a variety of stimuli (e.g., words, faces, shapes), but with a set of complex rules similar to those used in previous studies (e.g., "only respond to lower case letters"). Learning the task-relevant rules was associated with activation of an extended brain network including frontal (e.g., the inferior frontal sulcus, the pre-supplementary motor area, the anterior insular/frontal operculum, and rostral prefrontal cortex) and parietal brain areas (Dumontheil et al. 2011).

4.1.4 **Aging studies**

At present, few conclusions can be drawn in terms of the effects of healthy adult aging on the ability to maintain goals during the Goal Neglect Task. Whereas Duncan et al. (1996, 2008) provided evidence of goal neglect in middle-aged and older participants (Duncan et al. 1996, 2008), the performance of these participants on the Goal Neglect Task was not directly compared to that of younger individuals. Some support for the view that the ability to maintain task goals declines with age comes from studies involving other tasks that rely on goal maintenance. For example, during the Stroop Task, older participants are more likely to read the word rather than name the color of the ink that the word is printed in compared to younger adults (see Stroop Task in Section 3.4). In terms of anti-saccade tasks in which participants should suppress the tendency to attend automatically to a visually presented stimulus (i.e., cue) and direct their attention to the opposite location, older adults are less able to direct their attention away from the cue (e.g., Butler et al. 1999; Nieuwenhuis et al. 2000; 2004). Such a deficit has been attributed to a reduced ability to maintain the task goal in working memory (De Jong 2001). A more recent fMRI investigation (Hampshire et al. 2008) scanned younger (age range = 20–31 years) and older (age range = 46–77 years) adults as they were performing an attentional switching task. Participants were shown pairs of objects with each object consisting of a face and a building superimposed on top of one another. The participants' task was to identify the target object within the face/building combinations through trial and error, and to keep responding to it on successive trials. Similar to Reversal Learning (Section 4.2) and WCST (Section 4.4) paradigms, the target rule changed after six consecutive correct responses and participants were required to identify a new target. The results did not show an age effect on inhibitory control (i.e., older adults did not show an increased tendency to respond to a previously relevant target and did not commit more errors when a new target was identified). However, older individuals were more likely than younger adults to respond to a non-target object and to re-examine the objects they had already switched from. These results were interpreted as the reduced ability to maintain an efficient strategy. This was accompanied by reduced activation of the dorsolateral prefrontal cortex (BAs 9 and 46) and ventrolateral prefrontal cortex (BA 47), supporting a role for the lateral region of the prefrontal cortex in performing this goal maintenance task.

4.1.5 Summary

The work of Duncan et al. suggests that performance on the Goal Neglect Task is impaired following frontal lobe damage. However, no studies have examined the frontal subregions that might be involved. Some indirect evidence suggests that, although Goal Neglect Task performance correlates with neuropsychological tasks that tap the dorsolateral prefrontal cortex, an extended frontoparietal network is likely involved in maintaining task-relevant rules. Furthermore, some evidence suggests that the ability to implement efficient strategies during a goal maintenance task declines as people age, and that this decline is accompanied by reduced activity within the lateral areas of the prefrontal cortex.

4.2 Reversal Learning Task

4.2.1 Task description

The Reversal Learning Task (Rolls et al. 1994) is predominantly used to test behavioral flexibility; specifically, the ability to alter reward-based decision-making flexibly. Participants are asked to choose between two stimuli over a series of trials (e.g., everyday objects, abstract patterns). One stimulus is associated with a reward (e.g., real or abstract money in human studies, or a food reward in animal studies). The other stimulus is associated with some form of punishment (e.g., a loss of real or abstract money for humans, or an aversive stimulus for animals). Human participants are told that the objective is to make as many rewarding selections (e.g., earn as much money) as possible. Following the selection of one of the stimuli, feedback is given in the form of either reward or punishment. Individuals must use this information to identify which option is the rewarding stimulus in the subsequent trials; thus, in this initial learning phase, participants are able to build an initial stimulus–reward association. This learning phase ends when the participant makes a predetermined number of correct (rewarding) responses (which indicates successful encoding of the stimulus–reward relationship). The contingency between stimuli and outcomes is then reversed, such that selecting the previously rewarding stimulus now results in a loss or punishment, and selecting the previously aversive stimulus now results in a reward. Participants are required to "reverse" their initially learned stimulus–reward associations and choose the previously aversive but now rewarding stimulus. After the reversal has been made and a predetermined number of correct responses are achieved (which indicates that they have successfully identified the reversed contingency), the stimulus–reward association is switched or "reversed" again, and the same procedure is repeated. A schematic diagram of the Reversal Learning Task is presented in Figure 4.2.

The main outcome variable is the number of trials it takes for an individual to identify that the contingency has reversed, as measured by consistent correct responses to the new stimulus–reward association. Additional outcome measures include the amount of reward accrued and total number of incorrect responses (selection of aversive stimuli) made. In the original version of this test, developed to assess reversal learning in humans (Rolls et al. 1994), participants were also debriefed at the end, in order to gauge their understanding of the objectives using the following questions:

How could you gain and lose points in the test?

What were you thinking at the start of the test?

What happened later?

This debriefing interview takes place to determine whether individuals performing poorly on the Reversal Learning Task were doing so due to a failure to modify previously learned associations between stimuli and reward and punishment, or simply an impairment in the ability to understand the task objectives.

Commonplace variations of this task include the type of reward (e.g., virtual versus real money), type of stimuli used (e.g., real-world objects, abstract images), number of correct responses required for a stimulus–reward reversal, as well as the probability of each stimuli giving a reward or punishment. For example, the original version reported by Rolls et al. has become known as a deterministic contingency Reversal Learning Task because one image will always be associated with a win, and the other will always be associated with a loss. However, in probabilistic versions of the task, the probability with which the stimuli yields rewards and punishments can be manipulated (e.g., one stimuli has a reward:punishment ratio of 80:20 and the other has a

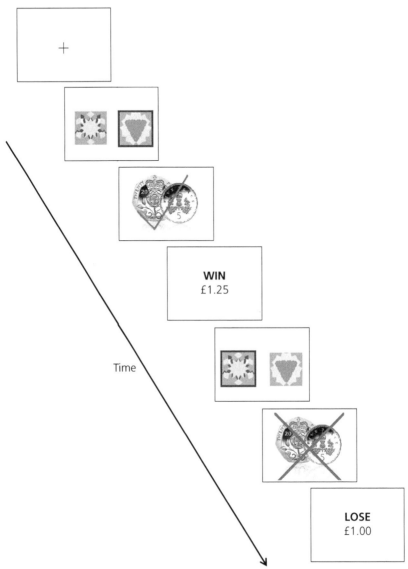

Fig. 4.2 Schematic of the Reversal Learning Task. A fixation point disappears after 500 ms, followed by a window of 2.5 s in which the participant can choose between two abstract stimuli. Here, the choice made is highlighted by the square surrounding the stimuli. Three seconds later, feedback is displayed, followed by the participant's running total (from their wins and losses) for 1 s, before the trial finishes and another one starts. Adapted from Alan N. Hampton, Peter Bossaerts, and John P. O'Doherty, The Role of the Ventromedial Prefrontal Cortex in Abstract State-Based Inference during Decision Making in Humans, *Journal of Neuroscience*, 26 (32), Fig. 1a, p. 8363. © 2006, The Society for Neuroscience.

reward:punishment ratio of 40:60). It is therefore more difficult to differentiate between stimuli because feedback must be integrated across multiple trials in order to correctly identify the more rewarding stimuli and make an overall monetary/reward gain. It also makes the contingency reversal more difficult to detect. This design was implemented to minimize the possibility of participants employing explicit verbal strategies rather than affective learning (Hornak et al. 2004). In light of this more challenging version of the test, researchers adopt a longer training phase to familiarize participants with the task and its requirements, and to reduce learning effects during the experimental phase.

The Reversal Learning Task has been compared to the Iowa Gambling Task (Bechara et al. 1994, see Section 9.2) as both tasks are thought to assess reinforcement learning (Fellows and Farah 2003). In the Iowa Gambling Task, participants should select cards from four decks of cards in order to maximize their profit on an initial sum of money: two "good" decks provide low immediate rewards but low punishment, and two "bad" decks provide high immediate rewards but high punishment. To make a profit over the 100 card selections, participants should choose more cards from the "good" decks. Given that the losses do not occur immediately, participants establish a prepotent response to select the "bad" decks with high immediate rewards. When the contingencies for the four decks change and the "bad" decks start leading to punishments, individuals tend to reverse their behavioral response and now choose from the "good" decks. Similarly, in the Reversal Learning Task, when the contingency between stimuli and reward/punishment is reversed, participants should now choose the previously aversive but now rewarding stimulus. Therefore, one might argue that both tasks can be failed due to an inability to inhibit prepotent behavioral responses (Rolls et al. 1994; Tomb et al. 2002; Fellows and Farah 2003; Maia and McClelland 2004; but see also Bechara et al. 2005).

4.2.2 Patient and lesion studies

The Reversal Learning Task was originally designed for non-human primate research in order to understand the neural underpinnings of flexible reward-based decision-making. It is hypothesized that the value of stimuli (positive or negative) and the ability to rapidly and flexibly reassign these values is represented in the orbitofrontal cortex, and there are several lines of evidence to support this theory from non-human primate studies (see Kringelbach and Rolls 2004). Cells in the orbitofrontal cortex have been shown to be sensitive to changing reward contingencies; for example, recordings from the macaque orbitofrontal cortex were shown to be sensitive to this reversal learning task, as cell-firing transferred from a previously rewarded stimulus to the newly rewarded one (Thorpe et al. 1983; Rolls et al. 1996). In addition, lesions to the orbitofrontal cortex in macaques have been shown to disrupt the alteration of stimulus–reward associations (Baxter et al. 2000).

In humans, the first study to examine regional specificity of the Reversal Learning Task within the frontal lobes compared a group of 12 patients with orbital frontal lesions with eight who had frontal lesions not involving this area (including two patients with dorsolateral prefrontal damage; Rolls et al. 1994). Patients with orbital lesions were unable to alter their behavior appropriately (i.e., change their stimulus–reward associations) compared to the lesion control group. Using a deterministic version of the Reversal Learning Task, the two frontal groups did not differ in their acquisition of the initial stimulus–reward relationship. However, the orbital patients took significantly more trials than their non-ventral counterparts to reach the criterion of nine consecutive correct responses after the contingency first changed. The contribution of the orbitofrontal cortex in reversal learning was replicated using a probabilistic Reversal Learning Task in patients with either orbital (BAs 10, 11, 12, and 25) or dorsolateral and dorsomedial (BAs 9, 46/8, 9, and 10) lesions (Berlin et al. 2004). This study reported that the orbitofrontal cortex group made significantly more overall errors (as measured by less money gained) and completed fewer reversals than either non-orbital lesion or healthy control groups.

Further research investigating localization of reversal learning processes within frontal subregions has been carried out in patients with dorsolateral or ventromedial prefrontal damage. Fellows and Farah (2005b) used another deterministic task in which one pack of cards consistently concealed a $50 win whereas the other yielded a $50 loss. Whereas both frontal groups were comparable to healthy controls in their ability to identify the initial stimulus–reward acquisition, only the ventromedial prefrontal group made significantly more reversal errors than the control group. Using a probabilistic version of the Reversal Learning Task, another study compared the performance of groups with circumscribed surgical frontal lesions involving different frontal subregions (Hornak et al. 2004). The key finding was that individuals with bilateral orbitofrontal lesions (or those with dorsolateral prefrontal lesions who did not attend to the crucial on-screen feedback, identified with post-test questions) exhibited significantly poorer performance than healthy controls. Patients with unilateral orbitofrontal lesions performed as well as healthy controls. Another study reported that a ventral group, in which each patient had some degree of bilateral orbital damage, was impaired in terms of Reversal Learning Task performance (Wheeler and Fellows 2008) and the authors ascribed their poor performance to an inability to learn from specifically negative feedback. Further, the performance of the orbitofrontal patients on this task was compared to that of individuals with psychopathy (which is associated with abnormalities in the ventromedial prefrontal cortex; Shamay-Tsoory et al. 2010) and healthy controls (Mitchell et al. 2006). Both experimental groups showed significant impairment in comparison to healthy controls.

It is therefore clear that the orbitofrontal cortex is a key processing center for the changing emotional valence of rewards and punishments and their effect upon subsequent behavior. However, it is also one part of a much larger network of regions, each making processing contributions to task performance (e.g., anterior cingulate cortex, dorsolateral prefrontal cortex, motor and premotor cortex, primary sensory areas, striatum, amygdala; Table 4.1). Williams et al. (2004) demonstrated a central role for the dorsal anterior cingulate cortex in integrating motor response with reward information. They showed increased firing of cells in human dorsal anterior cingulate cortex in response to diminished reward during a variant of the Reversal Learning Task. Moreover, following cingulotomy, the same patients made more response-selection errors than before surgery.

4.2.3 **Neuroimaging studies**

Evidence from the domain of functional imaging also supports a central role of the orbitofrontal cortex in reversal learning abilities (Table 4.2). Using a probabilistic

Table 4.1 Reversal Learning Task: Patient and lesion studies

Study	n	Patient/ Control Groups	Study type	Brodmann Areas	FP	DL	OF	ACC
Rolls et al. (1994)	12; 8	OF; non-OF	Lesion	–				✓
Berlin et al. (2004)	23; 20; 39	OF; non-OF; HA	Lesion	8, 9, 10, 11, 12, 25, 8/46	X	✓		
Hornak et al. (2004)	11; 11; 3; 6	OF; DL; DM; DF	Lesion	8, 9, 10, 11, 12, 25, 46	✓	✓		
Williams et al. (2004)	5	ACC	Lesion	–				✓
Fellows and Farah (2005b)	9; 11; 17; 14	VM; DL; HA1; HA2	Lesion	–		X	✓	
Wheeler and Fellows (2008)	11; 9; 24	VM; DL; HA	Lesion	–		X	✓	

FP = frontal pole; DL = dorsolateral prefrontal cortex; OF = orbitofrontal cortex; ACC = anterior cingulate cortex; HA = healthy adults; DM = dorsomedial prefrontal cortex; DF = diffuse frontal; VM = ventromedial prefrontal cortex; ✓ = frontal region damaged and impairment found; X = frontal region damaged but no impairment.

Table 4.2 Reversal Learning Task: Neuroimaging studies

Study	n	Patient/ Control Groups	Study type	Brodmann Areas	FP	DL	OF	ACC
O'Doherty et al. (2001)	9	HA	fMRI	10/11, 44/45, 10/32, 24/32			✓	✓
Cools et al. (2002a)	13	HA	fMRI	–			✓	✓
Kringelbach and Rolls (2003)	9	HA	fMRI	–			✓	✓
Remijnse et al. (2005)	27	HA	fMRI	–	✓	✓	✓	
Gläscher et al. (2009)	20	HA	fMRI	10, 11, 46	✓	✓		
Ghahremani et al. (2010)	16	HA	fMRI	–			✓	✓

FP = frontal pole; DL = dorsolateral prefrontal cortex; OF = orbitofrontal cortex; ACC = anterior cingulate cortex; HA = healthy adults; fMRI = functional magnetic resonance imaging; ✓ = frontal region involved.

version of the Reversal Learning Task, in which the magnitude of the reward itself was also varied, significant activation of the orbitofrontal cortex in relation to the receipt of a reward or a punishment was reported (O'Doherty et al. 2001). Although some lateral prefrontal activation was also reported, it was shown that predominantly medial orbitofrontal activation was positively correlated with the magnitude of the reward, and that lateral orbitofrontal activation was positively correlated with the magnitude of the punishment. The dorsal anterior cingulate cortex was also reported to be activated in response to punishment and uncertainty. The involvement of elevated orbital blood oxygenation level-dependent (BOLD) response on rewarding trials and dorsal anterior cingulate cortex response to punishment has been replicated elsewhere (Linke et al. 2010).

Significant activation of the lateral orbitofrontal cortex has also been reported during the acquisition of the new stimulus-reward contingency (i.e., when the participant changes response pattern; Cools et al. 2002a).[1] However, these studies have been criticized for their approach of a-priori selected regions of interest and the absence of an affectively neutral baseline—rather, fMRI contrasts were based on trials within the same task, and so it could be argued that processing

---

[1] Cools et al. (2002a) were unable to image the most ventral parts of the orbitofrontal cortex due to susceptibility artifacts.

relevant to the reversal was continuing beyond the reversal trial itself (Remijnse et al. 2005). In an attempt to address these shortcomings, Remijnse et al. used a task in which participants were told in advance which selection to make, and were given neutral feedback ("selection made"). Using this as a contrast baseline, they observed activation in the dorsolateral prefrontal cortex and anterior prefrontal cortex in addition to the orbitofrontal cortex, ventromedial prefrontal cortex and insula during general feedback processing, but only the orbitofrontal cortex and ventral striatum were explicitly activated by reward and punishment, corroborating their role in the processing of feedback regardless of whether it is positive or negative in nature (Remijnse et al. 2005).

The notion of the orbitofrontal cortex as being dissociable from dorsolateral and dorsal cingulate regions during Reversal Learning Task performance has subsequently been supported (Ghahremani et al. 2010). In order to identify the neural correlates specific to reversal learning compared to those of response inhibition, the authors compared frontal BOLD responses during a deterministic reversal learning paradigm with those during the stop-signal task. The stop-signal task is a test of response inhibition, which requires participants to respond using predefined stimulus–response associations apart from trials on which they are presented with the stop signal (in this case, an auditory tone). On such trials, responses to visually presented stimuli should be inhibited. Whereas the orbitofrontal cortex was engaged predominantly during the reversal of learned associations (in line with its suggested role in reformulating stimulus–reward associations based on emotional valence), the dorsal anterior cingulate cortex and inferior frontal gyrus were activated in more general response inhibition and thus are likely to guide the specific actions required by the pertinent contingency. Likewise, Gläscher et al. (2009) demonstrated that the ventromedial prefrontal cortex is activated during reversal learning, irrespective of whether the required response is action-based or stimulus-based. When participants decided to change their behavior from stay to switch, the dorsolateral prefrontal cortex became significantly active as well as the orbitofrontal cortex, possibly indicating a plan for the upcoming response which has been driven by identification of the extinct stimulus–reward contingency.

In an interesting variant of the Reversal Learning Task, Kringelbach and Rolls (2003) presented participants with a choice between the faces of two individuals. Once selected, the individual either smiled or looked angry; the task of the participant was to keep track of the mood of both faces by selecting the happy person as much as possible. The change in selection behavior at reversal, cued by the angry face of the previously happy person, was associated with activations in the orbitofrontal cortex and dorsal anterior cingulate cortex. Indeed, this was also the case when expressions other than anger were used to cue the reversal, suggesting that these areas may drive our ability to change behavior in social settings.

4.2.4 Aging studies

Among animals, some studies report age-related deficits on reversal learning paradigms (Bartus et al. 1979; Voytko 1999; Schoenbaum et al. 2002), whereas others do not show definitive effects of age (Rapp et al. 1990; Lai et al. 1995; Herndon et al. 1997). Studies examining age effects on Reversal Learning Tasks in humans are scarce (Table 4.3). Older participant groups have greater difficulty than younger adults in learning stimulus–reward associations, which remains significant even after controlling for deficits on executive type tasks (Marschner et al. 2005; Mell et al. 2005). Weiler et al. (2008) also reported that older participants showed poorer acquisition of the initial stimulus–reward association and impaired reversal learning when compared to a younger group. However, some propose that this is due to an alteration in the reward processing system outside the frontal cortex, such as the ventral striatum (Marschner et al. 2005; Schott et al. 2007). Comparing fMRI patterns between old and young, two studies have identified lower BOLD response in the ventral striatum during reward processing (Marschner et al. 2005; Schott et al. 2007), though Schott et al. did not report age-related differences in response accuracy concomitant with these fMRI group differences. In summary, the limited data in aging humans could indicate striatal changes with age that may be sufficient to alter the reward-processing network and hinder Reversal Learning Task performance. However, published aging studies suffer consistently from low group sizes ($n < 30$ in all cases). Hence, further research in larger groups is required to

Table 4.3 Reversal Learning Task: Aging studies

Study	n	Participant age groups (years)	Study type	Age effect
Marschner et al. (2005)	9; 9	Younger, mean = 24 Older, mean = 68	Cross-sectional (neuroimaging)	✓
Mell et al. (2005)	20; 20	Younger, mean = 23.15 Older, mean = 67.63	Cross-sectional (behavioral)	✓
Schott et al. (2007)	18; 19; 11	Younger, mean = 23.3 Older, mean = 69.0 PD, mean = 66.4	Cross-sectional (neuroimaging)	X
Weiler et al. (2008)	30; 30	19–33; 50–71	Cross-sectional (behavioral)	✓

PD = Parkinson's disease; ✓ = age effect found; X = age effect not found.

detect more reliably the presence and neural underpinnings of any age-related reversal learning deficits.

4.2.5 **Summary**

Overall, lesion and patient data support the hypothesis that the orbitofrontal cortex is required for the flexible acquisition and reassignation of stimulus–reward contingencies. Damage to this region consistently impairs performance on the Reversal Learning Task when compared to healthy control groups, and to those with lesions in other frontal areas. Equally, evidence from neuroimaging studies supports the central role of the orbitofrontal cortex during Reversal Learning Task performance. However, both patient and neuroimaging data also implicate other frontal (e.g., anterior cingulate cortex and dorsolateral prefrontal cortex) and non-frontal brain areas (e.g., the ventral striatum) in task-related processing—which may be complementary to, but not directly related to, the flexible assignation of stimulus–reward valence. Consequently, it has been suggested that the age effects on Reversal Learning Task performance may be explained by striatal rather than by orbitofrontal cortex changes with increasing age.

4.3 **Trail Making Test**

4.3.1 **Task description**

The Trail-Making Test is widely used to assess set-shifting ability and is a subtest from the Halstead–Reitan Neuropsychological Test Battery (Reitan and Wolfson 1985, 1993) and the Delis–Kaplan Executive Functions System (D-KEFS) battery (Delis et al. 2001). The task typically consists of two parts. In Part A, participants are presented with an A4 sheet of paper with circles each containing one number and which are randomly arranged on the page. Participants are required to draw a trail connecting the numbered circles in ascending numerical order as quickly and as accurately as possible but without lifting their pencil from the paper. In Part B, participants are given an A4 page with randomly arranged circles each containing either a number or a letter. The objective is to draw a trail connecting the numbers and letters in ascending numerical and alphabetical order, switching between the numbers and letters (e.g., 1… A… 2… B… 3… C, and so on) as quickly and as accurately as possible, again without lifting the pencil from the paper. The time taken to complete each part is recorded along with the number of errors made. Part A is often used as a baseline measure of motor and visual search speed, whereas Part B is used as a measure of set-shifting or switching. The difference between the time taken to complete Parts A and B is thought to quantify the complex set-shifting processes involved in Part B of the task.

However, it has been pointed out that Parts A and B differ not only in their reliance on set-shifting ability, but also in their visuomotor requirements. Gaudino et al. (1995) found that Part B completion times were longer, partly due to the greater physical distances between the consecutive stimuli than in Part A. The Trail Making Test from the D-KEFS includes four baseline conditions (i.e., visual scanning, number sequencing, letter sequencing, and motor speed) in place of Part A, which allows individual differences in both visuomotor and switching to be quantified, but resulting in a greater administration time.

4.3.2 Patient and lesion studies

The majority of lesion studies that have examined performance on the Trail Making Test have been concerned with the issue of whether performance might be: (i) more affected by frontal than by non-frontal lesions; and/or (ii) more dependent on left than on right frontal lobe integrity. Demakis (2004) conducted a large meta-analysis comparing Trail Making Test Part A and Part B performance in 321 frontal and 305 non-frontal patients and found that frontal patients were only significantly different compared to non-frontal patients in terms of Part A, not Part B. Moreover, Demakis (2004) noted that this difference would not be sufficient to discriminate reliably between frontal and non-frontal lesion types and no significant effect of lesion laterality was reported. In another study, Tamez et al. (2011) compared stroke patients' Trail Making Test performance with normative data in terms of completion times, reporting that the frontal ($n = 45$) and non-frontal ($n = 122$) lesion groups did not significantly differ on Parts A or B of the task. A similar finding was reported in 68 frontal and non-frontal traumatic brain-injured patients (Anderson et al. 1995).

In terms of lateralization, Heilbronner et al. (1991) examined patients with extensive lesions exclusively to either the left ($n = 27$) or right ($n = 29$) hemispheres, and those with lesions involving both hemispheres ($n = 31$) with a healthy control group ($n = 34$) performing the Trail Making Test. Heilbronner et al. (1991) reported that whereas the bilateral patient group were significantly slower than controls on Part A of the Trail Making Test, completion times in terms of Part B, Part B minus A (B–A) and Part B divided by A (B/A) were unable to discriminate accurately between the three patient groups. Channon and Crawford (2000) compared left and right anterior and posterior lesions with healthy controls performing the Trail Making Test, finding no effect of group or lateralization in terms of completion times. Other studies, however, have demonstrated that left frontal damage results in more errors and longer completion times on Part A and Part B than IQ-matched and non-brain-damaged controls (Gouveia et al. 2007). Hoerold et al. (2013) reported that a left frontal lesion group made significantly more errors on Part B than either left or right non-frontal patient groups, or controls. There was also a trend in the same direction for the right frontal group, but this did not reach significance.

In these laterality studies, specific lesion location *within* the frontal lobes has not been examined and therefore the extent to which frontal lobe damage is limited to a specific locus of interest is unclear. It is possible that combining patients with a variety of frontal lesions within the same frontal group obscured the localization of the processes associated with Trail Making Test performance. Few studies have examined localization of Trail Making Test processes (Table 4.4). In one of the few studies to suggest that there might be localization of Trail Making Test processes within frontal subregions, Stuss et al. (2001a) compared 49 patients with focal frontal lesions with 13 patients with non-frontal lesions and 19 healthy controls. They found that only frontal lobe patients made more than one error on Part B of the Trail Making Test, although not all frontal patients made errors. Those patients who were significantly impaired relative to controls had lesions in the dorsolateral prefrontal cortex, whereas the patients who made the fewest errors primarily had lesions in the inferior medial frontal areas. As the right frontal patients were not significantly different from controls, but left and right lesion groups were not significantly different from each other, this cannot be taken as direct evidence for laterality per se). Yochim et al. (2007) reported that patients with dorsolateral prefrontal lesions were disproportionately slower than controls on the D-KEFS Trail Making Test Part B, both as a raw score, and when accounting for the control conditions. The absence of a non-dorsolateral prefrontal lesion group precludes a direct inference that the dorsolateral prefrontal cortex is of particular functional relevance to Trail Making Test performance. Finally,

Table 4.4 Trail Making Test: Patient and lesion studies

Study	n	Patient/ Control Groups	Study type	Brodmann Areas	FP	DL	OF	ACC
Stuss et al. (2001a)	49; 13; 19	FL; non-FL; HA	Lesion	–		✓[a]		
Yochim et al. (2007)	12; 11	DL, HA	Lesion	–		✓		
Gläscher et al. (2012)	165; 179	FL; non-FL	Lesion (LSM)	–	X	X	X	✓

FP = frontal pole; DL = dorsolateral prefrontal cortex; OF = orbitofrontal cortex; ACC = anterior cingulate cortex; FL = frontal lesions; HA = healthy adults; LSM = lesion–symptom mapping; ✓ = frontal region damaged and impairment found; X = frontal region damaged but no impairment.

[a]The lesion groups were divided into three based on the number of errors. The two groups with the highest errors mainly comprised those with DL damage.

Gläscher et al. (2012) used lesion–symptom mapping among 344 individuals with focal lesions (165 frontal lesions) to identify areas required for successful Trail Making Test performance. They reported that the lesion locus in the rostral anterior cingulate cortex was associated with significantly poorer performance, but not in the dorsolateral prefrontal cortex, by contrast with the Stuss et al. (2001a) and Yochim et al. (2007) studies. The same area in the rostral anterior cingulate cortex was also significantly associated with a cognitive control factor derived from the Trail Making Test, the WCST, the Stroop test and the Controlled Oral Word Association test. Gläscher et al. (2012) claim that the activation in the rostral anterior cingulate cortex associated with Trail Making Test performance reflects set-shifting, whereas their dorsolateral prefrontal activation, which was associated with performance on the Stroop Test, reflects response inhibition.

In addition to the dorsolateral prefrontal cortex and anterior cingulate cortex, lesions in the cerebellum have also been reported to result in poorer Trail Making Test performance compared to controls (Exner et al. 2004; Gottwald et al. 2004; Alexander et al. 2012). Connectivity studies have suggested a confluence of functional connection between the frontal lobes and the contralateral posterior cerebellum (Allen et al. 2005). Although involving small numbers, patients with lesions due to stroke in the posterior inferior ($n = 6$)—but not the superior ($n = 5$)—cerebellar artery had longer completion times when compared to matched healthy controls ($n = 11$; Exner et al. 2004). Another report found that lesions to the right, but not left, side of the cerebellum resulted in slower completion on Parts A, B and B–A (Gottwald et al. 2004). However, a larger study found no significant difference in Part B performance between those with cerebellar lesions ($n = 32$) and controls ($n = 36$), though the authors did not examine cerebellar subregions (Alexander et al. 2012).

4.3.3 Neuroimaging studies

Few studies have examined performance on the Trail Making Test using functional neuroimaging, given the practical difficulties in adapting this paper-and-pencil task for inside the scanner (Table 4.5). One variant of the task required participants to articulate covertly the numbers for Part A, and the alternating letter–number sequence for Part B during fMRI (Moll et al. 2002c). Though the scoring method relied upon participants' self-report of the highest number/letter achieved (rather than the standard time-to-completion), Moll et al.'s (2002c) finding of left dorsolateral prefrontal (BAs 44 and 46) and medial frontal (BAs 6 and 32) activation is similar to results of another fMRI study using a different task design (Zakzanis et al. 2005). Rather than removing the visual and motor elements of the Trail Making Test for performance

Table 4.5 Trail Making Test: Neuroimaging studies

Study	n	Patient/ Control Groups	Study type	Task	Brodmann Areas	FP	DL	OF	ACC
Moll et al. (2002)	7	HA	fMRI	Covert articulation	6, 32, 44, 46		✓		✓
Zakzanis et al. (2005)	12	HA	fMRI	MRI stylus	–		✓		✓
Allen et al. (2011)	32	HA	fMRI	Covert search	–		✓		
Jacobson et al. (2011)	20	HA	fMRI	3-choice	47[a]		✓[a]		

FP = frontal pole; DL = dorsolateral prefrontal cortex; OF = orbitofrontal cortex; ACC = anterior cingulate cortex; HA = healthy adults; ✓ = frontal region involved.

[a]Activation found for Part B, but not when contrasted with Part A.

inside the scanner, Zakzanis et al. developed a task using an MRI-compatible stylus that converted the participants' movements over an acrylic tablet into cursor movements on the computer screen. In this study, activation in the left dorsolateral prefrontal cortex and anterior cingulate cortex was reported when the activation during Part A was subtracted from the activation during Part B. A more recent fMRI study contained only a Part B equivalent in which participants had to search covertly for the next item in the sequence and press a button once it was located (Allen et al. 2011). A line was then drawn between the previous and the correct subsequent item, which the authors argue acts as an effective error-correction approximation of the paper-and-pencil version. Nonetheless, Allen et al. (2011) acknowledge that this paradigm cannot ascertain participant compliance or the number of errors made, and they reported little frontal activation associated with Part B and did not have a Part A equivalent with which to contrast these results. They did, however, report that all 32 participants showed activation in the middle and superior frontal gyri (which comprise the dorsolateral prefrontal cortex; Rajkowska and Goldman-Rakic 1995), but registration to a template did not yield a single cohesive locus which could account for the absence of dorsolateral prefrontal activity in this study.

In an alternative paradigm, Jacobson et al. (2011) implemented a task in which participants were required to press one of three buttons to indicate whether a black box was on the left/above/right of the next number or letter in the sequence (see Figure 4.3). A black line would then be drawn to the target number/letter from the previous stimulus. Jacobson et al. (2011) reported

A 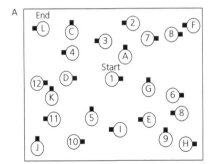 B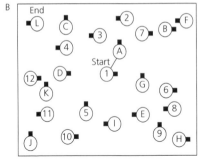

Fig. 4.3 Trail Making Test design from the functional magnetic resonance imaging study by Jacobson et al. (2011). Participants choose from three buttons to indicate whether the black box is to the left, above, or to the right of the next stimulus in the sequence. A trail is then drawn to that object (B). Reprinted from *Brain and Cognition*, 77 (1), Sarah C. Jacobson, Mathieu Blanchard, Colm C. Connolly, Mary Cannon, and Hugh Garavan, An fMRI investigation of a novel analogue to the Trail-Making Test, pp. 60–70, Copyright (2011), with permission from Elsevier.

activation in the right inferior middle frontal gyrus (BA 47) during Part B performance, and extensive left dorsolateral prefrontal activity at a liberal voxel-wise threshold ($P < 0.01$). However, they found no significant difference in BOLD response between Parts A and B in their version of the task. As Part A was stimulus-paced due to the inclusion of a compulsory delay between responses, participants were required to actively slow their responses and this may have resulted in the engagement of more controlled behaviors and subsequent dorsolateral prefrontal activation when also performing Part A.

4.3.4 **Aging studies**

A relatively large body of evidence indicates significant age effects on Trail Making Test performance, though these effects are less consistently reported in middle age (Table 4.6). Boll and Reitan (1973) did not find an effect of age on Trail Making Test performance in a sample of 244 healthy participants aged between 15 and 64 years. However, only 28 participants were aged >50 years, impairing the investigators' ability to comment reliably on age effects on the Trail Making Test beyond late middle-age. Rasmusson et al. (1998) explicitly examined cognitive performance among older participants aged 60–96 years. In their cross-sectional analysis of 667 non-demented participants, they found that slower Trail Making Test completion time was significantly associated with increasing age for Parts A and B. However, following up 385 of these participants two years later, Rasmusson et al. (1998) reported that there was significant slowing of their completion times for Part

Table 4.6 Trail Making Test: Aging studies

Study	n	Participant age groups (years)	Study type	Age effect
Rasmusson et al. (1998)	667	60–96	Cross-sectional (behavioral)	✓
Drane et al. (2002)	18; 39; 53; 46; 38; 36; 36; 19	<20; 20–29; 30–39; 40–49; 50–59; 60–69; 70–79; >80	Cross-sectional (behavioral)	✓
Hester et al. (2005)	130; 106; 79; 48	60–69; 70–74; 75–79; 80–89	Cross-sectional (behavioral)	✓
Hashimoto et al. (2006)	90; 53; 17	70–74; 75–84; ≥85	Cross-sectional (behavioual)	✓
Seo et al. (2006)	165; 349; 266; 149; 55; 13	60–64; 65–69; 70–74; 75–79; 80–84; 85–89	Cross-sectional (behavioral)	✓
Newman et al. (2007)	221	18–84	Cross-sectional (neuroimaging)	✓
Periáñez et al. (2007)	223	16–80	Cross-sectional (behavioral)	✓
Ashendorf et al. (2008)	152; 117	55–74; 75–98	Cross-sectional (behavioral)	✓
Hamdan and Hamdan (2009)	92; 66; 117; 43	18–34; 35–49; 50–64; 65–81	Cross-sectional (behavioral)	✓

✓ = age effect found; X = age effect not found.

B, but not Part A, with older groups showing the greatest change. Rasmusson et al. (1998) argue that these findings highlight the tendency for age effects to be more pronounced for complex cognitive tasks such as set-shifting (Salthouse 1991), as these tasks are thought to be subserved by the frontal lobes (e.g., Milner 1963; Luria 1969; Stuss and Benson 1986; Eslinger and Grattan 1993), which decline with age (Sullivan and Pfefferbaum 2007; Fjell et al. 2009; Burzynska et al. 2011). Drane et al. (2002) found that increasing age was significantly associated with poorer B–A scores and B:A ratio among 285 adults, aged between 18 and 90 years.

In another sample of 363 Australian participants aged between 60 and 89 years, Hester et al. (2005) found that although increasing age resulted in poorer Part A, Part B and B–A scores, there was no effect of age on the ratio score. This negative age effect on both direct and derived Trail Making Test measures was also found among 223 healthy controls in a mild cognitive impairment and dementia study (Ashendorf et al. 2008; Part A, Part B, Part

B error rate), 155 healthy Japanese participants aged >70 years (Hashimoto et al. 2006; Part A, Part B, B–A, B:A), 997 Korean volunteers aged between 60 and 90 years (Seo et al. 2006; Part A, Part B, derived scores not compared), a sample of 223 Spanish speakers aged between16 and 80 years (Periáñez et al. 2007; Part A, Part B, B–A, B:A), and 318 Brazilian participants aged between 18 and 81 years (Hamdan and Hamdan 2009; Part A, Part B, derived scores not compared).

The underlying neuroanatomical bases for these aging effects have also been widely studied. Pa et al. (2010) examined a sample of 160 participants who had either neurodegenerative disease, mild cognitive impairment, or were healthy older adults. Controlling for the Numbers component process in the D-KEFS Trail Making Test, they found that smaller volume of gray matter in the dorsolateral prefrontal cortex, frontal pole regions, and posterior parietal areas correlated with slower completion times. This effect disappeared when controlling for both the Numbers and Letter–Number measures. Pa et al. (2010) suggested that the true neural correlates of set-shifting were obscured when both control measures were used in the contrast because their correlates overlap to such a large degree. In addition, the analysis included all groups together; the implicit assumption being that poorer Trail Making Test performance was due to decrements in the same subregions in all participant groups, which may not have been the case. In a study that used voxel-based morphometry among 221 cognitively healthy adults (aged 18–84 years), Newman et al. (2007) reported a significant age effect on Part B performance, and an inverse relationship between Part B and gray matter volume in the right inferior frontal gyrus caudate, globus pallidus, and right posterior parietal lobe. However, the degree to which parcellation and non-linear registration were able to preserve gray matter characteristics to a non-aging-specific atlas suggests that such results should be interpreted with caution. This is something the authors themselves acknowledge when discussing the absence of dorsolateral prefrontal associations with Trail Making Test scores.

Several studies indicate that decrements in Trail Making Test performance may indicate more global age-related brain changes than simply those of the frontal lobes. Breteler et al. (1994) reported that both white matter lesion load and enlarged ventricles relative to brain size were significantly related to poorer Trail Making Test Part B performance among 90 older adults aged 65–84 years. Similarly, the presence of severe white matter hyperintensities in the whole brain of 845 older participants was linked to poorer Trail Making Test performance, though this was not true for individuals with a higher level of education (Dufouil et al. 2003). O'Sullivan et al. (2001) measured diffusion characteristics of white matter between 20 older and 10 younger participants.

The older group had significantly poorer white matter integrity, with the greatest group difference in the integrity of anterior white matter. Higher mean diffusivity (an index of poorer white matter integrity) was associated with a significantly greater difference between Trail Making Test Part A and Part B, suggesting that age-related decrements in white matter integrity may partially underlie age effects on the Trail Making Test. Another study compared relationships between Trail Making Test and visual ratings of periventricular hyperintensities, deep white matter hyperintensities and medial temporal lobe atrophy among 156 older participants (mean age = 68.4 years, SD = 8.9). Higher indices on all three general measures of brain aging were significantly associated with slower Part B completion times, and a greater B minus A difference. Controlling for a visual rating of general cortical atrophy did not alter this pattern of results. However, pertinent to each of the above studies is the criticism that without the direct comparison of Trail Making Test performance with both subregional frontal lobe measures and brain-wide indices of aging, it is unclear to what extent each directly/uniquely contributes to decrements in test performance above others. Currently, there is insufficient evidence to conclude the age-related degradation of the frontal lobes (and/or specific frontal subregions), rather than more global brain network disruption, is the primary driver of age-related decline in Trail Making Test performance.

4.3.5 Summary

Most lesion studies have been concerned with left/right frontal lobe dissociations in Trail Making Test performance, and these have yielded mixed results. As illustrated by the functional imaging literature and some recent lesion studies, assigning patients to either left or right frontal groups may lack the fidelity necessary to parse the functionally relevant (possibly the dorsolateral prefrontal cortex and anterior cingulate cortex) and less-relevant regions of the frontal lobes, though other non-frontal regions are also required for unimpaired Trail Making Test performance.

4.4 Wisconsin Card Sorting Test

4.4.1 Task description

The Wisconsin Card Sorting Test (WCST; Grant and Berg 1948; later modified by Nelson 1976) is a clinical test of set-shifting, attention, and inhibition widely used in both the patient and neuroimaging literature. Participants are presented with four target cards and two decks of 64 cards (one deck is presented at a time)—all of which depict shapes of a certain number and color (e.g., two red squares or three green triangles). Participants are required to sort the cards according to a rule set by the experimenter (e.g., color: a "green" pile, a "red" pile; shape: a "triangle" pile, a "circle" pile; number: a "2-item" pile, a "3-item" pile; see Figure 4.4) by drawing cards one-at-a-time from the deck of cards and matching each one with one of four target cards. In the most widely used form of the WCST, participants are not told the sort rule, and are required to discover the rule for themselves through trial and error. The experimenter gives the participants feedback after each card placement by simply saying "correct" or "incorrect". After a series of correct card placements, however, the sort rule changes without the participant's knowledge and the participant should work out what the new sort rule is. Performance is usually reported in terms of the number of contingencies (i.e., sorting rules) achieved and the number of perseverative errors made after the sorting rule changes (i.e., cards sorted according to the previous rule). However, other measures can also be reported (e.g., total correct card sorts, number of trials taken to achieve the initial sort rule). By contrast with perseverative errors, some studies also report non-perseverative error scores; these generally include occasions when, after the sort rule has changed, a response that is neither appropriate to the previous nor to the new sort rule is made, or when the sort rule has been followed correctly during one response but not during the subsequent response (i.e., failure to maintain the appropriate set).

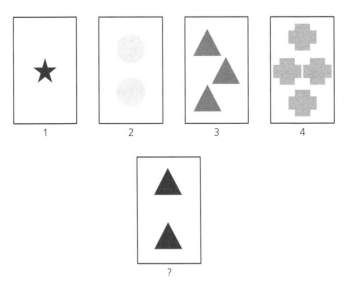

Fig. 4.4 Example of a trial in the Wisconsin Card Sorting Test. Sorted piles of cards are seen along the top, with the new to-be-sorted card at the bottom. The target card can be sorted by shape (pile 3), color (pile 1), or number (pile 2) according to the current sorting rule. Please see color plate section.

In the original version of the WCST, sorting could often be achieved by one of two coincidental dimensions. In the modified version of the task devised by Nelson (1976), ambiguity in the sorting rule is removed by ensuring that correct sorting can only be achieved using one dimension of the stimulus (e.g., color only, shape only). Participants are tested on two decks of 24 cards each, making it a shorter test overall than the original. A similar sort task, the Weigl Color–Form Sorting Task (Weigl 1927; Goldstein and Scheerer 1941), is often administered to patients who are more severely impaired, as it involves only two possible sorting dimensions (color and shape) and one sort rule change. Instead of sorting cards, stimuli are presented as physical wooden objects on a tabletop. The Weigl Color–Form Sorting Task has been modified to increase the number of sort dimensions (e.g., thickness of the shape; De Renzi et al. 1966) and to improve its sensitivity to dementia (e.g., Beglinger et al. 2008). However, due to the lack of evidence regarding specific prefrontal involvement when performing the task, the Weigl Color–Form Sorting Task will not be discussed further. Other modified card sort tasks also exist (e.g., 64-card WCST; Greve et al. 2001) but due to the infrequency of their use, they will not be discussed here.

4.4.2 Patient and lesion studies

Various patient studies have been carried out using the WCST since its inception in 1948. Left frontal lobe damage has been shown to increase the perseverative error rates (i.e., repeating a previous sort rule that is no longer appropriate) and to reduce the number of categories successfully sorted compared to right frontal, non-frontal and healthy control groups (Drewe 1974; Goldstein et al. 2004). In a single case study, patient MGS, who suffered right-sided ventromedial prefrontal damage after a penetrative brain injury in Vietnam, committed notably more perseverative errors than healthy normative data on the WCST. However, this was explained by the authors as inattention to feedback. After MGS had received feedback, he went on to achieve a similar number of categories to healthy controls (Dimitrov et al. 1999). However, other studies suggest that there is no effect of laterality on WCST performance. In the modified WCST, Nelson (1976) observed that patients with frontal lesions commit significantly more perseverative errors than those with non-frontal (including temporal, parietal, and occipital lobe) lesions, but that left and right frontal patients did not significantly differ in their performance. Impaired WCST performance has also been noted in a large meta-analysis of lesion studies, with frontal lesion patients performing more poorly than posterior lesion patients (Demakis 2003). However, no laterality effect was observed in the analysis, suggesting that right- and left-sided frontal lesions have similar implications.

Particular associations between poor WCST performance and dorsolateral prefrontal damage have been reported in various lesion studies. Milner (1963) observed that patients with cortical excisions involving the dorsolateral prefrontal cortex committed significantly more perseverative errors, but not non-perseverative errors, and achieved significantly fewer sorting categories than those with ventromedial prefrontal excisions or healthy controls. Furthermore, this difference was significant both pre- and postoperatively, with dorsolateral prefrontal excision patients committing more errors and achieving fewer sorting categories postoperatively compared to preoperatively. By contrast, those who underwent ventromedial prefrontal excisions did not show significant performance change postoperatively (Milner 1963). However, it should be noted that all of the patients were tested rather soon after intervention, when function was likely to be still recovering (Demakis 2003). Stuss et al. (2000) compared the performance of various patient groups with region-specific frontal lesions. Patients with dorsolateral prefrontal damage (with some additional frontal pole and anterior cingulate cortex involvement) performed significantly more poorly than other prefrontal patient groups (i.e., superior medial frontal or inferior medial frontal lesion groups), unilateral non-frontal lesion patients, and healthy controls on the WCST. Indeed, such patients achieved fewer sorting categories, and committed more perseverative errors during the task.

Frontal lobe-specific white matter lesions also have profound effects on WCST performance, with increasing error rates (including perseverative errors) and fewer categories achieved than either non-frontal patients or healthy controls (Hogan et al. 2006). Impaired event-related potential (ERP) correlates of error processing in the frontal white matter lesion group were reported and suggest that WCST deficits may be the result of disrupted communication between the dorsolateral prefrontal regions and other prefrontal regions normally associated with performance monitoring (Hogan et al. 2006).

The WCST impairment shown by many patients with dorsolateral prefrontal lesions can be contrasted with the unimpaired performance of patients with damage to the ventromedial prefrontal cortex. In a small sample of patients with lesions to the ventromedial prefrontal cortex, Bechara et al. (2001) noted no significant impairment in terms of perseverative errors or the number of sorting categories achieved when compared to healthy controls. However, many animal and human studies have noted WCST deficits associated with lesions in other frontal subregions. Indeed, whereas Dias et al. (1997) found that monkeys performed significantly more poorly on a task such as the WCST (in which target rules had to be learned and then shifted according to the change in the rule) after surgical dorsolateral prefrontal ablations, they also noted significantly reduced inhibitory control in ventromedial prefrontal lesion monkeys. In particular, monkeys with ventromedial prefrontal lesions made significantly more perseverative errors than either monkeys with dorsolateral prefrontal lesions or healthy control monkeys, but only after the first rule shift. Similarly, patients with ventromedial prefrontal lesions have also been found to commit more perseverative errors and achieve fewer sorting categories than posterior lesion patients or healthy controls in conditions where they are informed of the possible sorting rules before the task (i.e., shape, color, and number) but not warned that a rule switch may occur or not given the appropriate rule during the task (Stuss et al. 2000). The anterior cingulate cortex has also been implicated in WCST performance; patients with damage to both the dorsolateral prefrontal cortex and anterior cingulate cortex also exhibit an increased rate of perseverative, non-perseverative, and efficiency (shifting away from the correctly attained sorting rule) errors (Barceló and Knight 2002). Furthermore, in a positron emission tomography study, Sarazin et al. (1998) reported significant correlations between activation specifically within the dorsolateral prefrontal cortex and anterior cingulate cortex and WCST performance in patients with various frontal lesions including the dorsolateral prefrontal cortex, ventrolateral prefrontal cortex, ventromedial prefrontal cortex and frontal pole. However, it should be noted that, as well as the wide range of frontal damage included in their study, the activation observed by Sarazin et al. (1998) was averaged across both focal frontal lesion patients and patients with frontal variant frontotemporal dementia (fvFTD), limiting possible inferences about strict frontal lobe localization. Cortical thickness in the dorsolateral prefrontal cortex and anterior cingulate cortex has also been reported to correlate positively with the percentage of correct sorts on the WCST (Burzynska et al. 2011), although increasing numbers of perseverative errors have only been shown to correlate with caudate volume (Riley et al. 2011). Furthermore, cingulotomy patients have exhibited performance improvements postoperatively, suggesting that the anterior cingulate cortex is not required for successful WCST performance (Jung et al. 2006). Davidson et al. (2008) note that although patients with frontal lesions perform significantly more poorly than non-frontal patients, the location of damage within the frontal lobes (i.e., dorsolateral prefrontal cortex, ventromedial prefrontal cortex, frontal pole or anterior cingulate cortex) does not predict their WCST performance. Thus, it seems difficult to conclude that only damage to the dorsolateral prefrontal cortex results in WCST deficits in frontal lobe patients (Table 4.7).

4.4.3 Neuroimaging studies

A number of neuroimaging studies have investigated the neural correlates of WCST performance (Table 4.8). Early investigations of task-related activity

Table 4.7 Wisconsin Card Sorting Test: Patient and lesion studies

Study	n	Patient/ Control Groups	Study type	Brodmann Areas	FP	DL	OF	ACC
Milner (1963)	18; 33; 8; 5; 7	DL; TL; PL; PTOL; OTL	Lesion	–		✓	X	
Dias et al. (1997)	18	DL, OF, SHM	Lesion (monkey)	–			✓	
Stuss et al. (2000)	6; 6; 13; 10; 5; 6; 16	rDL; lDL; SM; IM; non-FL; HA	Lesion	6, 8, 9, 10, 11, 12, 24, 25, 32, 46	✓	✓		✓
Bechara et al. (2001)	41; 5; 40	SD; VM; HA	Lesion	–			X	X
Barceló and Knight (2002)	6; 8	DL; HA	Lesion	6, 8, 9, 44, 45, 46		✓		✓
Demakis (2003)	24 studies	FL; non-FL; rFL; lFL	Meta-analysis	–		✓		
Jung et al. (2006)	17	ACC	Lesion	–				X

FP = frontal pole; DL = dorsolateral prefrontal cortex; OF = orbitofrontal cortex; ACC = anterior cingulate cortex; TL = temporal lobe; PL = parietal lobe; PTOL = parieto-temporo-occipital lobe; OTL = orbital and temporal lobe; SHM = sham control monkeys; r = right; l = left; SM = superior medial frontal cortex; IM = inferior medial frontal cortex; FL = frontal lobes; HA = healthy adults; SD = substance-dependent participants; VM = ventromedial prefrontal cortex; ✓ = frontal region damaged and impairment found; X = frontal region damaged but no impairment.

implicated the dorsolateral prefrontal cortex. In a single-photon emission computed tomography (SPECT) study, Rezai et al. (1993) noted a significant increase in regional cerebral blood flow (rCBF) specifically within the left lateral prefrontal regions during the WCST. Similarly, Marenco et al. (1993) compared activation in healthy individuals associated with WCST performance and performance on a simple card-matching task. In particular, they subtracted the activation during the simple matching task from the WCST in order to investigate the unique activation related to the acquisition and shifting of rules. The authors observed significantly increased blood flow to the posterior dorsolateral prefrontal regions, suggesting that such areas are responsible for attention and set-switching.

However, associations between WCST performance and prefrontal activity are inconsistent, and several later studies have observed little or no involvement of the frontal regions. For example, in a SPECT study, rCBF changes within the inferior parietal cortex, but not the frontal regions, were associated

Table 4.8 Wisconsin Card Sorting Test: Neuroimaging studies

Study	n	Patient/ Control Groups	Study type	Brodmann Areas	FP	DL	OF	ACC
Rezai et al. (1993)	15	HA	PET	–		✓		
Marenco et al. (1993)	17	HA	SPECT	–		✓		
Berman et al. (1995)	40	HA	PET	8, 10, 11, 32/8, 44, 45/46, 46, 47	✓	✓	✓	✓
Nagahama et al. (1996)	18	HA	PET Number: Color: Shape:	6, 9, 10, 44, 45; 6, 9, 11; 6, 6/8, 9, 9/46, 10	✓ ✓	✓ ✓ ✓	✓	
Konishi et al. (1998a)	7	HA	fMRI	24/32, 44/45				✓
Fallgatter and Strik (1998)	10	HA	NIRS	–				
Sarazin et al. (1998)	13	FL	PET	8, 9, 45, 46		✓		
Konishi et al. (1999a)	7	HA	fMRI	9		✓		
Toone et al. (2000)	23; 11	schiz; HA	SPECT	–				✓
Monchi et al. (2001)	11	HA	fMRI Receiving negative feedback: Matching after negative feedback:	9/46, 32, 46, 47/12; 6, 6/8/44		✓	✓	✓
Periáñez et al. (2004)	16	HA	MEG	24, 32, 45, 47/12			✓	✓
Buchsbaum et al. (2005)	49 studies	HA	Meta-analysis	6/8, 10/11, 44, 47			✓	
Nagahama et al. (2005)	6; 12; 3; 51	OA; MCI; FTD; AD	SPECT	10	✓			

(continued)

Table 4.8 Continued

Study	n	Patient/ Control Groups	Study type	Brodmann Areas	FP	DL	OF	ACC
Carrie et al. (2006)	18; 10; 14	FLE; JME; HA	PET Cognitive shifting: Implementing shift:	6, 6/8/44, 9/46, 32, 46, 47/12; 6, 6/8/44		✓	✓	✓
Lie et al. (2006)	12	HA	fMRI	–		✓		✓
Wagner et al. (2006)	17	HA	rTMS	–		X		
Lumme et al. (2007)	32	HA	PET	–				✓
Ko et al. (2008)	10	HA	rTMS	46		✓		
Specht et al. (2009)	14	HA	fMRI	6, 8, 9, 10, 24, 32, 44, 45, 46, 47		✓		✓
Konishi et al. (2010)	48	HA	fMRI	–		✓		✓
Wilmsmeier et al. (2010)	28; 36	schiz; HA	fMRI	6, 9, 44/45, 46		✓		✓
Riley et al. (2011)	17; 9	TLE; HA	MRI	–		X		
Provost et al. (2012)	15	HA	fMRI	9, 9/46, 47/12		✓	✓	

FP = frontal pole; DL = dorsolateral prefrontal cortex; OF = orbitofrontal cortex; ACC = anterior cingulate cortex; HA = healthy adults; PET = positron emission tomography; SPECT = single-photon emission computed tomography; NIRS = near-infrared spectroscopy; FL = frontal lobes; schiz = schizophrenic patients; MEG = magnetoencephalography; OA = older adults; MCI = mild cognitive impairment; FTD = frontotemporal dementia; AD = Alzheimer's disease; FLE = frontal lobe epilepsy; JME = juvenile myoclonic epilepsy; rTMS = repetitive transcranial magnetic stimulation; ✓ = frontal region involved.

with recurrent perseverative error rates (in which individuals shift away from the correct sorting rule to make a previously valid response) across various dementia patients (including frontotemporal dementia and mild cognitive impairment) and healthy controls (Nagahama et al. 2005). Studies examining WCST performance and rCBF changes have primarily and consistently implicated non-frontal activity in regions such as the inferior temporal and inferior parietal lobes (Berman et al. 1995; Nagahama et al. 1996; Esposito et al. 1999;

Toone et al. 2000). Furthermore, transcranial magnetic stimulation (TMS) administered to the left dorsolateral prefrontal cortex did not affect WCST performance in healthy individuals (Wagner et al. 2006b).

Spectroscopy is a technique allowing researchers to investigate regional chemical concentrations within the brain, typically the oxygen content of the blood, which are indicative of integrity and activity. In the case of blood oxygenation, the presence of more oxygenated blood indicates greater activity of that particular region. In one such study, Fallgatter and Strik (1998) suggest that frontal blood oxygen concentration increases during the WCST. However, spectroscopy techniques have also suggested that the chemical concentration profiles associated with WCST performance appear to be different depending on the participant group used (Ohrmann et al. 2008). In particular, Ohrmann et al. noted a correlation between the concentration within the dorsolateral prefrontal cortex of a chemical associated with neuronal integrity and WCST performance in healthy individuals, but also a correlation between the concentration within the anterior cingulate cortex of chemicals associated with neuronal activity and WCST performance in schizophrenic patients.

More recent neuroimaging studies have helped to distinguish between the different stages of the WCST and their component processes. The sorting phase consists of several cognitive components. Working memory is required as individuals learn and maintain the current sort rule. When a change in the sort rule occurs, the ability to shift sets (similar to task-switching or mental flexibility) is required in order to implement the change. Inhibition is also required when the sort rule changes, in order to prevent perseverative responses. Finally, performance and error monitoring are required during the feedback phase in order to update the current response tendencies. In one study, Ko et al. (2008) compared the effects of applying TMS during the feedback and sorting phases of the WCST and found increased response times when TMS was applied to the right dorsolateral prefrontal cortex during the feedback phase, but not the sorting phase. This suggests a role for the right dorsolateral prefrontal cortex in performance monitoring but not set-shifting or inhibition. There was also a trend for an increase in total error rates after right dorsolateral prefrontal stimulation, but again only when applied during the feedback phase. In another study, Lumme et al. (2007) observed a positive correlation between error rates within the WCST and dopamine receptor binding within the anterior cingulate cortex, which was specifically associated with working memory and set-shifting, representing the importance of dopamine regulation in these processes. Consideration of the different phases of the task, and especially their component processes, rather than activation over the whole task, may help to clarify the involvement of particular prefrontal regions in WCST performance.

4.4.3.1 Set-shifting and inhibition

Using functional magnetic resonance imaging (fMRI), Konishi et al. (1998a) observed, within a small sample of healthy adults, a change in dorsolateral prefrontal activation during the sorting phase of the WCST. The researchers analyzed the activation at the time-point most associated with the set-shifting component of the task (i.e., when the sort-rule changes) compared to a control task that did not require set-shifting and noted dorsolateral prefrontal activation, which was accompanied by additional activation of the ventral prefrontal cortex and anterior cingulate cortex. Other neuroimaging studies have also demonstrated dorsolateral and more medial prefrontal activation associated with the set-shifting phase of the WCST (Konishi et al. 1998a; Periáñez et al. 2004). In a meta-analysis of neuroimaging studies involving the WCST, common activation was reported in the dorsolateral prefrontal cortex (BA 9), anterior cingulate cortex (BA 6), and ventrolateral prefrontal cortex (BAs 10, 11, and 47) across the whole task (Buchsbaum et al. 2005). In order to understand the component processes of the task, the authors then went on to analyze the overlap between activation in the WCST and two other tasks. Overlap between the activation reported in the WCST and task-switching studies was noted especially in the bilateral dorsolateral prefrontal cortex (BA 9), and this was thought to represent the set-shifting component of the tasks. By contrast, overlap between the brain regions associated with performance on the WCST and the Go/No-Go Task (thought to represent inhibition) was noted primarily in the right dorsolateral prefrontal cortex (BA 9) and anterior cingulate cortex (BAs 6 and 32). Other work has shown that the activation in the dorsolateral prefrontal cortex and anterior cingulate cortex increased only during the feedback phase after participants received negative feedback, not during the subsequent sort response (Wilmsmeier et al. 2010). This suggests a primary role for these regions in updating the response tendency but not the implementation of a switch. An fMRI study has instead implicated the ventrolateral prefrontal cortex (BAs 12 and 47) in set-shifting (Provost et al. 2012). Therefore it remains contentious as to whether the dorsolateral prefrontal cortex and/or the ventrolateral prefrontal cortex are involved in the decision to switch (Wilmsmeier et al. 2010; Provost et al. 2012), though several studies have demonstrated the involvement of the anterior cingulate regions in the resulting necessary inhibition of the previous response pattern (Buchsbaum et al. 2005; Wilmsmeier et al. 2010). The dorsolateral prefrontal cortex and the anterior cingulate cortex have additionally been implicated in the generation and implementation of a new response pattern only (Konishi et al. 2010)—with previously performed shifts associated with ventromedial prefrontal activation—as well as the subsequent performance monitoring (Monchi et al. 2001).

4.4.3.2 Set maintenance and working memory

Using fMRI, it has also been shown that there are significant activation changes within the dorsolateral prefrontal cortex when the working memory load within the task is reduced (by informing participants of the sort-rule to switch to prior to the switch; Konishi et al. 1999a). Indeed, Lie et al. (2006) compared fMRI activation over levels of working memory load within the WCST. Each participant received four blocks of trials—a baseline block, in which no set-shifting is required, a block in which participants are told the relevant rule before each trial, a block in which participants are only told the rule when a shift occurs, and a block in which no prompting is given. By subtracting activation observed during one block from another, the authors hoped to separate activation associated with increasing working memory load and that associated with set-shifting. In particular, the dorsolateral prefrontal regions were associated with working memory demands, but not for set-shifting. This would tie in with the notion that the dorsolateral prefrontal cortex is important for working memory abilities, as well as providing support for its role in the set-shifting phase where working memory is needed to store previous and current sort rules and to check the effectiveness of the current sort response (Konishi et al. 1999a). However, activation was not limited to the dorsolateral prefrontal regions, with additional difficulty-related activity in other prefrontal regions (e.g., the ventrolateral prefrontal cortex, anterior cingulate cortex) and non-frontal (e.g., temporal lobe, cerebellum) regions (Lie et al. 2006). Furthermore, a recent fMRI investigation demonstrates that prefrontal-wide activation persists during the WCST when controlling for working memory (Specht et al. 2009).

In summary, whereas there has been a great deal of research examining the various phases and cognitive components of the WCST, the extant data are insufficient for functional localization, either for the task overall or for the specific component processes of the task. Indeed, whereas dorsolateral prefrontal activation has been demonstrated throughout the majority of the phases of the task, this has not consistently been to the exclusion of other prefrontal regions.

4.4.4 **Aging studies**

The effects of healthy adult aging on WCST performance have been extensively examined (Table 4.9). Age effects have been demonstrated in terms of the ability to maintain the current rule (Hartman et al. 2001; Ashendorf and McCaffrey 2007) and the ability to switch rules (MacPherson et al. 2002; Ashendorf and McCaffrey 2007; Nagel et al. 2008; Gamboz et al. 2009; Adrover-Roig and Barceló 2010). Increasing age has been associated

Table 4.9 Wisconsin Card Sorting Test: Aging studies

Study	n	Participant age groups (years)	Study type	Age effect
Haaland et al. (1987)	10; 22; 25; 18	64–69; 70–74; 75–79; 80–87	Cross-sectional (behavioral)	✓
Fristoe et al. (1997)	48; 49	18–38, 60–86	Cross-sectional (behavioral)	✓
Nagahama et al. (1997)	6; 6	21–24; 66–71	Cross-sectional (neuroimaging)	✓
Lineweaver et al. (1999)	29; 84; 89; 27	45–59; 60–69; 70–79; 80–91	Cross-sectional and longitudinal (behavioral)	✓
Hartman et al. (2001)	Experiment 1: 85; 76 Experiment 2: 48; 48	Younger, mean = 19.7 Older, mean = 70.3 Younger, mean = 20.3 Older, mean = 69.8	Cross-sectional (behavioral)	✓
MacPherson et al. (2002)	30; 30; 30	20–38; 40–59; 61–80	Cross-sectional (behavioral)	✓
Ridderinkhof et al. (2002)	Experiment 1: 16; 24 Experiment 2: 30; 24	Younger, mean = 24.4 Older, mean = 68.1 Younger, mean = 22.1 Older, mean = 70.9	Cross-sectional (behavioral)	✓
Salthouse et al. (2003)	79; 112; 70	18–39; 40–59; 60–84	Cross-sectional (behavioral)	✓
Rhodes (2004)	Study 1: 34 studies Study 2: 34 studies	Younger, mean = 24.5 Older, mean = 71.3 Younger, mean = 24.8 Older, mean = 71.5	Meta-analysis (behavioral)	✓
Bugg et al. (2006)[a]	37; 20; 24; 16; 17; 52; 27	20s; 30s; 40s; 50s; 60s; 70s; 80s	Cross-sectional (behavioral)	✓
Ashendorf and McCaffrey (2007)	25; 19	18–22; 63–89	Cross-sectional (behavioral)	✓
Nagel et al. (2008)	164; 154	20–31; 60–70	Cross-sectional (genetic)	✓
Adrover-Roig and Barceló (2010)	40; 40	49–60; 61–80	Cross-sectional (behavioral)	✓

[a]Although n-values for the full samples are described here, the WCST was administered to only a subset of these individuals. The characteristics of this subsample are not described.

✓ = age effect found; X = age effect not found

with fewer sorting rules achieved, as well as an increase in perseverative and non-perseverative errors and the number of trials taken to achieve the first rule (Salthouse et al. 2003). An early study by Haaland et al. (1987) found that the oldest old-age group (aged 80–87 years) completed significantly fewer categories and committed significantly more perseverative errors than the youngest old-age group (aged 64–69 years), suggesting that WCST performance deteriorates rapidly in later life.

Lineweaver et al. (1999) conducted a study in which middle-aged and older adults (aged 45–91 years) were administered the modified WCST and then were tested again one year later. At initial test, middle-aged participants achieved significantly more sorting rules and made fewer non-perseverative errors than the oldest participants. Interestingly, though non-perseverative error rates in middle-aged and older adults improved when assessed a year later, perseverative error rates and the number of rules completed did not. Given that some older adults did show longitudinal increases in non-perseverative errors whereas others did not, Lineweaver et al. (1999) propose that the number of categories achieved and perseverative errors are more reliable and sensitive markers of cognitive change with age. Ridderinkhof et al. (2002) noted that older adults exhibited problems switching between rules even when the shift was explicitly cued, suggesting that the ability to switch is the underlying cause of increasing perseverations with age. By contrast, older adults were able to sort once the initial rule was established, and once the subsequent shifts had been achieved. In terms of brain activation in older adults performing the WCST, Nagahama et al. (1997) demonstrated a significantly lower level of dorsolateral prefrontal activation in older adults (aged 66–71 years) compared to younger adults (aged 21–24 years), which was associated with an increased number of perseverative errors.

Declines in processing speed may explain a large proportion of the age-related declines in WCST performance (see Fristoe et al. 1997; Bugg et al. 2006). Similarly, level of education (Rhodes 2004) and genetic factors associated with the integrity of the dopaminergic system (Nagel et al. 2008) have also been implicated in age-related WCST decline. Therefore, it may be difficult to separate the specific contribution of working memory and executive processes to WCST performance in older adults from additional factors, such as processing speed.

4.4.5 Summary

There is a great deal of literature implicating the prefrontal cortex in WCST performance. However, the evidence from patient and lesion studies regarding further localization within the prefrontal cortex is somewhat mixed, with studies reporting dorsolateral prefrontal cortex, ventromedial prefrontal cortex, and anterior cingulate cortex involvement. Neuroimaging studies have recently aimed to clarify these different findings by allowing the investigation of different phases and component processes of the WCST. Although the dorsolateral prefrontal cortex appears to be recruited for set-shifting and working memory aspects of the task, other prefrontal regions (including the ventrolateral prefrontal cortex and anterior cingulate cortex) have also been implicated in these same processes. As there is limited consensus, more research is required in order to identify specific regions of the prefrontal cortex involved in the different processes inherent in the WCST. Finally, although age-related impairments have been noted on the WCST in terms of perseverative errors and number of sort rules achieved, due to the multi-factorial nature of the task it is difficult to interpret which processes may be most affected by age. Similarly, there is evidence to suggest that such impairments may be explained by declines in other abilities, such as speed of information processing, rather than the frontal executive functions required by the WCST per se.

Chapter 5

Multi-tasking

5.1 Six Elements Task and Multiple Errands Task

5.1.1 Six Elements Task

The Six Elements Task (Shallice and Burgess 1991b) is a task used to assess strategy-application disorder—a disorder characterized by difficulty carrying out everyday tasks that involve planning and multi-tasking such as shopping or cooking a meal. In the Six Elements Task, participants attempt to perform six open-ended tasks (three tasks with Parts 1 and 2) within a fixed 15 min period of time. Participants score points not only for how much of a single task they perform, but also for how many of the six tasks they attempt. The tasks commonly require the participant to dictate a previous and intended route, solve arithmetical problems, and write down the names of pictures of objects (Shallice and Burgess 1991b; see also Wilson et al. 1996), or, in more recent versions, copy abstract pictures, shapes, or patterns in the place of the dictation tasks (e.g., Levine et al. 1998; see Figure 5.1). Participants are told that: they should attempt all of the task elements; they cannot perform Parts 1 and 2 of a given task consecutively; earlier items will be awarded more points than later items; errors will be penalized. The Six Elements Task highlights the importance of task-switching and time management if participants hope to achieve the highest score possible.

5.1.2 Multiple Errands Task

A similar but less frequently used task is the Multiple Errands Task (Shallice and Burgess 1991b). In this real-world version of the Six Elements Task, participants are asked to walk around a small shopping district with the aim of completing certain subtasks set by the experimenter beforehand (see Box 5.1). These subtasks can be as simple as buying a particular item. However, they can be more complex, such as expecting participants to be at a certain place 15 min after the task has started—requiring them to plan ahead and monitor their performance so that they arrive on time. Another, somewhat more demanding, task involves participants writing down four specific pieces of information (such as the exchange rate of a certain currency) on to a postcard and sending it back to the experimenter at the end of the task. This requires participants to plan in advance where to go to obtain these pieces of information (e.g., a Bureau de

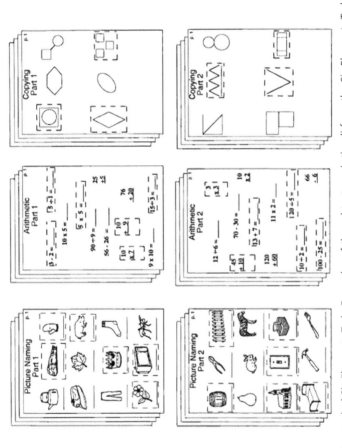

Fig. 5.1 Subtests involved in a typical Six Elements Task. Examples of the subtests and stimuli from the Six Elements Task. Upper row, from left to right: Parts 1 of a picture-naming task, an arithmetic task, and an abstract shape and pattern-copying ask. Lower row, from left to right: Parts 2 of a picture-naming task, an arithmetic task, and an abstract shape and pattern-copying task. Reproduced from Brian Levine, Donald T. Stuss, William P. Milberg, Michael Paxson Alexander, Michael Schwartz, and Ron MacDonald, The effects of focal and diffuse brain damage on strategy application: Evidence from focal lesions, traumatic brain injury and normal aging, *Journal of the International Neuropsychological Society*, 4 (3), pp. 247–264, Figure 1. © 1998, Cambridge University Press.

Box 5.1 Example of instructions and rules given to participants before the Multiple Errands Task

Tasks for Multiple Errands Task

1. Buy a brown loaf.
2. Buy one package of throat pastilles.
3. Buy one packet of tissues.
4. Buy one postcard.
5. Buy one bookmark.
6. Buy one bar of soap.
7. You must be at a certain place 15 min after starting.
8. You must gather the following pieces of information and write them down on the postcard:

   a. The name of the shop in the street likely to have the most expensive item.

   b. The price of a pound of tomatoes.

   c. The name of the coldest place in Britain yesterday.

   d. The rate of the exchange of the French franc yesterday.

Rules for Multiple Errands Task

- You are to spend as little money as possible (within reason).
- You are to take as little time as possible (without rushing excessively).
- No shop should be entered other than to buy something.
- Please tell the experimenter when you leave a shop what you have bought.
- You are not to use anything not bought on the street (other than a watch) to assist you.
- You may do the tasks in any order.

Data from Tim Shallice and Paul W. Burgess, Deficits in strategy application following frontal lobe damage in man. *Brain*, **114**(2): pp. 727–741. doi: 10.1093/brain/114.2.727, 1991.

Change) as well as remembering online both to collect the information and to return the postcard. In most cases, participants are only provided with a watch and must purchase all other items necessary to complete the task. Several rules are provided to participants before they begin. These include instructions to spend as little money as possible, to take as little time to complete all of the subtasks as possible, and not to enter a shop without the intention of buying something within. These rules encourage participants to be clear which shop they are going into in relation to a specific subtask, and not to enter shops unnecessarily. The overall rationale behind this task is to assess an individual's ability to perform a number of open-ended tasks in order to achieve an overall goal in normal, everyday life, using a task thought to have better ecological validity than more traditional, laboratory-based assessments. However, caution must be used when adopting this paradigm, as it has been suggested that some patients may exhibit errors based on misinterpretation of the rules rather than disorganized thought per se (Alderman et al. 2003). Though both tests are designed to assess strategy application disorder,[1] successful performance on the two tests may rely upon different abilities. The Six Elements Task requires participants to have a basic plan to efficiently switch between set subtasks at different time intervals, and to monitor both their performance and the total task time so as to modulate the strategy online. Additionally, the Six Elements can measure perseveration using both the number of subtasks attempted and the total time spent on individual subtasks. In contrast, the Multiple Errands Task requires not only the formation of a basic plan, but also consideration of the most efficient route and retrospective memory ability to hold this route in mind. There are also several subtasks which require prospective memory. Due to its real-word setting, the Multiple Errands Task also requires the plan to be flexible in the face of unforeseen difficulties encountered on the participant's travels. Furthermore, the ability to monitor time is only important for one subtask in the Multiple Errands Task. Unlike the Six Elements Task, the Multiple Errands Task also gives an opportunity for the social and affective impairments often seen in frontal patients to manifest (e.g., climbing onto an outside fruit display to see the price of tomatoes inside a shop; Goldstein et al. 1993).

The instructions (tasks to complete) and rules given to participants before starting the Multiple Errands Task are demonstrated in Box 5.1 (reproduced from Shallice and Burgess 1991b). For a more recent version, see Tranel et al. (2007).

5.1.3 **Patient and lesion studies**

The original experiment performed by Shallice and Burgess (1991b) investigated the performance of three frontal lobe patients on the Six Elements Task.

---

[1] Other tasks, such as the Greenwich Task (Burgess et al. 2000) or the Hotel Task (Manly et al. 2002), have also been used to assess strategy application deficits and multi-tasking deficits. However, given that the Multiple Errands Task and Six Elements Task have been more extensively researched and are commonplace in clinical settings, only these two tasks and their variants will be discussed here.

Each of these patients presented with impaired organizational skills in everyday living despite performing within normal limits on the majority of traditional neuropsychological tasks they were assessed on. By comparing their performance with that of healthy controls, the authors hoped to capture this everyday functional deficit within a laboratory-based setting. Indeed, they found that two of the three frontal patients attempted significantly fewer subtasks on the Six Elements Task than healthy controls, and that all three patients spent longer on any one subtask. Similarly, on a second testing session three weeks later, each of the three patients performed fewer tasks and spent longer on a single task than healthy controls.

Shallice and Burgess (1991b) also tested the same participants using the Multiple Errands Task described above and all three patients committed more errors than healthy age-matched controls. Interestingly, when the errors were broken down into the types of errors made, the patients committed significantly more "inefficiencies" (e.g., entering a single shop more than once) and "rule-breaks" (e.g., leaving a shop without buying anything) than healthy controls. Notably, the patients also had problems adhering to two additional timing tasks which required participants to stop task performance after a given amount of time. This suggests problems with the process of performance monitoring may be related to failure to adhere to time-regulated subtasks of the Multiple Errands Task (e.g., meeting the experimenter 15 min after starting). This may also help explain why frontal patients seem unable to switch between subtasks when performing the Six Elements Task (Shallice and Burgess 1991b). Shallice and Burgess (1991b) suggest that a selectively impaired ability to monitor and evaluate performance may explain the number and type of errors committed by frontal patients.

5.1.4 Localization of the processes associated with Six Elements Task performance

A handful of studies have examined how patients with lesions in distinct frontal subregions perform on the Six Elements Test (Table 5.1). Levine et al. (1998) administered a modified Six Elements Task to patients with frontal lobe lesions where certain subtasks were worth substantially more points than others. This required participants to prioritize their time and perform the most rewarding tasks. Additionally, the dictation subtasks from the original Shallice and Burgess (1991b) Six Elements Task were replaced with block-design subtasks in which participants had to arrange wooden blocks to create set geometric shapes. The performance of patients with focal frontal lesions was compared to that of patients with focal non-frontal lesions, and similarly traumatic brain injury (TBI) patients' performance was compared to that of

Table 5.1 Six Elements Task: Patient and lesion studies

Study	n	Patient/ Control Groups	Study type	Task	Brodmann Areas	FP	DL	OF	ACC
De Zubicaray et al. (1997)	1	HFI	Lesion (single case)	Six Elements	–		X		
Burgess et al. (2000)	60; 60	Cerebral lesions; HA	Lesion	Greenwich	–				
				Retrospective Memory:	24				✓
				Planning:	8, 9, 46		✓		
				Rule-breaks and switches:	8, 9, 10	✓			
Baird et al. (2006)	2	ACC; ACC + OF	Lesion (single case)	Six Elements	8, 11, 12, 24, 25, 32			X	X
Tranel et al. (2007)	9; 8; 17; 20	VM; other FL; non-FL; HA	Lesion	Six Elements	10, 11, 12, 25, 32	X		X	X
Roca et al. (2011)	7; 8; 25	FP; other FL; HA	Lesion	Hotel	10	✓			

FP = frontal pole; DL = dorsolateral prefrontal cortex; OF = orbitofrontal cortex; ACC = anterior cingulate cortex; HFI = hyperostosis frontalis interna; HA = healthy adults; VM = ventromedial prefrontal cortex; FL = frontal lobe; ✓ = frontal region damaged and impairment found; X = frontal region damaged but no impairment.

matched healthy controls (Levine et al. 1998). TBI patients were found to perform significantly worse than their healthy counterparts, accumulating fewer points and attempting fewer of the more rewarding tasks. However, the authors observed that although the majority of focal frontal lesion patients accumulated very few points, their performance was not significantly different to that of non-frontal lesion patients with both groups showing marked inefficiencies. Furthermore, patient IK who had sustained only subcortical and brainstem lesions, exhibited severe inefficiencies on a Six Elements Task-like task (Breakfast Task; see Craik and Bialystok 2006), spending more time on individual subtasks and neglecting others (West et al. 2007). These impairments are unlikely to be caused by attention or processing speed deficits as patient IK exhibited no accompanying impairments—in terms of errors or response times—on other frontal tasks (such as the Wisconsin Card Sorting Test) when compared to age-matched healthy controls. Such disorganized behavior, then, suggests cortical lesions (such as in the dorsolateral prefrontal cortex) are not necessary for impaired strategy application. In line with this, several studies have failed to find significant differences between frontal patients with lesions in the anterior cingulate cortex and medial prefrontal cortex (Baird et al. 2006) or ventromedial prefrontal lesions (Tranel et al. 2007) and control groups on the Six Elements Task.

One explanation for such conflicting findings is that strategy application and multi-tasking may be further localized to specific frontal regions. For example, Gouveia et al. (2007) observed that left frontal patients who predominantly had dorsolateral prefrontal lesions scored fewer points and committed more rule-breaks in the Six Elements Task than either right frontal patients mainly with dorsolateral prefrontal lesions or healthy controls. Interestingly, this impairment did not extend to the number of tasks completed or performance on any one subtask with the patient groups not significantly differing from the control group on these measures. Meanwhile, the right frontal patients performed within the normal range on all Six Elements Task measures. It should be noted, however, that some of the frontal patients also had lesions involving medial and orbital regions, making specific localization of Six Elements Task performance through this patient group problematic. Roca et al. (2011) examined multi-tasking in patients with frontal lesions including or excluding the frontal pole (BA 10). They administered the Hotel task (Manly et al. 2002)—a task similar to the Six Elements Task in which the activities relate to running a hotel—and found that those patients whose lesions involved the frontal pole attempted fewer tasks and spent longer on each subtask than healthy controls. In contrast, the performance of frontal patients with lesions sparing the frontal pole exhibited similar performance to healthy controls (though the two patient groups also did not significantly differ in terms of performance). Moreover, both lesion groups performed notably worse than healthy controls on tests of executive function (e.g., inhibition), suggesting both that the poor multi-tasking in patients with BA 10 lesions is not due to disproportionate executive dysfunction, and that executive dysfunction per se is not sufficient to cause multitasking impairments (Roca et al. 2011).

Interpretation of this literature requires some methodological considerations to be taken into account. The profiles of the three patients examined by Shallice and Burgess (1991b) are rather varied in terms of etiology, presenting symptoms, and lesion location. Similar issues can be seen in other such studies (e.g., Levine et al. 1998; Gouveia et al. 2007) in which localization beyond the "frontal" lobes cannot be made due to the varied etiology of the lesions examined and the relatively small sample sizes utilized. In the case of Shallice and Burgess (1991b), the performance of the three patients on the Self-Ordered Pointing Task (Petrides and Milner 1982)—a commonly employed task of dorsolateral prefrontal cortex function—and various other frontal function tasks is mixed, and makes implicating particular frontal subregions in strategy application disorder difficult. Patient AP who had the more clearly circumscribed lesion out of the three patients had a lesion involving the frontal pole (BAs 10 and 11; Burgess et al. 2000). In contrast, the single case described by Goldstein and colleagues did not exhibit any impairment on traditional neuropsychological tasks commonly associated with frontal subregions, such as the Self-Ordered Pointing Task (Petrides and Milner 1982), despite a large left frontal lobectomy (Goldstein et al. 1993).

5.1.5 Localization of the processes associated with Multiple Errands Task performance

Few patient studies have examined the localization of the processes associated with performance on the Multiple Errands Task (Table 5.2). The patient described by Goldstein et al. (1993) provides evidence which dissociates Six Elements Task and Multiple Errands Task performance. In particular, the patient exhibited behavioral impairments including increased levels of lethargy and indecision, resulting from the removal of a large portion of the left frontal lobe. Interestingly, although damage was noted within both dorsolateral and ventromedial prefrontal regions, no corresponding functional deficit was found using classical neuropsychological tests such as the Wisconsin Card Sorting Task and verbal fluency. Similar to the previously discussed observations of Levine et al. (1998), Goldstein et al. (1993) observed that the patient made as many errors as controls on the Six Elements Task, and even performed better in allocating their time among the tasks by spending less time on any one task than healthy controls. In contrast, the patient in question showed significant impairments in Multiple Errands Task performance. Goldstein et al. (1993) noted both formal errors such as entering the same shop twice

Table 5.2 Multiple Errands Task: Patient and lesion studies

Study	n	Patient/ Control Groups	Study type	Task	Brodmann Areas	FP	DL	OF	ACC
Tranel et al. (2007)	9; 8; 17; 20	VM; other FL; non-FL; HA	Lesion	Multiple Errands	10, 11, 12, 25, 32	✓	X	✓	✓

FP = frontal pole; DL = dorsolateral prefrontal cortex; OF = orbitofrontal cortex; ACC = anterior cingulate cortex; VM = ventromedial prefrontal cortex; FL = frontal lobe; HA = healthy controls; ✓ = frontal region damaged and impairment found; X = frontal region damaged but no impairment.

(i.e., inefficiencies) and leaving the designated street (i.e., rule-breaks) as well as more social errors such as arguing with shopkeepers and climbing on shop displays. More importantly, these errors were made despite the patient knowing and understanding all the Multiple Errands Task rules both before and after the task. Goldstein et al. (1993) suggested that, in contrast to the Six Elements Task, the Multiple Errands Task is particularly useful for measuring strategy application disorder due to its improved ecological validity. De Zubicaray et al. (1997) reported similar findings from observations of patient EW, a patient with predominantly left dorsolateral prefrontal damage due to hyperostosis frontalis intern, who showed no significant deficit in Six Elements Task performance. Patient EW did not commit rule breaks and attempted five out of six tasks during the allotted time. Furthermore, Tranel et al. (2007) observed no significant impairment on any Six Elements Task measure when comparing a large variety of lateral frontal patients—including those with dorsolateral prefrontal damage—to healthy controls. Thus, lateral prefrontal damage does not necessarily result in deficits on the Six Elements Task.

A simplified version of the Multiple Errands Task was administered to a group of lesion patients who experienced traumatic brain injury, stroke or excision of a brain tumor and similarly aged healthy controls with the aim of investigating the validity of the task (Alderman et al. 2003). By removing any ambiguity from the task rules and providing participants with an instruction sheet which they were explicitly told to read and complete during the task,[2] Alderman et al. (2003) hoped to reduce the number of errors resulting from interpretation problems or misunderstandings. In particular, Alderman et al. clarified existing rules—such as specifying an exact spending limit—and added rules—such as not to re-enter a shop already visited. Using this simplified version of the Multiple Errands Task, the researchers found that patients not only made more errors than healthy participants but also made different types of errors—including task errors (failing to record a piece of information) and social rule breaks (committing a socially inappropriate action). Interestingly, and in comparison to earlier studies (e.g., Shallice and Burgess 1991b; Goldstein et al. 1993), patients did not commit significantly more inefficiencies than healthy controls. Nonetheless, patients did commit more rule-breaks and were noted to commit more task failures (i.e., where a particular task is not completed satisfactorily). These results suggest that when the Multiple Errands Task instructions are less clear, inefficiencies might be due to the misinterpretation of instructions (Alderman et al. 2003).

---

[2] In the original Shallice and Burgess (1991b) study, participants were not encouraged to write down information.

Knight et al. (2002) conducted a similar study in which patients with acquired damage to the frontal lobes were given an Multiple Errands Task set within the boundaries of a hospital. The authors used rules similar to those of Alderman et al., again designed to clarify the task instructions (e.g., specifying a spending limit, outlining location boundaries). Those with frontal lobe damage committed significantly more rule breaks and task failures than healthy matched controls. Similar to Alderman et al. (2003), patients and healthy individuals did not differ in terms of the number of inefficiencies made. However, it is worth noting that Alderman et al. (2003) did not investigate the specific location of damage within their neurological patients, nor did they state whether the damage involved frontal lobe structures. Knight et al. (2002) only recruited patients with acquired frontal lobe damage, but did not report any attempts to localize the damage in their patients or compare effects with non-frontal lesion controls. Thus, although this study demonstrates the utility of the Multiple Errands Task as a method of assessing real-life strategy application impairments with more sensitivity than the Six Elements Task, it provides no evidence that it recruits specific frontal subregions.

The previously mentioned study conducted by Tranel et al. (2007) did, however, attempt to look at Multiple Errands Task performance in relation to lesion location. Tranel et al. recruited ventromedial prefrontal lesion patients in addition to other prefrontal lesion patients, non-frontal lesion patients, and healthy controls. They administered the Multiple Errands Task within the confines of an indoor shopping center, making sure that all participants understood and could recall the various rules and tasks before beginning the experiment. Tranel et al. (2007) found that ventromedial prefrontal lesion patients failed significantly more of the tasks than the non-prefrontal lesion patients and the healthy controls, as well as committing more total errors. The ventromedial prefrontal lesion patients also attempted fewer tasks than healthy controls and completed fewer tasks than both healthy controls and non-prefrontal lesion patients; of those that were completed, fewer were done error-free. Thus, unlike the pattern of performance reported by Tranel et al. (2007) in the Six Elements Task, ventromedial prefrontal lesion patients seem to perform more poorly than non-prefrontal lesion patient groups on the Multiple Errands Task—with more errors committed and fewer tasks completed successfully by those with ventromedial prefrontal lesions. However, it is important to note that the ventromedial prefrontal lesion patients did not significantly differ from other prefrontal patients in terms of Multiple Errands Task performance. The other prefrontal patients are described as having lesions that do not encroach upon ventromedial prefrontal regions (Tranel et al. 2007 describe the ventromedial prefrontal cortex as encompassing BAs 10, 11, 25, and 32, though no similar definition of other prefrontal regions is supplied). Since both the ventromedial prefrontal lesion group and the other prefrontal lesion group perform equally poorly on the Multiple Errands Task, it is unclear whether successful task performance, or strategy application more generally, involves multiple frontal regions. Such recruitment of multiple regions could be interpreted as the additional involvement of other prefrontal-related functions (such as working memory), but may also reflect the importance of multiple frontal regions for strategy application itself. In support of this, when the Greenwich Task (a task similar to the Six Elements Task) was administered to 90 neurological patients, distinct frontal subregions were associated with different strategy-application disorder impairments (Burgess et al. 2000). In this study, left anterior cingulate lesions were associated with retrospective memory problems, the right dorsolateral prefrontal cortex was associated with planning difficulties, and the left medial prefrontal cortex was associated with poor overall multi-tasking performance due to rule breaks. Whether the types of error made and the performance on particular subtasks can help discriminate between ventromedial prefrontal and dorsolateral prefrontal lesions remains to be seen, as there are insufficient studies utilizing the Multiple Errands Task in patient populations at the current time.

Logie et al. (2010) identified several limitations of the original Multiple Errands Task. First, although the test is widely used to assess patients with frontal damage, healthy individuals often perform at or near ceiling on the task. Second, the administration of the Multiple Errands Task can be problematic both in terms of the time and expense associated with setting up the task and monitoring participants, and the lack of control the researcher has over the real-world environment (see Logie et al. 2010 for a brief discussion). Instead, many studies of strategy-application disorder have used "virtual" versions of the Multiple Errands Task (e.g., McGeorge and Phillips 2001; Morris et al. 2002; McDermott and Knight 2004; Farrimond et al. 2006). "Virtual" versions of the Multiple Errands Task have been shown to bear a close resemblance to the real-life version, with both correlations between the "virtual" and "real-life" versions, as well as shared associations with activities of daily living and executive functions (Rand et al. 2009). Furthermore, brain injury patients have been shown to complete fewer errands and form more disorganized plans on both a real-life and a virtual Multiple Errands Task (McGeorge et al. 2001). Through the use of such "virtual" environments, Law et al. have shown performance to be sensitive to spatial working memory interference as well as executive load (Law et al. 2013). Rand et al. (2009) administered a version of the Multiple Errands Task in which videos of various locations within a shopping center were presented to the participant in such a way that they felt as though they were exploring the shopping center (i.e., the videos were triggered when participants chose to visit a specific location on the map in order to complete a given task). Rand et al. (2009) found that a group of stroke patients performed significantly more poorly than healthy controls, committing significantly more errors including inefficiencies, rule breaks, and task failures. Furthermore, the authors found strong correlations between stroke patient performance on the real-life Multiple Errands Task and its virtual counterpart. However, Rand et al. do not supply information as to the localization of damage for the stroke patients; therefore, conclusions about specific regional involvement cannot be made. Similarly, in a virtual Multiple Errands Task-type task, Morris et al. (2002) noted that prefrontal lesion patients commit significantly more rule violations than healthy controls. Prefrontal lesion patients also exhibited problems primarily in the time-based accuracy of a particular action (i.e., the degree to which participants were too early or late in initiating a task) rather than in absolute task-failures (Morris et al. 2002).

5.1.6 Neuroimaging studies

Due to the practical demands of the Six Elements Task and the Multiple Errands Task, neuroimaging investigations have been difficult to conduct. Generally, researchers have traded the ability to perform online functional investigations of brain activation for the ecological validity afforded by the real-life setting.

5.1.7 Aging studies

A number of studies in the cognitive aging literature have examined the effects of healthy adult aging on performance on the Six Elements Task (Table 5.3) and the Multiple Errands Task (Table 5.4) and similar tasks. Levine et al. (1998) observed no significant effect of healthy adult aging on Six Elements Task performance, though they did note a tendency for younger participants to score higher than their older counterparts. Similar results have been observed when

Table 5.3 Six Elements Task: Aging studies

Study	n	Participant age groups (years)	Study type	Task	Age effect
Levine et al. (1998)	20; 20	18–39; 63–79	Cross-sectional (behavioral)	Six Elements	X
Kliegel et al. (2000)	31; 31	20–48; 62–83	Cross-sectional (behavioral)	Six Elements	✓
Garden et al. (2001)	20; 20	31–46; 53–64	Cross-sectional (behavioral)	Six Elements	X
Craik and Bialystock (2006)	30; 30	18–30; 60–80	Cross-sectional (behavioral)	Breakfast	✓

✓ = age effect found; X = age effect not found

Table 5.4 Multiple Errands Task: Aging studies

Study	n	Participant age groups (years)	Study type	Task	Age effect
Garden et al. (2001)	20; 20	31–46; 53–64	Cross-sectional (behavioral)	Multiple Errands	X
Rand et al. (2009)	20; 20	20–33; 53–81	Cross-sectional (behavioral)	Multiple Errands	✓
McAlister and Schmitter-Edgecombe (2013)	50; 50	18–33; 60–74	Cross-sectional (behavioral)	Day Out	✓

✓ = age effect found; X = age effect not found

comparing middle-aged participants with younger controls (Garden et al. 2001). Indeed, although Garden et al. note that younger individuals seem to complete more subtasks than middle-aged individuals, there is no significant difference in other Six Elements Task measures such as number of tasks attempted or time spent on any one task. These results taken together suggest that the Six Elements Task is perhaps not sensitive to age-related declines in frontal function, though task fidelity could be improved by increasing the number of subtasks (Garden et al. 2001). However, in another study in which a modified Six Elements Task emphasizing prospective memory was administered to younger and older adults, older adults developed less complex plans, and were less likely to start and complete the proposed actions than younger adults. Yet, the two age groups did not differ in their ability to retain and carry out the plan (Kliegel et al. 2000). Furthermore, older adults have been shown to commit more errors and to spend longer on subtasks than younger individuals on the Breakfast Task (Craik and Bialystok 2006). Interestingly, older adults who scored highly on a battery of tests designed to measure frontal functions (e.g., the Wisconsin Card Sorting Test, Backwards Digit Span) also performed well on a time-based prospective memory task similar to the "stop" subtask of the Six Elements Task[3] (McFarland and Glisky 2009). Studies in mice have related such age impairments on time-sensitive prospective memory tasks to neuronal changes in the medial prefrontal cortex and the reduction of sensitivity during encoding (Caetano et al. 2012).

---

[3] McFarland and Glisky (2009) administered a task in which participants were required to respond every 5 min during a task. In the original Six Elements Task (Shallice and Burgess 1991b) participants were asked to stop completion of a task either 1.25 or 2.5 min after starting. McFarland and Glisky (2009) also administered a task requiring participants to respond only when they thought 10 s had elapsed.

Recent evidence seems to suggest that performance on the Multiple Errands Task, particularly the virtual version, can distinguish between older and younger age groups. Rand et al. (2009), as well as testing stroke patients, also administered the virtual Multiple Errands Task to older individuals. Older individuals seemed to commit more inefficiencies and task failures than their younger counterparts. Notably, the participant groups tended to form a continuum of performance, with stroke patients committing more errors of most types than older participants, who committed more errors of most types than younger participants. However, the use of inappropriate strategies did not differ between younger and older participants, despite the greater number of efficiency errors made by older adults. In a task similar to the original Multiple Errands Task (i.e., a non-virtual environment), older adults have been shown to exhibit strategy-application deficits (McAlister and Schmitter-Edgecombe 2013). In particular, older adults commit more inefficiency-type errors and poorer task sequencing than younger adults, despite similar task-switching performance.

5.1.8 Summary

The Six Elements Task and Multiple Errands Task do appear to have clinical relevance, as certain patient groups do seem to perform poorly on both tests. Likewise, there is some evidence to suggest that both the Six Elements Task and Multiple Errands Tasks are sensitive to age-related cognitive decline (with possible specificity to frontal function), at least in terms of efficiency. However, when considering the actual specific brain damage or disorder associated with poor multi-tasking and strategy-application performance, the existing literature is distinctly lacking. Moreover, frontal localization using the Six Elements Task deserves particular caution, as even extensive damage to both dorsolateral and ventromedial prefrontal structures does not seem to elicit dissociable profiles of task performance. Although both the Six Elements Task and the Multiple Errands Task were designed to capture frontal dysfunction not observable on classical tests (Shallice and Burgess 1991b), this presents problems when attempting to associate strategy application disorders with other measures of executive dysfunction (Levine et al. 1998). The Multiple Errands Task has been shown to be both more ecologically valid than the Six Elements Task, as well as somewhat more reliable in identifying performance deficits in lesion patients (Rand et al. 2009). Furthermore, the initial difficulties posed by performing the task in a real-life setting are being overcome with the use of virtual environments that will no doubt prove fruitful for much-needed future research, particularly the current absence of functional neuroimaging evidence (Logie et al. 2010).

Chapter 6

Problem-solving and judgment

6.1 Cognitive Estimation Task

6.1.1 Task description

The Cognitive Estimation Task (CET; Shallice and Evans 1978) was devised to assess the ability to estimate measures likely to be unknown to the participants (e.g., "What is the length of an average man's spine?"). This ability is necessary for activities in everyday life such as estimating how much food to cook for dinner guests or estimating the weight of one's luggage before going on a flight. The CET requires participants to: recognize and decide upon a suitable cognitive set (e.g., the spine is a component of the human body, so knowledge and estimates of body parts could be used); employ and manipulate specific information from that cognitive set (e.g., an average man's height is ~1.75 m, minus the sum of head height (~0.25 m) and leg length (~0.75 m)); examine how suitable their estimate is (e.g., 0.75 m) and perform the same procedure again if a better estimate can be achieved. Executive processes are thought to play an important role in generating suitable cognitive estimates, hence the CET is widely used as a test of executive dysfunction (Strauss et al. 2006). However, cognitive estimation has also been shown to rely upon other cognitive abilities such as working memory (e.g., Levinoff et al. 2006), semantic knowledge (e.g., Della Sala et al. 2004), and naming and arithmetical abilities (e.g., MacPherson et al. 2014). Therefore, the CET can be failed for a number of reasons in addition to executive dysfunction.

The original version of the CET (Shallice and Evans 1978) includes both quantitative (e.g., "How fast do race horses gallop?") and qualitative (e.g., "What is the largest fish in the world?") items where responses are scored in relation to a control group. Since then, other versions of the CET have been devised which include fewer items (e.g., O'Carroll et al. 1994) or items suitable for use in American populations (e.g., Axelrod and Millis 1994) or Italian populations (Della Sala et al. 2003), as well as more up-to-date parallel forms of the CET for use with British populations (MacPherson et al. 2014). The *Test zum kognitiven Schätzen* is a version of the CET for German populations which also provides a picture of the question-related object (see Figure 6.1) to reduce the mnemonic load (Brand et al. 2002) whereas the Biber Cognitive Estimation

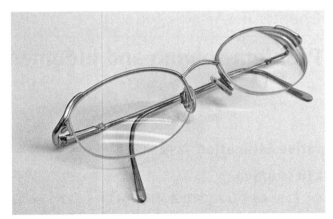

Fig. 6.1 Example of the stimuli from the Test zum kognitiven Schätzen. Reproduced from Matthias Brand, Elke Kalbe, and Josef Kessler, *Test zum kognitiven Schätzen (TKS)*. Figure 1, Hogrefe Verlag GmbH & Co. KG, Göttingen. © 2002, Hogrefe Verlag GmbH & Co. KG.

Test (Bullard et al. 2004) also stipulates the unit of measurement that should be used to answer each item.

6.1.2 **Patient and lesion studies**

Shallice and Evans (1978) observed that patient JS, who had a right frontal lesion, was impaired when asked questions such as, "What is the length of an average man's spine?" He would produce estimates such as 1.4 m and did not seem to be aware that his responses were bizarre, even defending them when challenged. Thus, Shallice and Evans (1978) administered the CET to 45 frontal patients and 51 patients with posterior lesions not involving the frontal lobes. Frontal patients produced significantly more extreme responses than the posterior patients, suggesting that poor CET performance is associated with frontal lobe damage. Several studies subsequently have also demonstrated deficits in CET performance in patients with frontal lobe lesions. Della Sala et al. (2004) administered an Italian version of the CET (Della Sala et al. 2003) to 21 patients with frontal lobe lesions due to traumatic brain injury or stroke and 21 healthy controls. Again, it was found that patients with frontal lobe lesions produced significantly more extreme responses than healthy controls. One example of a bizarre answer in response to the item, "How heavy is a pair of stiletto shoes?" is a frontal patient responding 5000 g, whereas the mean response for the control group was 416 g with the highest control response at 2000 g. Stanhope et al. (1998) administered the original version of the CET to 15 patients with frontal lobe lesions, 14 patients with temporal lobe lesions, 15 patients with diencephalic lesions, and 20 healthy controls. The frontal patients produced significantly more bizarre estimates than the temporal group and the healthy controls. MacPherson et al. (2014) devised two new nine-item parallel forms of the CET which contain more up-to-date items. Twenty-four patients with frontal lesions were administered the CETs and their error scores compared with those of 48 healthy controls. In line with the previous studies, the frontal group produced significantly higher error scores than controls on both versions of the CET.

Nonetheless, CET deficits have not exclusively been related to frontal pathology. Taylor and O'Carroll (1995) administered a shortened version of the CET to a large group of 370 neurological patients and 150 healthy controls. When the authors examined the performance of a subset of 15 patients with focal frontal and 17 patients with focal non-frontal lesions, these patient subgroups did not significantly differ. However, the performance of these patient groups was not compared against a control group. Thus, it is unclear from this study whether either brain lesion type had a significant bearing on normal CET performance.

Few studies have examined the localization of CET processes within frontal subregions, and the extant reports have not reached a consensus (Table 6.1). Leng and Parkin (1988) compared the CET performance of seven patients with alcoholic Korsakoff syndrome and five patients with herpes simplex encephalitis as well as patient JB who had suffered a ruptured anterior communicating artery aneurysm. Both of the patients with herpes simplex encephalitis and the anterior communicating artery aneurysm patient performed poorly on the CET compared to the Korsakoff patients. As patient JB had orbitofrontal cortex damage and as herpes simplex encephalitis is thought to involve predominantly the orbitofrontal cortex (unlike Korsakoff syndrome), Leng and

Table 6.1 Cognitive Estimation Task: Patient and lesion studies

Study	n	Patient/ Control Groups	Study type	Brodmann Areas	FP	DL	OF	ACC
Eslinger and Damasio (1985)	1; 14	OF; HA	Patient (single case)	–			X	
Leng and Parkin (1988)	7; 5; 1; 7	KS; HS; ACoAA; HA	Patient	–				
Shoqeirat et al. (1990)	16; 10; 5; 31	KS; HS; ACoAA; HA	Patient	–				

FP = frontal pole; DL = dorsolateral prefrontal cortex; OF = orbitofrontal cortex; ACC = anterior cingulate cortex; HA = healthy adults; KS = Korsakoff syndrome; HS = herpes simplex encephalitis; ACoAA = anterior communicating artery aneurysm; ✓ = frontal region damaged and impairment found; X = frontal region damaged but no impairment.

Parkin (1998) claimed that this was evidence of the CET being sensitive to orbitofrontal damage. Yet, in a larger study involving patients with the same three etiologies, Shoqeirat et al. (1990) found that deficits in the CET were not specific to patients with orbitofrontal-related pathology. All three patient groups performed poorly on the task. Moreover, patient EVR, who had a bilateral orbitofrontal lesion due to the resection of a meningioma, has also been reported to perform normally on the CET (Eslinger and Damasio 1985).

6.1.3 Neuroimaging studies

There do not appear to be any neuroimaging studies in the literature that have directly examined the neural correlates of the CET. However, there is a large neuroimaging literature that has focused on examining the estimation of time intervals between stimuli. These studies have consistently reported activation in the basal ganglia, supplementary motor area and cerebellum, and in the inferior frontal gyrus when healthy participants are asked to explicitly estimate durations (for a review, see Coull et al. 2011). As the processes involved in time estimation are clearly different, whether this frontal activation would also be reported during the CET remains to be seen.

6.1.4 Aging studies

Aging studies examining the effects of healthy adult aging on the CET suggest that estimation abilities do not decline with age (Table 6.2). Axelrod and Millis (1994) devised a modified version of the original CET which they administered to 164 healthy American volunteers. On subdividing the participants into four age groups (17–29, 30–39, 40–49, and 50–95 years), no significant difference was found between the groups in terms of the cognitive estimates produced. Della Sala et al. (2003) administered an Italian version of the CET to a young group of 18–39-year-olds, a middle-aged group of 40–59-year-olds and an older group of 60–87-year-olds. Again, there was no significant difference between the estimates from the three age groups. Similarly, studies involving correlational analyses have not found significant effects of age on CET performance (O'Carroll et al. 1994: 150 participants aged 17–91 years; Crawford et al. 2000: 123 participants aged 18–75 years; Gillespie et al. 2002: 101 participants aged ≥55 years). When MacPherson et al. (2014) administered both their versions of the CET to 184 British participants aged between 18 and 79 years with 9–22 years of education, increasing age and years of education were found to be significantly correlated with successful CET performance as well as gender, intellect, naming, arithmetic, and semantic memory abilities. Therefore, the literature seems to agree that CET performance does not deteriorate with age but only MacPherson et al. (2014) have reported improved age-related performance.

Table 6.2 Cognitive Estimation Task: Aging studies

Study	n	Participant age groups (years)	Study type	Age effect
Axelrod and Millis (1994)	45; 42; 25; 29	17–29; 30–39; 40–49; 50–95	Cross-sectional (behavioral)	X
Della Sala et al. (2003)	70; 52; 53	18–39; 40–59; 60–87	Cross-sectional (behavioral)	X
O'Carroll et al. (1994)	150	17–91	Cross-sectional (behavioral)	X
Crawford et al. (2000)	123	18–75	Cross-sectional (behavioral)	X
Gillespie et al. (2002)	101	≥55	Cross-sectional (behavioral)	X
MacPherson et al. (2014)	184	18–79	Cross-sectional (behavioral)	✓

✓ = age effect found; X = age effect not found

6.1.5 Summary

While the CET is commonly used as a test of frontal lobe dysfunction and has generally been found to be sensitive to frontal lobe lesions, there is little evidence of localization of cognitive estimation processes within frontal subregions. Both future patient and neuroimaging studies are needed to examine whether the task processes are associated with specific regions within the frontal lobes. By contrast, there is generally agreement in the aging literature that CET performance does not decline with age. Therefore, age-related CET deficits reported in individuals might suggest pathological rather than healthy adult aging.

6.2 Recency and temporal order discrimination

6.2.1 Task description

The recency discrimination task measures the ability to retrieve the relative temporal order of two items (e.g., words or pictures; Milner et al. 1991). In one version of the task (i.e., within list tasks), participants are instructed to study a series of items. They are then presented with a pair of stimuli from the studied list, and asked to indicate which stimulus in the pair was presented most recently (e.g., Zorrilla et al. 1996; Cabeza et al. 1997). In another version of the task (i.e., between list tasks), participants are presented with two lists of stimuli. At test, participants are presented with pairs of stimuli from both lists and asked to indicate which one was encountered in the list shown more recently (e.g., Suzuki et al. 2002). The temporal order discrimination task can also be considered as a recency discrimination task since participants are first presented with either one or two different lists of stimuli. During the test phase, participants are instructed to indicate which item occurred earlier in a previously studied list (within list task; e.g., Amiez and Petrides 2007) or to indicate in which list the items were presented (between list task; e.g., Nyberg et al. 1996; Johnson et al. 1997; Kopelman et al. 1997) (see Figure 6.2).

6.2.2 Patient and lesion studies

Few lesion studies have investigated the effect of focal frontal damage on recency discrimination (Table 6.3). Some early lesion studies have reported no association between focal frontal damage and task performance. For example, Kopelman (1989) found that the performance on a temporal order discrimination task involving two sequences of pictures taken from magazines presented 45 min apart did not correlate with neuroradiological measures of frontal atrophy in patients with Korsakoff syndrome. Similarly, Butters et al. (1994) found that unilateral or bilateral frontal lesions did not impair performance on a temporal order discrimination task using everyday objects. Some studies, however, suggest that task performance does decline following midlateral prefrontal damage. In one such study, Milner et al. (1991) compared

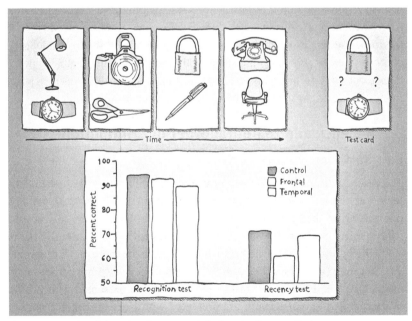

Fig. 6.2 Example of the stimuli presented during the Recency Task.

Table 6.3 Recency and temporal order discrimination: Patient and lesion studies

Study	n	Patient/ Control Groups	Study type	Task type	Brodmann Areas	FP	DL	OF	ACC
Milner et al. (1991)	36; 23; 20	FL; FTL; HA	Lesion	Recency	–		✓		
Johnson et al. (1997)	1; 3; 3	ACoAA; FL; HA	Lesion	Temporal order	–				
Kopelman et al. (1997)	15; 14; 13; 20	FL; TL; dienc; HA	Lesion	Temporal order	–				✓

FP = frontal pole; DL = dorsolateral prefrontal cortex; OF = orbitofrontal cortex; ACC = anterior cingulate cortex; FL = frontal lobe; FTL = frontotemporal lobe; HA = healthy adults; ACoAA = anterior communicating artery aneurysm; TL = temporal lobe; dienc = diencephalic; ✓ = frontal region damaged and impairment found; X = frontal region damaged but no impairment.

the performance of a group of patients with widespread frontal damage following frontal excision ($n = 36$) or fronto-temporal cortical removal ($n = 23$) with that of 20 healthy controls on three versions of recency discrimination tasks (i.e., concrete words, representational drawings, and abstract drawings). The frontal damage involved the mid-lateral prefrontal region in 44 of the 59 frontal patients whereas this area was spared in the remaining 15 patients. Although no significant difference emerged on the verbal item recognition task, the researchers demonstrated poorer performance on verbal recency discrimination in patients with excision of the mid-lateral prefrontal cortex, especially when the removal involved the left hemisphere. By contrast, performance on the picture versions of the task, especially the abstract designs, was impaired compared to healthy controls only in those patients with right frontal removal, suggesting hemispheric specialization for verbal and pictorial information.

Some evidence that the dorsolateral prefrontal cortex is important in making recency discrimination judgments is provided by a study comparing temporal order memory in frontal patients with either dorsolateral prefrontal damage or non-dorsolateral prefrontal damage compared to healthy controls (Kopelman et al. 1997). Participants were presented with two sequences of line drawings, with an interval of 45 min. At test, participants were shown a list of items presented one at a time and instructed to indicate whether they had seen the item before (i.e., a recognition memory task) and in which list (i.e., temporal memory). Patients with dorsolateral prefrontal damage were impaired on the temporal memory task, whereas the performance of those patients with medial frontal damage sparing the dorsolateral prefrontal cortex did not differ from that of healthy controls. Another study by Johnson et al. (1997) also suggests that the medial prefrontal cortex may not play a role in performing recency discrimination tasks. The researchers administered a verbal and a pictorial version of a temporal order discrimination task—similar to the one employed by Kopelman et al. (1997)—to patient GS, who had suffered the rupture of an aneurysm of the anterior communicating artery. Computerized tomography showed a bifrontal medial prefrontal lesion. Patient GS performed similarly to healthy controls on both versions of task. Taken together, the results of these studies suggest that the lateral but not the medial prefrontal cortex is important for retrieving temporal order information.

6.2.3 Neuroimaging studies

Several studies have investigated the neural correlates of recency discrimination (Table 6.4). An early functional magnetic resonance imaging (fMRI) study demonstrated that the dorsolateral prefrontal cortex was activated when performing the task (Zorrilla et al. 1996). The researchers compared the fMRI activation during a recency discrimination task and a non-mnemonic visual-matching task. Participants were first instructed to study a list of words presented, one at time, on a computer screen. During the recency discrimination task, participants were presented with two words from the studied list and instructed to indicate which word had appeared most recently. During the visual matching task, a pair of non-studied words was presented on the screen. One of the two words was repeated and presented again in the middle of the screen. The participants' task was to choose the word in the pair that did not match the one presented in the middle. The fMRI results showed bilateral activation of the dorsolateral prefrontal cortex (Brodmann Area (BA) 9) associated with the recency discrimination task, which the authors interpreted in terms of working memory (e.g., monitoring, manipulation) and episodic memory retrieval. Similar results emerged in a positron emission tomography (PET) study that compared brain activity associated with item recognition memory and recency discrimination (Cabeza et al. 1997). In this investigation, after studying a list of words, participants were presented with a pair of words. In the item recognition task, one word was new (non-studied) and one was old (studied), and participants were instructed to indicate which word they saw in the previous list. In the recency discrimination task, both words were old and participants indicated which one they saw most recently. Subtracting activation during the item recognition memory task from the recency discrimination task showed activation of the dorsolateral prefrontal cortex (BA 9).

It has been argued that contrasting the activation associated with item recognition and recency discrimination may mask the activation specifically associated with recency discrimination, as the brain activation common to

Table 6.4 Recency and temporal order discrimination: Neuroimaging studies

Study	n	Patient/Control Groups	Study type	Task type	Brodmann Areas	FP	DL	OF	ACC
Zorrilla et al. (1996)	7	HA	fMRI	Recency	6, 9		✓		
Cabeza et al. (1997)	12	HA	PET	Recency	6, 9		✓		
Konishi et al. (2002)	16	HA	fMRI	Recency	9, 45/44, 10/46, 32		✓		✓
Dobbins et al. (2003)	11	HA	fMRI	Recency	6, 8, 9, 10, 13	✓	✓	✓	
Rajah and McIntosh (2006)	8	HA	fMRI	Recency	9, 45		✓		
Amiez and Petrides (2007)	17	HA	fMRI	Temporal order	9/46, 46, 47/12		✓		✓
Dudukovic and Wagner (2007)	18	HA	fMRI	Recency	6/8, 10, 9/46	✓	✓		
St Jacques et al. (2008)	17	HA	fMRI	Recency Recollection: 6, 32, 46			✓		✓
				Familiarity: 6, 9			✓		
Jimura et al. (2009)	31	HA	fMRI	Recency	9, 45, 47		✓		
Oztekin et al. (2008)	15	HA	fMRI	Recency	6, 9, 45		✓		
Kimura et al. (2010)	73	HA	fMRI	Recency	6, 8, 9/45, 32, 45, 47		✓		✓
Rajah et al. (2011)	16	HA	fMRI	Recency	9, 10, 46, 47	✓	✓		

FP = frontal pole; DL = dorsolateral prefrontal cortex; OF = orbitofrontal cortex; ACC = anterior cingulate cortex; HA = healthy adults; fMRI = functional magnetic resonance imaging; PET = positron emission tomography; ✓ = frontal region involved.

both tasks is subtracted out (Konishi et al. 2002). Instead, Konishi et al. (2002) investigated fMRI activation associated with two verbal recency discrimination tasks, which varied in their memory demands (i.e., high versus low). In the low-demand task, there was considerable temporal distance between the two words presented (i.e., separated by eight different words during encoding). In contrast, in the high-demand task, the temporal distance between the two words was small (i.e., separated by three words at encoding). The results showed activation of the bilateral frontal area (BA 9), as well as the left inferior lateral prefrontal area (BA 45/44) and the left anterior prefrontal region (BA 10/46) associated with high task demands. These findings support the view that the lateral prefrontal cortex is important for retrieving temporal information under high demands. Amiez and Petrides' (2007) fMRI study extended the results to visual stimuli. In this task, participants were presented with four abstract designs and instructed to encode the order of presentation of the stimuli. At test, they were presented with pairs of stimuli and instructed to indicate which stimulus appeared earlier in the sequence. The fMRI result showed that the dorsolateral prefrontal cortex (BAs 9/46 and 46) was recruited to a greater extent during the retrieval of mid-position stimuli compared to stimuli presented at the beginning or end of the sequence, suggesting a greater involvement of this area when making more demanding judgments.

A different line of research has shown that the brain network associated with the temporal order retrieval of stimuli presented in one list (within list items; e.g., Zorrilla et al. 1996) may differ from the retrieval of stimuli presented in separate lists (between list items; e.g., Cabeza et al. 1997). In an fMRI study, Suzuki et al. (2002) presented their participants with two different lists of images depicting everyday objects. One list was studied in the morning and one in the afternoon. Participants were then shown pairs of images from one list (within list) or images from separate lists (between lists). Their task was to indicate which images they saw most recently. The results showed that both tasks activated lateral prefrontal brain areas, which included BAs 44/9, 45, and 46 as well as the ventrolateral prefrontal cortex (BA 47). Further analysis showed that the inferior frontal gyrus (BA 44/45) was specifically activated during between-list items, whereas the middle frontal gyrus (BA 8/9) was activated during within-list items. This differential activation was explained in terms of different cognitive strategies being required to perform the two types of recency discrimination tasks. As the between-list items were studied at different times (one in the morning and one in the afternoon), the researchers suggested that the retrieval of temporal information would be driven by contextual information in addition to the temporal order information. By contrast, the retrieval of within-list items would rely on temporal order information only.

The involvement of the dorsolateral prefrontal cortex in recency discrimination has been associated with executive demands such as strategic information processing (e.g., the ability to organize information) or information monitoring (e.g., the ability to verify that the information is appropriate for the task). For example, in an fMRI study, Rajah and McIntosh (2006) investigated the neural correlates associated with item recognition memory and recency discrimination with a non-mnemonic strategic control task (i.e., a reverse alphabetizing task) which is thought to require the strategic ordering of information. The control task instructed participants to order three words in reverse alphabetical order. The fMRI results showed greater activation of the right dorsolateral prefrontal cortex (BA 9) during the performance of the recency discrimination task and the strategic control task compared to the item recognition memory task. Further analysis revealed that this region was not differentially activated in the recency discrimination and strategic control task. In a later study, Rajah et al. (2008) employed two modified versions of the recency discrimination task and manipulated strategic ordering, selection, and motor control processes. The strategic ordering process was manipulated by varying the number of stimuli presented in the list while the selection and motor-controlled processes were manipulated by varying the number of responses required. Participants were first shown a series of photographs of faces followed by a recognition memory task that manipulated the number of stimuli but maintained the number of responses required. Specifically, participants were presented with either two or three faces and instructed to indicate whether they recognized one face (i.e., one motor response) or which face they recognized (i.e., one motor response). The recency task manipulated both the number of stimuli and number of responses. Participants were presented with either two or three faces and asked to indicate the face they saw most recently (i.e., one response) or to indicate the reverse temporal order in which the faces were seen during the encoding phase (i.e., three motor responses). In the control ordering task, participants were presented with two or three images and asked to indicate the youngest face (i.e., one motor response) or to order the faces according to their age (i.e., three motor responses). The fMRI results showed greater dorsolateral prefrontal (BA 9) activity associated with recency judgments compared to the control task. Furthermore, activation of the dorsolateral prefrontal cortex correlated with the accuracy on the recency task but not on the control task. Further analysis showed that the left dorsolateral prefrontal cortex was associated with selection and motor response processes (e.g., stimulus–response mapping) whereas the right dorsolateral prefrontal cortex was associated with cognitive control process (e.g., monitoring). In fact, greater right dorsolateral prefrontal cortex emerged during retrieval (recognition and recency) compared to the ordering task. As the delay between encoding and retrieval was short (i.e., 30 s), the authors claimed that the right dorsolateral prefrontal cortex was recruited during the retrieval of information from working memory, and they interpreted its activity as being important in retrieval-related executive processes. These findings suggest that activation of the dorsolateral prefrontal cortex during recency judgments is associated with the executive demands of the task including strategic ordering.

Neuroimaging studies have also investigated the role of hemispheric lateralization when making recency judgments (Dobbins et al. 2003; Dudukovic and Wagner 2007; St Jacques et al. 2008; Oztekin et al. 2008). For example, in an fMRI study, Dudukovic and Wagner (2007) compared brain activation associated with item novelty detection and recency discrimination. Participants were first shown a series of words and instructed to make an abstract/concrete judgment for each presented word. At test, they were presented with three words at a time (i.e., two old, previously studied words, and one new). Their task was to indicate either the most recently seen word or the novel word. The results showed greater left dorsolateral prefrontal activation (BA 8, 9/46) associated with correct recency discrimination compared to item recognition. However, Dudukovic and Wagner (2007) also found right dorsolateral prefrontal activation associated with incorrect relative to correct temporal judgments. It was concluded that the left prefrontal cortex was associated with making recency judgments, whereas the right prefrontal cortex was related to cognitive effort associated with monitoring the task demands.

Some researchers have proposed that two main mechanisms might underlie temporal judgments: recollection and familiarity (Dobbins et al. 2003; St Jacques et al. 2008). The former is effortful in that it requires participants to remember contextual details associated with the memory that guides the retrieval of temporally close events. By contrast, the familiarity-based processes are related to the strength of the memory trace and play a central role in making judgments related to temporally distant events. These two processes have been shown to recruit different brain networks. Dobbins et al. (2003) employed a paradigm that required participants to retrieve detailed contextual information or to discriminate the items on the basis of their familiarity in the fMRI scanner. Participants were first presented with a series of words and instructed to indicate whether the word was pleasant/unpleasant or abstract/concrete. In a subsequent memory test, they were presented with pairs of words and instructed to indicate which word they performed a source recognition judgment (i.e., pleasant versus unpleasant) about and which word they performed a recency judgment (i.e., the word they saw most recently) about. The results showed that source recognition judgments (i.e., recollection) were associated with left prefrontal activity whereas the recency judgment task (i.e., familiarity) recruited the right prefrontal region. Similar results were reported in an fMRI study that investigated brain activation associated with recency judgments regarding autobiographical material (St Jacques et al. 2008). The researchers assumed that greater effort is required to discriminate between events that occurred near in time. Therefore, effortful recollective processes would guide the retrieval of close events. By contrast, the familiarity-based processes related to the strength of the memory trace would play a central role in making judgments regarding distant events. Participants first took a series photographs at different campus locations following a pre-set order. During the test phase, they were shown pairs of images taken in different locations and were instructed to indicate which picture they took first. The temporal distance between photographs was manipulated to obtain pairs of photographs with short, medium, and long temporal distances. fMRI showed greater right dorsolateral prefrontal (BA 9) activation associated with recency judgments for temporally distant images compared to short temporal distances. There was also greater left dorsolateral prefrontal (BA 46) activation associated with the retrieval of temporally close compared to distant images. These findings support the view that activation of the right prefrontal cortex is associated with familiarity-based judgments, whereas the left prefrontal cortex is recruited during the performance of more effortful tasks that require recollection of contextual details.

Activation of the ventrolateral prefrontal cortex during recency discrimination tasks has also been reported (Suzuki et al. 2002; Rajah and McIntosh 2006; Jimura et al. 2009; Kimura et al. 2010; Rajah et al. 2011). The role of this region has been associated with semantic and phonological processing during task performance. For example, Rajah and McIntosh (2006) found a similar pattern of ventrolateral prefrontal activity across three tasks: item recognition, recency judgments and strategic control, suggesting that this area of the prefrontal cortex may be recruited to support more general semantic/phonological processing of verbal material.

Several of the neuroimaging studies discussed above also reported activation of the anterior prefrontal cortex (BAs 10 and 10/46) during recency discrimination (Konishi et al. 2002; Suzuki et al. 2002; Dobbins et al. 2003; Rajah and McIntosh 2006; Dudukovic and Wagner 2007) as well as BA 13 (Dobbins et al. 2003). The role of BA 10 during recency discrimination has been linked to successful or contextual retrieval processes. For example, Suzuki et al. (2002) found left BA 10 activation during the recognition of within-list items. More recently, Rajah et al. (2011) suggested that the recruitment of BA 10 might be related to successful retrieval. In this fMRI study, the researchers presented their participants with a series of photographs of human faces. The memory test consisted of easy and difficult conditions: in the easy task, participants were instructed either to select the face that appeared in a specific position or the face that they saw most recently. In the difficult task, participants were instructed to order three faces from right to left or from the most to the least recently seen. fMRI showed that several prefrontal areas were activated during both tasks, including the dorsolateral prefrontal cortex (BAs 9 and 46), the ventrolateral prefrontal cortex (BA 47), as well as the anterior prefrontal cortex (BA 10). Greater activation of BA 10 emerged during the easy compared to the difficult condition in both the spatial and the recency tasks. As participants performed better on the easy than on the difficult task, the researchers suggested that its activation may be related to successful retrieval. It must be considered, however, that no correlation between accuracy and activation of BA 10 was apparent.

Altogether, the findings from the neuroimaging studies reveal a network of brain regions within the frontal lobes associated with recency discrimination performance, which includes the lateral prefrontal (i.e., the dorsolateral and ventrolateral prefrontal cortex) as well as the anterior prefrontal cortex (BA 10). Whereas the dorsolateral prefrontal cortex is thought to be important for retrieving temporal order information, the ventrolateral prefrontal cortex is thought to reflect semantic and phonological processing, with activation of the anterior prefrontal cortex related to the retrieval of contextual details.

6.2.4 Aging studies

Age effects on the ability to process temporal order information have been investigated using both within- and between-list tasks (Table 6.5). Although some early studies did not report any age effect on task performance (Fozard and Weinert 1972; Perlmutter et al. 1981; McCormack 1982), several more recent investigations have shown a decline in the ability to process temporal information as people become older (Mittenberg et al. 1989; Parkin et al. 1995; Daum et al. 1996; Fabiani and Friedman 1997; Cabeza et al. 2000; Wegesin et al. 2000; Newman et al. 2001; Bastin and Van der Linden 2005; Czernochowski et al. 2008; Rajah and McIntosh 2008, Rajah et al. 2010).

Newman et al. (2001) compared the performance of younger (mean age = 23.1 years) and older (mean age = 66.5 years) adults on a pictorial recency discrimination task involving a series of images of common objects. At test, participants were shown pairs of stimuli, containing either one old and one novel image or two old images. Participants were instructed to indicate which stimulus in the pair they had seen before (item recognition) or which stimulus they had seen more recently (recency discrimination). Older adults performed more poorly on both the item and the recency tasks than younger adults. The performance of younger adults did not differ across the two tasks, whereas the older group performed more poorly on recency discrimination compared to item recognition. These findings suggest a stronger age effect on memory for temporal information than item retrieval. This view is further supported by other studies reporting impaired temporal context memory in older adults, even when item recognition does not show age-related declines (e.g., Fabiani

Table 6.5 Recency and temporal order discrimination: Aging studies

Study	n	Participant age groups (years)	Study type	Task type	Age effect
Fozard and Weinert (1972)	21	25–73	Cross-sectional (behavioral)	Recency	X
Perlmutter et al. (1981)	32; 32	18–24; 60–69	Cross-sectional (behavioral)	Recency	X
McCormack (1982)	50; 50	17–29; 59–76	Cross-sectional (behavioral)	Recency	X
Mittenberg et al. (1989)	68	20–75	Cross-sectional (behavioral)	Recency	✓
Parkin et al. (1995)	30; 29	18–25; 74–95	Cross-sectional (behavioral)	Temporal order	✓
Daum et al. (1996)	50	20–29; 30–39; 40–49; 50–59; 60–69	Cross-sectional (behavioral)	Temporal order	✓
Fabiani and Friedman (1997)	14; 14	22–28; 65–88	Cross-sectional (behavioral)	Recency	✓
Cabeza et al. (2000)	12; 12	20–28; 60–78	Cross-sectional (neuroimaging)	Recency	✓
Wegesin et al. (2000)	24; 23; 24	17–30; 63–73; 74–87	Cross-sectional (behavioral)	Temporal order	✓
Newman et al. (2001)	10; 10	Younger, mean = 23.1 Older, mean = 66.5	Cross-sectional (behavioral)	Temporal order	✓
Bastin and Van der Linden (2005)	48; 48	18–26; 60–70	Cross-sectional (behavioral)	Temporal order	✓
Czernochowski et al. (2008)	15; 15	18–26; 65–82	Cross-sectional (behavioral)	Recency	✓
Rajah and McIntosh (2008)	8; 8	21–35; 62–80	Cross-sectional (neuroimaging)	Recency	✓
Rajah et al. (2010)	21; 21	19–35; 60–80	Cross-sectional (neuroimaging)	Recency	✓

✓ = age effect found; X = age effect not found

and Friedman 1997; Cabeza et al. 2000; Czernochowski et al. 2008; Rajah and McIntosh 2008; Rajah et al. 2010).

The age effect on the ability to process temporal context information has been related to retrieval rather than to encoding deficits. In one experiment, Bastin and Van der Linden (2005) investigated the effect of incidental and intentional encoding on temporal context memory in younger and older participants. Some participants were explicitly asked to encode the item and the order of its presentation (intentional encoding), whereas others were given no specific instruction (incidental encoding). Older adults performed more poorly than younger adults regardless of the encoding instructions; the different encoding instructions did not affect the task performance of either younger or older participants. On the basis of these results, Bastin and Van der Linden proposed that the age effect associated with recency discrimination may reflect a deficit in retrieval processes. In a second experiment, Bastin and Van der Linden (2005) investigated whether the age effect was specific to temporal discrimination or whether older adults were impaired in retrieving contextual information associated with the encoding phase. Participants were first presented with two sets of faces associated with different contextual information: in one set, participants indicated how intelligent the face looked, whereas in the other set, they indicated how honest the face appeared. At test, half of the participants were asked to indicate whether they recognized the face and in which set it appeared; the other half were encouraged to remember the judgment they previously made to remember in which list the face appeared. Based on the results of a post-task questionnaire which instructed participants to indicate what strategy they used to discriminate between the two lists, younger and older adults were divided into those who retrieved the contextual information (i.e., intelligence or honesty judgment) to decide whether they saw the face in the first or second list, and those who instead relied on temporal distance processes (e.g., a feeling of recency). Older participants were impaired compared to younger adults when they used contextual retrieval strategies but not when they used temporal distance information, suggesting that the latter process may be unaffected by age.

A different line of research has investigated whether age effects on recency discrimination are associated with a decline in frontal lobe functions such as flexibility. Correlational studies have found that performance on recency and list discrimination tasks significantly correlated with performance on tasks thought to measure frontal executive abilities such as the Wisconsin Card Sorting Test (WCST) and verbal fluency (e.g., Parkin et al. 1995; Fabiani and Friedman 1997; Czernochowski et al. 2008). Parkin et al. (1995) found that temporal discrimination was negatively associated with increasing age for an older ($n = 29$; mean age = 81.6 years; SD = 4.8) compared to younger ($n = 30$; mean age = 21.5 years; SD = 2.2) group of participants. Temporal discrimination performance decreased with age on a series of verbal and non-verbal fluency tasks (e.g., category fluency, alternate animal and country names, and design fluency). Fabiani and Friedman (1997) employed a verbal and a pictorial task to investigate the contribution of frontal functions on item recognition and recency discrimination in younger (mean age = 24.5 years) and older (mean age = 72.43 years) adults. The older group was significantly impaired compared to younger participants on both the verbal and the visual recency tasks, whereas a decline with age on recognition task emerged for verbal but not for visual material. The performance on the recency tasks correlated with scores on the WCST. In particular, the performance of younger adults on the visual recency task correlated positively with the number of correct responses on the WCST, whereas the performance of older adults on the pictorial recency task was negatively correlated with several scores on the WCST (i.e., number of trials to complete the task and to complete the first category, number of total errors, number of perseverative responses, number of perseverative and non-perseverative errors). The performance of older participants on the verbal recency task was negatively correlated with the failure to maintain set on the WCST. None of the measures derived from the WCST correlated with recognition of either words or pictures. These results might suggest that the ability to make recency judgments may be mediated by executive abilities, but they could also suggest that the WCST and recency judgment performance rely on separate cognitive abilities which are similarly affected by increasing age.

Further support for the view that the frontal lobes are involved in processing temporal information comes from a series of aging studies that have investigated brain activation during recency discrimination tasks. In a PET study, Cabeza et al. (2000) investigated age differences in the brain activation associated with recency judgments. Participants were also administered neuropsychological tests thought to measure functions associated with the dorsolateral prefrontal cortex (i.e., the Self-Ordered Pointing task and the WCST). The behavioral results revealed that the older group performed significantly more poorly than younger adults on the Self-Ordered Pointing task and the WCST and there was a trend for older adults to perform more poorly than younger participants on the recency task ($P = 0.06$). The PET results showed that both groups recruited the left dorsolateral prefrontal cortex (BA 9) to a greater extent during the recency compared to the item recognition task. Further analysis revealed greater right anterior prefrontal (BA 10) activation associated with recency judgments compared to item recognition in younger but not older participants, whereas no age difference emerged in the dorsolateral prefrontal activation while performing the two tasks. This suggests that reduced right prefrontal activation accompanies the age decline in performance on the temporal order discrimination task. Further analysis, however, revealed greater activation of the left prefrontal cortex (BA 10) in older adults during item recognition compared to recency judgments; this was interpreted as compensatory activation associated with retrieval impairments.

Other studies have found that the performance of older adults on the recency discrimination task may be accompanied by increased frontal activation compared to younger individuals (Czernochowski et al. 2008; Rajah and McIntosh 2008; Rajah et al. 2010). This increased brain activation represents the recruitment of compensatory processing to supplement the function of brain networks that experience age-related decline in efficiency. For example, Rajah et al. (2010) scanned younger and older participants using fMRI while they were performing three tasks: item recognition, spatial recognition and recency discrimination. The results showed that performance decreased as a function of task difficulty, item recognition being the easiest task (i.e., fastest response times and most accurate responses), followed by the spatial task. The recency discrimination task was the most difficult (i.e., slowest response times and lowest accuracy) for both younger and older participants. Older participants were impaired on the spatial and temporal tasks compared to younger adults, whereas no age effect emerged on the item recognition task. These behavioral results were accompanied by differential brain activation. The young group showed a linear increase in the activation of the right dorsolateral prefrontal cortex across the item recognition, spatial, and then recency tasks. Activation of the right dorsolateral prefrontal cortex (BA 46) correlated with performance on all tasks, especially the recency discrimination task. By contrast, older participants did not show such a linear trend of right dorsolateral prefrontal involvement, with no significant difference in activation during the temporal task compared to the spatial task. Right dorsolateral prefrontal activation did not correlate with the performance on the temporal task in older adults. Instead, the recency task performance of older but not younger participants correlated with the left dorsolateral prefrontal cortex (BA 46) and the right anterior prefrontal cortex (BA 10). The researchers concluded that older adults exhibit a deficit associated with right dorsolateral prefrontal functions (e.g., performance monitoring) and that the activation of left dorsolateral prefrontal cortex and the right anterior prefrontal cortex reflects compensatory processing for age-related decline in right dorsolateral prefrontal functions.

Other studies suggest that the increased brain activation in older participants may not be sufficient to compensate for the functional decline with age. For example, Rajah and McIntosh (2008) used fMRI to examine younger and older participants performing item recognition and recency discrimination tasks. Performance on the recency task but not the item recognition task declined with age. Although both age groups showed bilateral dorsolateral prefrontal (BA 9) and bilateral anterior prefrontal (BA 10) activation during the memory tasks, older adults showed greater recruitment of these same areas in the right hemisphere. To determine whether such an increased brain activity would compensate for age-related cognitive decline, the researchers examined the relationship between brain activation and task performance. Increased brain activation in older participants was correlated with increased item recognition but not with recency discrimination accuracy. The authors concluded that the increased prefrontal activation in older participants was not sufficient to compensate for the decline in temporal information processing.

Other researchers have suggested that compensatory brain activation might emerge only in older adults with higher socio-economic status (i.e., education and occupation). It has been claimed that educational and occupation achievements might facilitate the use of compensatory or alternative cognitive strategies as people age, and that therefore these strategies might protect older adults from cognitive decline associated with aging. For example, in one ERP study, Czernochowski et al. (2008) found that performance on recency discrimination in high socio-economic status older adults did not differ from that of younger participants, and that both groups outperformed the low socio-economic status older group. Larger frontal ERPs were associated with the recency performance of the high socio-economic status older group only. The researchers concluded that older individuals with high socio-economic status may use different strategies and recruit additional neural resources to compensate for any age-related memory decline.

These cognitive aging studies suggest that the ability to make accurate recency judgments declines with age. Furthermore, this age effect has been interpreted in terms of deterioration of cognitive functions associated with the frontal lobe, especially the dorsolateral prefrontal cortex, although the cognitive decline associated with age may be compensated for by the use of alternative strategies.

6.2.5 Summary

Whereas few patient and lesion studies have investigated the role of focal frontal damage on recency discrimination, the evidence suggests that the ability to make temporal judgments relies on a brain network that includes the lateral as well as the anterior areas of the prefrontal cortex. The role of the lateral prefrontal cortex has been associated with executive and working memory task demands. Furthermore, the ability to make recency discriminations decreases as people age. However, other factors, such as the level of education, might reduce the negative effect of age on task performance.

6.3 Tower Tests

6.3.1 Task description

There is a range of tasks that fall under the heading of Tower Tests. Such tasks are thought to tap planning and self-monitoring abilities, and include the

Tower of London (Shallice 1982), Tower of Hanoi (Byrnes and Spitz 1977), the Stockings of Cambridge subtest from the Cambridge Neuropsychological Test Automated Battery (CANTAB; Sahakian et al. 1988; Owen et al. 1990) and the Tower subtest from the Delis–Kaplin Executive Function System (D-KEFS; Delis et al. 2001). Balls or disks are arranged on pegs (or as socks suspended from a beam in the case of the Stockings of Cambridge) to form the "start state," and these balls or disks must be moved (either manually or on a computer) from location to location in order to configure them into a target arrangement or "goal state" (see Figure 6.3). The manipulations are subject to a set of rules that are explicitly outlined to participants at the start of the test (e.g., only move one ball or disk at a time) and should be clearly displayed throughout testing to reduce the influence of memory on task performance.

There are subtle differences between the various versions of the Tower Tests that are worth noting. Tests such as the Tower of Hanoi and the D-KEFS Tower are similar: they present participants with a series of disks of graded sizes and three pegs of uniform length. The rules are that only one disk may be moved at a time, and a larger disk can never be placed on top of a smaller one. The Tower of London and Stockings of Cambridge tests provide pegs or "socks" of differing length that can carry 3, 2, or 1 colored balls of the same size. Some versions of the Tower Test initially present simple problems requiring a small number of moves to achieve the goal before incrementally increasing the minimum number of moves required. Others begin with a fully constructed tower which has to be moved to a different location from the very first problem. A planning phase is sometimes included, in which participants are encouraged either to predict the moves they will make in advance of carrying them out, or to identify the minimum number of moves required to complete the task without physically attempting the problem. However, some evidence suggests that humans performing the Tower Test are not effective planners beyond a certain number of steps (Phillips et al. 2001), calling into question the validity of a planning phase for more complex problems.

The main outcome measure for the Tower Test is the number of moves taken to achieve the goal state (aggregated over a series of trials of increasing difficulty) with a broad time limit often imposed. In some studies, number of rule-breaks and time-to-completion have also been used as indices of performance. Further measures may be calculated (such as mean first-move time or move:accuracy ratio) although it is less clear from the literature how these metrics relate to the structural integrity and metabolism of the frontal lobes. It has also been demonstrated that problem difficulty can be manipulated through the ambiguity of goal priorities (Newman et al. 2009) where the optimal path is obvious (unambiguous) or unclear (ambiguous). Ambiguous problems have been shown to be more

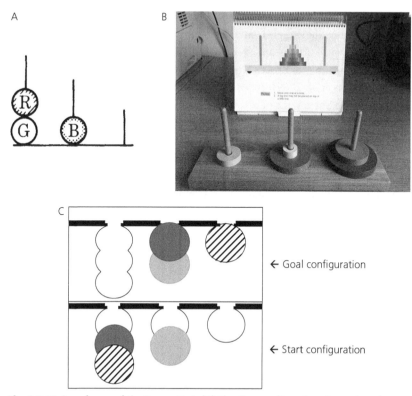

Fig. 6.3 Various forms of the Tower Test. (A) The Tower of London. Reproduced from T. Shallice, Specific Impairments of Planning, *Philosophical Transactions B*, 298 (1089), pp. 199–209, Figure 2, doi:10.1098/rstb.1982.0082. Copyright © 1982 The Royal Society (B) D-KEFS Tower, Data from Delis, D. C., Kaplan, E., & Kramer, J., *Delis Kaplan Executive Function System*, The Psychological Corporation, 2001. (C) Stockings of Cambridge. Reproduced from Deborah Feldmann, Daniel Schuepbach, Bettina von Rickenbach, Anastasia Theodoridou, and Daniel Hell, Association between two distinct executive tasks in schizophrenia: a functional transcranial Doppler sonography study, *BMC Psychiatry*, 6 (25), Figure 2, doi:10.1186/1471-244X-6-25. © 2006 Feldmann et al.; licensee BioMed Central Ltd.

difficult than unambiguous problems, while keeping the overall number of moves required at a constant level. Thus, the authors suggest that total number of moves should not be used as the only index of difficulty for relevant variants of this task.

6.3.2 Patient and lesion studies

Early lesion studies suggest the sensitivity of the Tower Tests to frontal lobe lesions (Shallice 1982; Owen et al. 1990; Owen et al. 1995), with more recent lesion evidence pointing to the specific involvement of the dorsolateral prefrontal cortex (Table 6.6). Lesion studies suggest that Tower performance is affected by dorsolateral prefrontal lesions when compared to the performance of patients with orbital and ventromedial prefrontal lesions (Manes et al. 2002) and healthy controls (Mavaddat et al. 1999; Gomez-Beldarrain et al. 2004; Yochim et al. 2009). By contrast, patients with ventromedial prefrontal lesions due to aneurysms of the anterior communicating artery (Hornak et al. 1996; Cicerone and Tanenbaum 1997; Mavaddat et al. 1999) and cerebrovascular hemorrhage or tumor resection (Manes et al. 2002) do not appear to show poor Tower performance. In apparent contradiction to these findings, Vietnam Veterans with dorsolateral prefrontal and ventromedial prefrontal lesions did not significantly differ in their Tower overall score (Krueger et al. 2009), and

Table 6.6 Tower tests: Patient and lesion studies

Study	n	Patient/ Control Groups	Study type	Brodmann Areas	FP	DL	OF	ACC
Hornak et al. (1996)	12; 11	VM; non-VM	Lesion	–			X	
Cicerone and Tanenbaum (1997)	1	TBI	Lesion (single case)	–			X	
Mavaddat et al. (1999)	45; 20	ACoAA; HA	Lesion	–			X	
Manes et al. (2002)	5; 4; 5; 5	OF; DL; DM; Mix	Lesion	–		✓	X	✓
Schmidtke et al. (2002)	20; 56	DL; HA	Lesion	6, 8, 9, 10, 24, 32, 45, 46	✓	✓		✓
Gomez-Beldarrain et al. (2004)	14; 6; 20	OF; DL; HA	Lesion	10, 11, 12, 25, 32; 9, 46		✓	X	
Mazza et al. (2007)	18; 20; 20	FL; schiz; HA	Lesion	9, 10, 11, 12, 25, 46			✓	
Krueger et al. (2009)	17; 21; 29	DL; VM; HA	Lesion	–		X	X	X
Yochim et al. (2009)	12; 12	DL; HA	Lesion	–		✓		

FP = frontal pole; DL = dorsolateral prefrontal cortex; OF = orbitofrontal cortex; ACC = anterior cingulate cortex; VM = ventromedial prefrontal cortex; TBI = traumatic brain injury; ACoAA = anterior communicating artery aneurysm; HA = healthy adults; DM = dorsomedial prefrontal cortex; Mix = dorsal and ventral prefrontal cortex; FL = frontal lobes; schiz = schizophrenic patients; ✓ = frontal region damaged and impairment found; X = frontal region damaged but no impairment.

patients with right ventromedial prefrontal lesions performed significantly more poorly than controls (Mazza et al. 2007).

However, the interpretation of these findings should be undertaken with caution, given that the categorization of the ventromedial and lateral frontal groups by Krueger et al. (2009) both explicitly included BAs 9 and 46, and no formal tests were performed to compare performance of either group with controls (though all three groups' scores appear similar). Likewise, Mazza et al. (2007) included damage to BAs 10, 11, 12, 25 as well as 9 and 46 in their definition of their ventromedial prefrontal lesion group. Finally, one study evaluated Tower of London performance in patients with focal frontal lesions in comparison to that of age- and education-matched healthy controls (Andrés and Van der Linden 2001). Although patients' responses were generally slowed, there was no significant difference in the number of moves or time taken to solve three- or five-move problems. However, it should be noted that despite having information on specific lesion foci for the patient group, analysis examining group differences based on frontal lesion locus was not undertaken, possibly due to limitations of statistical power (frontal patients, $n = 15$), though seven out of 15 patients had orbitofrontal lesions. Thus, these data cannot speak directly to the question of localization of function within the frontal lobes.

6.3.3 Neuroimaging studies

Neuroimaging studies have proposed that there is some degree of hemispheric specialization in the frontal lobes associated with Tower Test performance, with the right hemisphere being involved in the planning aspects of the task, in contrast to the left hemisphere which is implicated in the execution of that plan (Newman et al. 2003; see Newman et al. 2009 for a review). More specifically, a considerable number of the fMRI and PET studies involving healthy participants have shown active clusters in the dorsolateral prefrontal cortex during performance of Tower Tests with a consistent absence of orbital activation (Baker et al. 1996; Owen et al. 1996a, 1998a; Elliott et al. 1997; Dagher et al. 1999, 2001; Lazeron et al. 2000; Rowe et al. 2001; Fincham et al. 2002; Beauchamp et al. 2003; Cazalis et al. 2003; Newman et al. 2003; Schall et al. 2003; van den Heuvel et al. 2003; Lazeron et al. 2004; Unterrainer et al. 2004; Rasser et al. 2005; Unterrainer et al. 2005; van den Heuvel et al. 2005; Boghi et al. 2006; Cazalis et al. 2006; Wagner et al. 2006a; Just et al. 2007; den Braber et al. 2008; Fitzgerald et al. 2008; de Ruiter et al. 2009; Newman et al. 2009). The dorsolateral prefrontal cortex is also known to receive extensive dopaminergic projections from the ventral tegmental area (Lewis and O'Donnell 2000), and patient groups in which reduced dopamine is a defining characteristic have been shown to perform significantly more poorly than controls on the Tower of London (Morris et al. 1988; Owen et al. 1995; Owen 1997a; Culbertson et al. 2004). Indeed, one study examined the performance of Parkinson's disease patients on and off L-dopa medication and reported that the administration of L-dopa significantly increased the blood oxygen level-dependent (BOLD) response in the dorsolateral prefrontal cortex and significantly improved Tower of London performance (Cools et al. 2002b).

It is also prudent to note that certain other brain regions are often identified as being involved in Tower performance. Activation of the dorsal anterior cingulate cortex has been reliably reported in neuroimaging studies, though it is not clear whether this activation is indicative of processing specific to Tower task performance. For example, Dagher et al. (1999) identified some additional task-related anterior cingulate cortex activation, although this was shown to correlate with hand movements (right hemisphere; BAs 24 and 32) and task complexity (both hemispheres; dorsal BA 24). Other studies have also attempted to explain reported anterior cingulate involvement by comparing the activation patterns of superior and normal performers (Cazalis et al. 2003, 2006). The authors found that only normal performers showed increased activation of the anterior cingulate cortex. These findings are consistent with some of the proposed roles of the anterior cingulate cortex in autonomic regulation (which may be affected during a period of cognitive challenge), and some portions of the anterior cingulate cortex are connected with motor areas and its proposed role in autonomic regulation. Thus, it is currently unclear whether anterior cingulate cortex BOLD responses during the Tower Test reflect more general cognitive processes that, although elicited by the task, are not essential for unimpaired performance. Table 6.7 provides a summary of the frontal subregions activated during Tower Test performance.

Beyond the frontal lobe, the basal ganglia have also been identified as a potential contributor to Tower Test performance (Dagher et al. 1999; Rowe et al. 2001; Beauchamp et al. 2003; van den Heuvel et al. 2003; Newman et al. 2009). Whereas it is currently unclear what contributions to task performance this region might make, it is thought to facilitate rule deduction and application during taxing reasoning tasks such as the Tower Test (Melrose et al. 2007; Newman et al. 2009).

6.3.4 Aging studies

Several studies report that older adults perform more slowly and less accurately than younger adults on the Tower Test (Allamanno et al. 1987; Charness 1987; Robbins et al. 1998; D-KEFS Technical Manual, Wecker et al. 2000; Table 6.8). The presence of age differences on Tower Test performance is a consistent finding, and some literature has attempted to identify which of the

Table 6.7 Tower tests: Neuroimaging studies

Study	n	Patient/ Control Groups	Study type	Brodmann Areas	FP	DL	OF	ACC
Baker et al. (1996)	6	HA	PET	9, 10, 24, 46	✓	✓		✓
Owen et al. (1996a)	12	HA	PET	9, 10, 24/32, 46	✓	✓		✓
Elliott et al. (1997)	6	HA	PET	9, 10, 24, 46	✓	✓		✓
Owen et al. (1998a)	6; 6	PD; HA	PET	6, 45, 47		✓		
Dagher et al. (1999)	6	HA	PET	8, 9, 10, 24, 32, 44, 46, 47	✓	✓		✓
Lazeron et al. (2000)	9	HA	fMRI	–		✓		✓
Dagher et al. (2001)	6; 6	PD; HA	PET	9/46, 10, 32	✓	✓		✓
Rowe et al. (2001)	10	HA	PET	9/46, 10, 11, 32, 46	✓	✓		✓
Cools et al. (2002b)	11	PD	fMRI	–		✓		
Fincham et al. (2002)	8	HA	fMRI	6, 8, 9, 24, 44		✓		✓
Beauchamp et al. (2003)	12	HA	PET	6, 9/46, 10, 25	✓	✓		✓
Cazalis et al. (2003)	11	HA	fMRI	–		✓		✓
Newman et al. (2003)	12	HA	fMRI	8, 9, 10, 11, 45, 46	✓	✓		
Schall et al. (2003)	6; 6	HA; HA	PET + fMRI	8, 9, 10, 32, 46	✓	✓		✓
van den Heuvel et al. (2003)	22	HA	fMRI	9, 10, 32, 46	✓	✓		✓
Lazeron et al. (2004)	23; 18	MS; HA	fMRI	–		✓		
Unterrainer et al. (2004)	22	HA	fMRI	9, 10, 32, 46	✓	✓		✓

(continued)

Table 6.7 Continued

Study	n	Patient/ Control Groups	Study type	Brodmann Areas	FP	DL	OF	ACC
Rasser et al. (2005)	10; 10	schiz; HA	fMRI	6, 9, 10, 44, 46	✓	✓		
Unterrainer et al. (2005)	20	HA	fMRI	9, 32, 46		✓		✓
van den Heuvel et al. (2005)	22; 22	OCD; HA	fMRI	9, 32, 46		✓		✓
Boghi et al. (2006)	18	HA	fMRI	6, 8, 32, 44, 46		✓		✓
Cazalis et al. (2006)	10; 11	TBI; HA	fMRI	–		✓		✓
Wagner et al. (2006a)	17	HA	fMRI	6, 8, 10, 46, 47	✓	✓		
Just et al. (2007)	18; 18	ASDhf; HA	fMRI	–		✓		
den Braber et al. (2008)	12; 12	OCD; TC	fMRI	6, 9, 10	✓	✓		
Fitzgerald et al. (2008)	13; 13	MDD; HA	fMRI	–		✓		✓
de Ruiter et al. (2009)	19; 19; 19	PG; Sm; HA	fMRI	–		✓		✓
Newman et al. (2009)	30	HA	fMRI	6, 8, 10, 32	✓	✓		✓

FP = frontal pole; DL = dorsolateral prefrontal cortex; OF = orbitofrontal cortex; ACC = anterior cingulate cortex; HA = healthy adults; PET = positron emission tomography; PD = Parkinson's disease; fMRI = functional magnetic resonance imaging; MS = multiple sclerosis; schiz = schizophrenic individuals; OCD = obsessive compulsive disorder; TBI = traumatic brain injury; ASDhf: autism spectrum disorder (high functioning); TC = twin controls without ASD; MDD = major depressive disorder; PG = problem gamblers; Sm = smokers; ✓ = frontal region involved.

cognitive processes required for Tower Test performance might be affected by age. For example, Gilhooly et al. (1999) found an age effect on the initial planning phase (during which they required participants to reason out loud prior to attempting to solve the problem), but found no differences in the number of moves taken to solve the problems once the strategy had been planned out. The authors took these findings to reflect age-related deficits in working memory, given that the planning phase took place in the absence of

Table 6.8 Tower tests: Aging studies

Study	n	Participant age groups (years)	Study type	Age effect
Allamanno et al. (1987)	8; 12; 17; 14; 19; 13; 19; 15; 5; 9	40–45; 46–50; 51–55; 56–60; 61–65; 66–70; 71–75; 76–80; 81–85; 86–88	Cross-sectional (behavioral)	✓
Charness (1987)	45	21–71	Cross-sectional (behavioral)	✓
Robbins et al. (1998)	77; 49; 36; 61; 83; 35	<55; 55–59; 60–64; 65–69; 70–74; 75–79	Cross-sectional (behavioral)	✓
Gilhooly et al. (1999)	20; 20	17–25; 60–76	Cross-sectional (behavioral)	✓
Andrés and Van der Linden (2000)	47; 48	Younger, mean = 22.8 Older, mean = 65.0	Cross-sectional (behavioral)	✓
Wecker et al. (2000)	112	20–79	Cross-sectional (behavioral)	✓
Phillips et al. (2003)	36; 36	18–30; 60–76	Cross-sectional (behavioral)	✓
Salthouse (2005)	254	18–95	Cross-sectional (behavioral)	✓
Phillips et al. (2006)	78	22–80	Cross-sectional (behavioral)	✓

✓ = age effect found; X = age effect not found

visuospatial support from the stimuli themselves. Phillips et al. (2003) subsequently employed a dual task paradigm to selectively load different components of working memory (see Baddeley 2012) while performing the Tower of London. Younger and older adults were asked to perform a secondary task while performing the Tower of London: either articulatory suppression to tap the phonological loop, spatial pattern tapping to tap the visuospatial sketchpad, or random number generation or spatial random tapping to assess the central executive. Phillips et al. (2003) found that all four secondary tasks disrupted performance on the Tower Test in older individuals, whereas only those tasks that primarily loaded on executive functioning disrupted performance in younger adults.

Andrés and Van der Linden (2000) found that Tower of London performance was significantly poorer in older ($n = 48$) than younger ($n = 47$) participants for problems requiring three and five moves. Older adults took significantly more moves to solve problems, took more time to initiate the first move, and more overall time to solve the problem on average. In a group-wide analysis, individual differences in processing speed explained the majority of the variance in Tower of London performance, suggesting that processing speed may be an important mediator between age and Tower of London performance. By contrast, Salthouse (2005) reported that age effects on the Tower of Hanoi among 254 participants aged between 18 and 95 years were attenuated to non-significance when accounting for general cognitive abilities such as reasoning and memory, with no load on speed of processing. Phillips et al. (2006) found that age effects (n = 78, range = 22–80 years) on Tower of London total moves to completion were largely attenuated by measures of processing speed (assessed using digit symbol substitution) and years of education. However, 17% of the initial effects of age on Tower of London performance were unaccounted for by processing speed and education.

6.3.5 **Summary**

Overall, there exists a substantial literature from both patient and neuroimaging studies to suggest that the dorsolateral prefrontal cortex is important for Tower Test performance, in contrast to the orbital and ventromedial prefrontal regions. Neuroimaging studies also report BOLD response in the anterior cingulate cortex during this task, but the absence of lesion studies addressing the significance of anterior cingulate cortex integrity for Tower Test performance makes it difficult to judge the role played by this frontal region. There are also consistent reports of associations between increasing age and higher errors, longer time, and higher moves to completion. There remains some debate as to whether (and to what degree) aging per se affects the specific abilities required to carry out the Tower task successfully over and above the effect of covariates such as years of education or general age-dependent slowness in processing speed, as these appear to account for a significant proportion of the Tower Test variance.

Chapter 7

Working memory

7.1 Digit Span Backwards Task

7.1.1 Task description

Digit Span Backwards often forms a component of a neuropsychological test battery, including the Wechsler Memory Scale—III (WMS-III; Wechsler 1997) and Wechsler Adult Intelligence Scale—IV (WAIS-IV; Wechsler 2008), where it is typically administered together with Digit Span Forwards. The researcher or clinician reads out loud a list of single digits at a rate of one digit per second, which participants should recall back either in the same (digit forwards) or reverse (digit backwards) order as the digits were previously presented.[1] In the widely used WMS-III and WAIS-IV versions of the task, two trials are given at each list length (from two to eight digits) until the participant fails to get either trial correct, and performance is measured as the total number of digit sequences correctly recalled. In other studies, the discontinue rule is omitted and participants perform all trials (e.g., Aleman and van't Wout 2008). Digit Span Backwards can be scored in terms of the proportion of correctly recalled sequences, the maximum sequence length recalled, or a discrepancy score (the difference between Digit Span Forwards and Digit Span Backwards). Whereas Digit Span Forwards and backwards both assess short-term memory, Digit Span Backwards is also conceived to require focused attention and manipulation within working memory (Baddeley 1992), and so is often thought to measure executive abilities (Robbins 1996). Indeed, there are some suggestions that Digit Span Backwards is associated more with the executive component of working memory than storage and rehearsal per se (e.g., Hale et al. 2002).

---

[1] Various other span tasks exist which also tap verbal working memory abilities. Common examples include reading span—in which participants remember words presented at the end of sentences—and computational span—in which participants remember numbers presented at the end of maths problems. However, in comparison to digit span tasks these tests are relatively recent, and so much less lesion and neuroimaging work has been carried out using them.

7.1.2 **Patient and lesion studies**

One of the difficulties with examining localization of the processes involved in Digit Span Backwards is that it is often included as a background measure of frontal executive function rather than as the focus of a patient or lesion study. Although this means that a vast number of studies have administered the task to a variety of lesion patients, the majority of them do not directly compare Digit Span Backwards performance between groups. For example, Schnyer et al. (2004) conducted a study of episodic memory in diffuse frontal lesion patients. Although Digit Span Backwards was used as a measure of working memory (i.e., maintenance and manipulation of information), the performance of the lesion group was not directly compared either to healthy controls or to normative data, and was instead used along with other tasks to calculate composite "frontal" scores. Of the lesion studies that have directly contrasted Digit Span Backwards performance across patient groups, there has been mixed evidence for frontal involvement. In a study designed to assess Trail Making Task performance in patients with diffuse frontal lesions, Stuss et al. (2001a) noted that patients with lesions involving either the left or bilateral frontal lobe tended to perform more poorly on the Digit Span Backwards Task than healthy controls achieving fewer correct sequences, though this trend was not significant. Parkin et al. (1996) described the case of patient JB who presented with damage to the left frontal lobe and caudate due to a ruptured anterior communicating artery aneurysm. JB was notably impaired on the Digit Span Backwards Task when compared to normative data from the Wechsler Memory Scale—Revised (WMS-R; Wechsler 1984). Similarly, in another study, whereas patients with left unilateral or bilateral lesions involving the frontal lobe successfully completed fewer Digit Span Backwards trials than healthy controls, patients with right unilateral lesions (involving the frontal lobe) were also impaired relative to controls (Heilbronner et al. 1991). Ischemic stroke patients with frontal lobe lesions have also exhibited poorer Digit Span Backwards performance when compared to non-frontal lesion patients or healthy controls, with the non-frontal group performing as well as healthy controls (Leskelä et al. 1999). These results suggest that the Digit Span Backwards Task can be used to discriminate between dysfunction caused by frontal and posterior lesions.

This same pattern of frontal lobe impairment has not been observed for Digit Span Forwards. Canavan et al. (1989) demonstrated a dissociation between Digit Span Backwards and Digit Span Forwards performance when comparing frontal patients to Parkinson's disease patients, temporal lobe lesion patients, and healthy controls, leading the authors to suggest that the two tasks are differentially sensitive to frontal dysfunction. In addition, the Digit Span Forwards

Task does not appear to distinguish between frontal and more posterior damage. Black and Strub (1978) noted that whereas both frontal and posterior lesion patients performed more poorly than healthy controls, performance between the two groups did not significantly differ. Heilbronner et al. (1991) observed that patients with diffuse (frontal and posterior) lesions and healthy controls did not differ in terms of their Digit Span Forwards performance; Stuss et al. (1998) noted that frontal lesion, non-frontal lesion, and healthy control groups did not significantly differ in terms of Digit Span Forwards performance.

However, not all studies have observed impaired Digit Span Backwards performance in patients with frontal lobe damage. Indeed, whereas diffuse frontal and parietal damage following traumatic brain injury (TBI) appears to impair performance on Digit Span Backwards (but not Digit Span Forwards) compared to TBI patients without signs of damage on computerized tomography, TBI patients with focal frontal contusions affecting both the orbital and medial prefrontal cortices exhibit intact Digit Span Backwards performance (Fork et al. 2005). Only mild Digit Span Backwards deficits using the Wechsler Adult Intelligence Scale—Revised (WAIS-R; Wechsler 1981) have been noted in adult patients with prefrontal damage acquired in early childhood (Price et al. 1990). In an early study by Black and Strub (1978), frontal and posterior lesion patients, as well as healthy control participants, did not differ in terms of Digit Span Backwards performance. Stuss et al. (2001a) noted the same pattern of intact Digit Span Backwards performance when comparing frontal lobe lesion patients either to non-frontal lesion or to healthy control groups.

In terms of further localization within the frontal lobes, D'Esposito and Postle (1999) reviewed the studies examining performance on Digit Span Backwards in patients with prefrontal lesions. When examining the lesion overlap, the authors noted that impaired digit span performance was associated with dorsolateral prefrontal damage. However, several of the reviewed studies only reported combined Digit Span Forwards and Digit Span Backwards scores, making it difficult to conclude that dorsolateral prefrontal involvement was specific to Digit Span Backwards. Moreover, several studies have shown that damage to frontal regions not involving the dorsolateral prefrontal cortex may also result in Digit Span Backwards impairments. For example, an early patient study by Wallesch et al. (1983) observed impaired performance on digit span tasks in patients with medial prefrontal lesions, but not those with dorsolateral prefrontal lesions. Notably, the neuroanatomical classification of each patient group is somewhat unclear, as some medial prefrontal patients exhibited damage involving Brodmann Area (BA) 9 among other non-dorsolateral prefrontal regions (see Figure 3 in Wallesch et al. 1983). Wallesch et al. used a combined Digit Span Forwards and Digit Span Backwards measure, again making it difficult to focus on Digit Span Backwards specifically. However, Leimkuhler and Mesulam (1985) described a patient with a tumor affecting the medial aspects of the frontal lobe who also exhibited impaired performance on both Digit Span Forwards and Digit Span Backwards. The patient also exhibited impaired performance on other reverse tasks, such as saying the months backwards, suggesting that the medial prefrontal cortex may be involved in either the re-ordering of information within working memory or the inhibition of the forward sequence.

Impaired Digit Span Backwards performance can also result from damage to regions outside the frontal lobe. For example, Van der Werf et al. (1999) described a patient with damage to the caudal intralaminar nuclei of the thalamus, an area with strong projections to frontal cortices. The patient scored within the normal range on the Digit Span Forwards Task, but exhibited a marked impairment on the Digit Span Backwards Task without performing poorly on other short- and long-term memory tests. On a similar note, Silveri et al. (1998) described the case of an 18-year-old boy presenting with a cerebellar lesion who exhibited impaired Digit Span Backwards Task performance both immediately before and after surgery to remove a lesion from the right cerebellar hemisphere, with a span estimate of around three digits. By contrast, around six months after surgery, the patient's digit span estimate had increased to seven.

Evidence from patient and lesion studies has predominantly pointed towards the importance of the dorsolateral prefrontal cortex in the performance of the digit span tasks, with damage resulting in poorer performance and fewer lists recalled correctly (Table 7.1). However, whether dorsolateral prefrontal damage specifically impairs Digit Span Backwards (rather than Digit Span Forwards) performance is less clear. There is some limited evidence to suggest that patients with damage to medial or posterior regions may also exhibit problems on the digit span tasks, though this is likely for different reasons than those with dorsolateral prefrontal damage.

7.1.3 Neuroimaging studies

Several neuroimaging studies have examined the localization of processes associated with performance on Digit Span Backwards (Table 7.2). Hoshi et al. (2000) demonstrated significant and predominantly right-sided activation within BAs 9 and 46 in healthy individuals performing the Digit Span Backwards Task; a dorsolateral prefrontal pattern that the authors suggest represents the manipulation of working memory. Furthermore, individuals exhibiting activation of the right dorsolateral prefrontal cortex could recall significantly longer backwards digit sequences than those exhibiting left dorsolateral prefrontal

Table 7.1 Digit Span Backwards: Patient and lesion studies

Study	n	Patient/Control Groups	Study type	Brodmann Areas	FP	DL	OF	ACC
Wallesch et al. (1983)	18; 18; 14	DL; ML; P	Lesion	–		✓		✓
Leimkuhler and Mesulam (1985)	1	ML	Lesion (single case)	–				✓
D'Esposito and Postle (1999)	8 studies	Lateral FL	Meta-analysis (lesion)	9, 46		✓		
Fork et al. (2005)	11; 11; 17	TBI-DAI; TBI-FL; TBI-C	Lesion	–	✓	✓		

FP = frontal pole; DL = dorsolateral prefrontal cortex; OF = orbitofrontal cortex; ACC = anterior cingulate cortex; ML = medial prefrontal cortex; P = parietal cortex; FL= frontal lobe; TBI-DAI = traumatic brain injury with diffuse axonal injury (but no focal lesions); TBI-FL = traumatic brain injury with focal lesions (but no diffuse axonal injury); TBI-C = traumatic brain injury control participants (without focal lesions or diffuse axonal injury); ✓ = frontal region damaged and impairment found; X = frontal region damaged but no impairment.

Table 7.2 Digit Span Backwards: Neuroimaging studies

Study	n	Patient/Control Groups	Study type	Brodmann Areas	FP	DL	OF	ACC
Hoshi et al. (2000)	8	HA	NIrOT	8/9, 9, 9/46, 46/45		✓		
Owen et al. (2000)	8	HA	PET	9, 11, 24, 47		✓	✓	✓
Gerton et al. (2004)[a]	14	HA	PET	6, 9, 10, 32, 44, 46;	✓	✓		✓
O'Sullivan et al. (2005)	18	CADASIL	DTI	6/8, 8, 9/44, 9, 10	✓	✓		
Sun et al. (2005)[b]	10; 10	YA; OA	fMRI	9, 44/45		✓		
Fitzgerald et al. (2006)	25; 25	DP-AT; DP-SH	rTMS	–		✓		
Aleman and van't Wout (2008)	7	HA	rTMS	–		✓		
Luerding et al. (2008)	20	FM	MRI (VBM)	6, 24, 32				✓

FP = frontal pole; DL = dorsolateral prefrontal cortex; OF = orbitofrontal cortex; ACC = anterior cingulate cortex; HA = healthy adults; NIrOT = near-infrared optical tomography; PET = positron emission tomography; CADASIL = participants with cerebral autosomal dominant arteriopathy with subcortical infarcts and leukoencephalopathy; YA = younger adults; OA = older adults; DTI = diffusion tensor imaging; fMRI = functional magnetic resonance imaging; rTMS = repetitive transcranial magnetic stimulation; DP-AT = depression active treatment group; DP-SH = depression sham stimulation group; FM = individuals with fibromyalgia; VBM = voxel-based morphometry; ✓ = frontal region involved.

[a] This summary describes a combination of both Experiment 1 and Experiment 2.

[b] Younger adults reported only.

activation (Hoshi et al. 2000). Owen et al. (2000) conducted a positron emission tomography (PET) investigation of the regions activated during Digit Span Backwards Tasks, using healthy middle-aged participants. Importantly, they also administered a Digit Span Forwards Task, and contrasted the two tasks in order specifically to localize the executive demands of the Digit Span Backwards Task. When compared to activation during a control task (in which participants repeated a string of five identical digits), the Digit Span Backwards Task resulted in increased brain activity in the dorsolateral prefrontal cortex (BA 9/46) and ventrolateral prefrontal cortex (BA 47). However, when compared to the activation baseline for Digit Span Forwards, significant regional cerebral blood flow changes were observed only in the dorsolateral prefrontal regions (Owen et al. 2000). In another study, the dorsolateral prefrontal cortex (BA 9) and occipital region (BA 17/18/19) show greater activation and blood oxygen level-dependent (BOLD) signal change during the recall phase of a Digit Span Backwards Task when contrasted to a Digit Span Forwards Task (Sun et al. 2005). By comparison, when contrasted to Digit Span Backwards Task performance, Digit Span Forwards Task performance resulted in greater activation only in the inferior frontal gyrus (BA 44/45). Likewise, Gerton et al. (2004) found evidence of bilateral dorsolateral prefrontal activation in healthy individuals undergoing PET imaging during a Digit Span Backwards Task, but they also noted inferior parietal lobule (BA 40) and inferior frontal gyrus (BA 44) activation when contrasted with a Digit Span Forwards baseline.

Using repetitive transcranial magnetic stimulation (rTMS), Fitzgerald et al. (2006) observed that stimulation applied to the dorsolateral prefrontal cortex (to both right and left sides sequentially) of clinically depressed individuals resulted in significantly improved Digit Span Backwards performance. By contrast, rTMS centered over the right dorsolateral prefrontal cortex has been noted to impair digit span performance in healthy individuals, although the impairment did not appear to differ between Digit Span Forwards and Digit Span Backwards Tasks (Aleman and van't Wout 2008). This suggests that even Digit Span Forwards performance relies on some degree of function associated with the dorsolateral prefrontal cortex, in particular the executive control of working memory through rehearsal and maintenance of the items within. Transcranial direct current stimulation (tDCS)—a method similar to rTMS which is designed to excite neurons within a region—applied to the left dorsolateral prefrontal cortex, alongside a concurrent working memory training task, has been shown to improve performance on Digit Span Forwards, but not Digit Span Backwards (Andrews et al. 2011). Notably, the difference between these two studies may be as simple as the region targeted (right versus left dorsolateral prefrontal cortex respectively). This suggests that while the right dorsolateral prefrontal cortex may represent the storage processes common to both Digit Span Forwards and Digit Span Backwards, the left dorsolateral prefrontal cortex may be much more involved in the processes particular to Digit Span Forwards.

Diffusion tensor imaging (DTI) carried out by O'Sullivan et al. (2005) has also linked Digit Span Backwards performance to the structural integrity of the dorsolateral prefrontal cortex, particularly the white matter integrity of the left inferior frontal gyrus. However, O'Sullivan et al. (2005) also observed an association between the orbitofrontal cortex and medial prefrontal white matter integrity (BAs 10 and 6 respectively) and Digit Span Backwards performance. In another study, Luerding et al. (2008) examined the neural correlates of Digit Span Backwards performance in fibromyalgia patients (a condition whose etiology is unclear, but which is characterized by chronic pain and tiredness) using voxel-based morphometry. They reported positive associations between performance on the Digit Span Backwards Task and gray matter volume in medial prefrontal regions including the supplementary motor area (BA 6), anterior cingulate cortex, and white matter volume in the cingulum. Although behavioral performance on the Digit Span Backwards Task was not significantly different between the fibromyalgia patients and normative data from healthy controls, there was a trend towards poorer performance in the patient group. Given the small sample recruited by Luerding et al. (2008), the generalizability of these findings is limited.

There is also evidence that other brain regions are activated during Digit Span Backwards performance. A PET study by Gerton et al. (2004) found evidence of medial occipital cortex activation during the Digit Span Backwards Task, even when participants wore blindfolds to reduce visual stimulation. This may indicate the use of visual imagery strategies while performing Digit Span Backwards. In order to complete a Digit Span Backwards Task, participants are likely to employ both the manipulation of visuospatial (as the numbers appear on the page or in a mental representation) and verbal information (as the numbers are read out or rehearsed; Larrabee and Kane 1986).

7.1.4 **Aging studies**

The evidence for age-related declines in performance on Digit Span Backwards Tasks is mixed (Table 7.3). Several studies of performance across the lifespan have reported age-related impairment on both Digit Span Forwards and Digit Span Backwards (e.g., Dobbs and Rule 1989; Clark et al. 2004). However, a meta-analysis of span tasks conducted by Bopp and Verhaeghen (2005) found that the Digit Span Backwards Task demonstrated stronger age-related differences than basic span tasks (such as the Digit Span Forwards Task or the word

Table 7.3 Digit Span Backwards: Aging studies

Study	n	Participant age groups (years)	Study type	Age effect
Dobbs and Rule (1989)	228	30–39; 40–49; 50–59; 60–69; ≥70	Cross-sectional (behavioral)	✓
Verhaeghen et al. (1993)	10 studies	16–30; 61–81	Meta-analysis	X
Hedden et al. (2002)	64; 64	Younger (mean = 21.2) Older (mean = 67.9)	Cross-sectional (behavioral)	✓
Park et al. (2002)	48; 48; 48; 47; 57; 49; 48	20–29; 30–39; 40–49; 50–59; 60–69; 70–79; 80–89	Cross-sectional (behavioral)	X
Clark et al. (2004)	140; 160; 150; 100	11–20; 21–30; 31–50; 51–70	Cross-sectional (behavioral)	✓
Hester et al. (2004a)	67; 80; 85; 75; 96; 80; 79; 88; 80; 88; 90; 63; 59	16–17; 18–19; 20–24; 25–29; 30–34; 35–44; 45–54; 55–64; 65–69; 70–74; 75–79; 80–84; 85–89	Meta-analysis	✓
Lamar and Resnick (2004)	23; 20	20–40; 60–80	Cross-sectional (behavioral)	X
Bopp and Verhaeghen (2005)	57 studies	16–29, 60–77	Meta-analysis	✓
Sun et al. (2005)	10; 10	19–27; 60–72	Cross-sectional (neuroimaging)	✓
Zimmerman et al. (2006)	148	21–76	Cross-sectional (behavioral)	✓
Logie and Maylor (2009)	73018	18–79	Cross-sectional (behavioral)	✓

✓ = age effect found; X = age effect not found

span task), suggesting that the manipulation rather than storage is the prominent working memory deficit affected by age. Furthermore, the ability to hold and manipulate the contents of working memory as measured by span tasks (both backwards and forwards) appears to decline linearly between young and old age (Bopp and Verhaeghen 2005).

Whereas other span tasks (e.g., reading span) and processing speed tasks (e.g., digit–symbol substitution from the WAIS-IV) show more pronounced decline in comparison to long-term memory measures (e.g., Benton Visual Retention Test; Sivan 1992), Digit Span Backwards appears to be more resilient, with very little change in terms of score between age 20 and 80 years (Park et al. 2002). This relative stability of Digit Span Backwards performance over the lifespan has been replicated in other studies (e.g., Logie and Maylor 2009; see also Verhaeghen et al. 1993). Hester et al. (2004a) observed that the rate of age-related decline in Digit Span Backwards performance was equivalent to that of Digit Span Forwards performance. When they conducted a large re-analysis of 1030 participants from across the lifespan who took part in the standardization of the Wechsler Adult Intelligence Scale—III (WAIS-III; Wechsler 1997b) and WMS-III (Wechsler 1997a), Hester et al. (2004a) noted that Digit Span Backwards and Digit Span Forwards decline at very similar rates across the lifespan, and to a much lesser extent than spatial span measures. This suggests that both Digit Span Backwards and Digit Span Forwards Tasks may tap very similar abilities, and that such verbal working memory abilities may be relatively resistant to age-related decline in comparison to other domains of working memory. Indeed, the similarity between forward and backward span measures remained, even after controlling for gender and education (Hester et al. 2004a).

Lamar and Resnick (2004) reported no age-related impairment in terms of Digit Span Backwards performance. However, given the much smaller sample size (43 participants in total) than those in the studies noted above, lack of power may explain the failure to detect previously reported age effects. Lamar and Resnick (2004) themselves reported notably better task performance in both younger and older participants when contrasted to other studies (e.g., Dobbs and Rule 1989; Clark et al. 2004; Bopp and Verhaeghen 2005)— suggesting a particularly high-functioning sample. Sun et al. (2005) also found similar behavioral performance between younger and older adults on a Digit Span Backwards Task, but observed significantly greater right inferior frontal gyral activation (BA 44/45) for older adults when compared to younger adults. The authors suggested that this represented a compensatory mechanism in response to the increased demand placed on executive functioning by the Digit Span Backwards Task (Sun et al. 2005). This ties in well with suggestions that the right dorsolateral prefrontal cortex is recruited to compensate for age-related impairments in verbal memory function (see Park and Reuter-Lorenz 2009; de Chastelaine et al. 2011). Zimmerman et al. (2006) used functional magnetic resonance (fMRI) to investigate the regional gray matter changes associated with age and their relationship with Digit Span Backwards Task performance, as well as other frontal executive measures. Performance on the executive tests including Digit Span Backwards was predicted by age, and by concomitant reductions in dorsolateral prefrontal cortex volume. By contrast, performance on Digit Span Forwards was included as an attentional measure; performance on these tasks was predicted separately by age and by dorsolateral prefrontal and orbitofrontal gray matter volume (Zimmerman et al. 2006).

Performance on the Digit Span Backwards Task has been shown to be influenced by cultural effects with age (Hedden et al. 2002). In particular, Hedden et al. noted that Chinese individuals outperformed individuals from the USA, but that this effect was only significant in the younger adult group. Older adults did not show such a cultural effect. Interestingly, the culture effect was significant in older adults on the Digit Span Forwards Task, with Chinese older adults achieving more correctly recalled trials than American older adults. This suggests that care should be taken when administering digit span tasks—especially forwards—to older adults, as cultural differences may prevent direct comparisons between older and younger adult groups. It is unclear whether these changes in cultural sensitivity emerge specifically in older age, or whether Digit Span Backwards in middle-aged individuals is also less susceptible to cultural effects.

7.1.5 Summary

Although most studies describing the performance of frontal lesion patients on Digit Span Backwards have noted impairments when compared to healthy controls, patients with focal damage not encroaching upon the frontal lobe also exhibit poor performance. It is likely that Digit Span Backwards Task impairments in non-frontal groups are due to the disruption of processes other than manipulation and storage, such as speech production and preparation. Further localization based on lesion evidence alone is problematic, as Digit Span Backwards deficits have been described in a variety of patients with focal prefrontal lesions, including either dorsolateral prefrontal cortex or medial prefrontal cortex, and studies often combine both Digit Span Forwards and Backwards performance. Neuroimaging studies, on the other hand, have tended to suggest the involvement of dorsolateral prefrontal regions in healthy task performance, yet several studies have also reported the involvement of other prefrontal (e.g., BAs 6 and 44) and non-frontal (e.g., BAs 22 and 40) regions. Contrasting Digit Span Forwards and Digit Span Backwards indicates dorsolateral prefrontal involvement on Digit Span Backwards but not Forwards. The research suggests that Digit Span Backwards performance (in terms of behavioral performance or brain activation) should be contrasted to that of Digit Span Forwards, as considering the pattern of behavior across both tasks may help in identifying dorsolateral prefrontal dysfunction. Finally, the evidence for age effects in the Digit Span Backwards Task is somewhat inconsistent, and even when age effects have been observed, these are often weaker than the decline in the performance of other span tasks, such as reading span or visual pattern span. If the right dorsolateral prefrontal cortex may help to compensate for age-related impairments in the Digit Span Backwards Task, this might explain the comparatively subtle age effects on digit span task performance when compared to more pronounced age effects on other tasks thought to involve the dorsolateral prefrontal cortex.

7.2 Target/response delay tasks

7.2.1 Task description

There are several tasks based on the concept of maintaining a target or response in mind over a period of time. Such tasks include the Delayed Response Task, the Delayed Alternation Task, the Delayed Match to Sample Task, and the Delayed Non-Match to Sample Task. The majority of these tasks originated from the study of non-human primates and rodents, and employ a variety of stimuli dimensions and modalities. The early non-human Delayed Response Tasks (e.g., Jacobsen 1935; Finan 1942) involved the baiting of one of several locations with food, during which the animal is allowed to watch. An opaque screen or hood is lowered to cover the animal's view of the locations for a set period of time. Once the screen is raised again, the animal is free to retrieve the food from the target location (see Figure 7.1). In this way, the correct response is cued beforehand and the animal is required to maintain a motor plan over the course of the delay. The Delayed Alternation Task generally involves a similar set-up with two locations, food being hidden in one of the locations. On choosing the correct location, a screen covers the animal's view for a specified delay period. During this delay, the other location is then baited so that the animal must switch its response in order to obtain more food (e.g., Mishkin 1957). The Delayed Match to Sample Task frequently involves animals viewing an array of illuminated buttons, one of which turns green. The animal is required to touch the illuminated button, which then switches off for a delay period. After the delay, the animal is given the choice of two buttons that are illuminated in different colors and it is required to pick the button matching the color of the target light (e.g., Bauer and Fuster 1976; Penetar and McDonough 1983). In the Delayed Non-Match to Sample Task, participants are asked to pick the stimulus which does not match the target (i.e., the novel stimulus, rather than the familiar one; e.g., Mishkin and Delacour 1975). These various tasks have been adapted for use in humans, with variants using spatial stimuli, object (shape or color) stimuli, face stimuli, etc. (e.g., Baldo and Shimamura 2000; Lamar and Resnick 2004; Olsen et al. 2009; see also Teuber 2009).

In target/response delay tasks, three specific functions attributed to the prefrontal cortex have been identified as key to performance: working

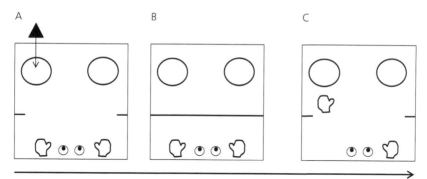

Fig. 7.1 Example of a classic spatial Delayed Response Task trial. (A) A reward (represented by a triangle) is placed in a well in full view of the participant (either monkey or human); (B) a screen covers the participant's view for a set period of time (the delay); (C) the screen is removed and the participant is allowed to pick a well (in this case the participant chooses the rewarded well).

memory, inhibition, and executive control of attention (Fuster 1999). During the delay period, two distinct executive working memory processes can be identified—one maintaining the sensory information from the recent past, and one maintaining the intended motor plan (Fuster 2000). Goldman-Rakic et al. (1990) have used evidence from the Delayed Response Task to support the notion that the prefrontal cortex maintains task-related information online across delays.

7.2.2 Patient and lesion studies

Most early evidence regarding frontal involvement in target/response delay tasks comes from non-human primate lesion studies. In the study by Finan, two mangabey monkeys who underwent the removal of BAs 8, 9, 10, 11, and 12 were shown to be impaired on the Delayed Response Task (Finan 1942; see also Gross and Weiskrantz 1962). By contrast, performance on a discrimination learning task using similar materials was relatively intact. In a later study by Glickstein et al. (1963), rhesus monkeys were tested using the Delayed Response Task after three stages of surgery. After the first stage—a unilateral optic tract section intended to restrict visual input to one hemisphere—monkeys could still perform the task over all delay conditions, including the longest one of 15 s (Glickstein et al. 1963). After the second stage of surgery, in which unilateral ablations were made to the prefrontal cortex to restrict fronto-occipital connections to the commissural system only, monkeys showed a marked deficit in performance, but only if the prefrontal lesion was contralateral to the damaged optic tract. Whereas the contralateral lesion monkeys failed to achieve the longest delay condition (often achieving only a 10–12 s delay), ipsilateral lesion monkeys continued to perform as well as they did preoperatively. In the third stage, in which the anterior commissure was cut, this had the effect of reducing Delayed Response Task performance in contralateral lesion monkeys even further. Indeed, when the view of contralateral lesion monkeys with a commissurotomy was obscured in this way, they could only perform well over much shorter 3–4 s delays (Glickstein et al. 1963). In another study, Funahashi et al. (1993) noted that unilateral lesions to the prefrontal cortex of rhesus monkeys may lead to accuracy impairments on a memory-guided saccade task with a delayed response, but not on an oculomotor control task without a memory component. Also, saccades were disproportionately impaired after longer delay periods, when the cue stimulus was presented to the visual field contralateral to the prefrontal lesion (Funahashi et al. 1993). Malmo (1942) examined the Delayed Response Task performance of a rhesus monkey and a mangabey monkey before and after removal of the frontal cortex, which included BAs 6 and 8, 9, 10, 11, and 12. Malmo noted surprisingly intact accuracy post surgery in both monkeys after a standard 10 s delay period. The only decrement in performance was found when, postoperatively, the monkeys were given visual interference (a bright light) during the delay period (Malmo 1942). This suggests that the frontal lobes may not support memory rehearsal mechanisms, but instead they may play an important role in protecting the motor plan to be stored from interfering stimuli and processes. Similarly, Orbach and Fischer (1959) administered a Delayed Response Task in which bright lights were used as interference during the delay period. The authors observed that rhesus monkeys with frontal lesions exhibited impaired performance when the interference was presented, even in the minimal delay conditions. Orbach and Fischer (1959) suggested that frontal regions may not be integral in maintaining the response over the delay, but that again it may play a role in protecting against interference at any length of delay.

Whereas the architecture of monkey and human frontal lobes is fairly similar, the degree to which associations between complex cognition and brain in monkeys may be related with those in humans is not entirely clear (e.g., Diamond and Goldman-Rakic 1989; Ungerleider et al. 1998; Levy and Goldman-Rakic 2000; Ongür and Price 2000). Thus, Freedman and Oscar-Berman (1986) conducted an early study administering these same delay tests to human patients with frontal lobe lesions. They examined the performance of frontal patients with and without memory impairment and control patients with no evident brain damage but with significant memory impairment (e.g., due to Korsakoff syndrome) on a Delayed Response Task and a Delayed Alternation Task. Rather than including a healthy control group, the authors compared the performance of the three patient groups to participants with a history of alcohol abuse but no presentation of memory impairments (i.e., alcoholic non-amnestic controls). This was to account for the effects of alcohol abuse on Delayed Response and Delayed Alternation Task performance. Similar to the non-human primate studies discussed above, the tasks required participants to monitor a reward (in this case money) being placed into a specific well, before the view of the wells was covered for a set period of time. The Delayed Response Task had four delay conditions—one with no delay (0 s), one with a 10 s delay, one with a 30 s delay, and one with a 60 s delay. The Delayed Alternation Task, on the other hand, involved only a 5 s delay. After this time, participants were free to choose the well in which they thought the reward was present. For the Delayed Response Task, the reward contingencies were predetermined, whereas the contingencies were switched on the Delayed Alternation Task when participants achieved a number of correct responses in a row. Freedman and Oscar-Berman noted that, compared to alcoholic non-amnestic controls, the frontal lesion group committed more errors on both the Delayed Response Task and the Delayed Alternation Task. The Korsakoff group (memory impairments in the absence of frontal damage) committed significantly more errors than the controls on the Delayed Alternation Task only (Freedman and Oscar-Berman 1986). Interestingly, the researchers observed that both frontal patients with and without amnesia exhibited difficulty on the tasks, suggesting that the deficit seen especially on the Delayed Response Task may be due to frontal executive dysfunction rather than memory impairment (Freedman and Oscar-Berman 1986). However, there is some doubt about the importance of the prefrontal cortex during the delay in target/response delay tasks. For example, using a Delayed Response Task, Baldo and Shimamura (2000) noted that there was no interaction between participant group and delay, suggesting that those with frontal lesions were not disproportionately affected by increasing delays. There is also some evidence that lesions in specific brain regions beyond the prefrontal cortex also impair performance on target/response delay tasks. For example, patients with medial temporal lobe epilepsy also appear to be impaired on the Delayed Match to Sample Task (Stretton and Thompson 2012).

Attempts have also been made to further localize prefrontal involvement in the Delayed Response Task by considering subdivisions within the prefrontal cortex. Mishkin (1957) investigated the effect of various localized prefrontal lesions (ventral, inferior lateral, midlateral, or superior lateral lesions) on Delayed Alternation Task performance in rhesus monkeys. Only the "midlateral" lesion group exhibited significant decline in performance, mostly committing perseverative errors with the inferior frontal lesion group also showing some signs of impairment. Furthermore, Oscar-Berman (1975) investigated performance on the Delayed Response Task in rhesus monkeys after receiving either dorsolateral or ventrolateral/orbitofrontal lesions. Dorsolateral prefrontal lesion monkeys showed the poorest performance on a visual Delayed Response Task and performed significantly more poorly than the ventrolateral/orbitofrontal lesion group, who themselves performed significantly more poorly than healthy control monkeys. An auditory Delayed Response Task was not able to discriminate between the lesion groups, with both lesion groups performing more poorly than controls but not each other (Oscar-Berman 1975).

Localization of the functions involved in Delayed Response Task performance has also been examined within the human prefrontal cortex (Table 7.4). Bechara et al. (1998) examined the performance of both dorsolateral/dorsomedial prefrontal patients and ventromedial prefrontal patients on both the Delayed Response Task and the Delayed Non-Match to Sample Task. Interestingly, there was significantly poorer accuracy overall and with increasing delay than healthy controls in both the ventromedial prefrontal patient group and the right dorsolateral/dorsomedial prefrontal patients, but not the left dorsolateral/dorsomedial prefrontal patients (Bechara et al. 1998). However, the posterior ventromedial prefrontal lesion group was associated with delay problems on both tasks (Bechara et al. 1998). A similar lesion study conducted by Vérin et al. (1993) noted that dorsolateral prefrontal lesion patients committed more errors than posterior lesion patients and healthy controls on the Delayed Response Task, and committed more perseverative errors than either posterior lesion patients or healthy controls on the Delayed Alternation Task. Similarly, rTMS applied to either the right or left dorsolateral prefrontal cortex during the 5 s delay period of a spatial Delayed Response Task created significantly higher error rates than stimulation of the motor cortex or no stimulation (Pascual-Leone and Hallett 1994). The degree of damage to BA 46 correlates positively with the number of errors committed by unilateral frontal lesion patients, and such a patient group has been shown to perform more poorly on a spatial oculomotor Delayed Response Task than healthy controls (Baldo and Shimamura 2000).

A meta-analysis of human lesion studies conducted by D'Esposito and Postle (1999) created composite lesion maps from 10 studies that administered spatial variants of the Delayed Response Task. The integrity of BAs 8, 9, and 46 was found to be important for performance under normal delay conditions and when distracters were presented during the delay (D'Esposito and Postle 1999). In the few studies that have looked at specific prefrontal involvement on Delayed Response Tasks, the integrity of BA 46 was found to be important for resisting distracters while maintaining the motor plan (D'Esposito and Postle 1999). However, both patients with lesions involving BA 46 and healthy

Table 7.4 Target/Response Delay Tasks: Patient and lesion studies

Study	n	Patient/Control Groups	Study type	Task	Brodmann Areas	FP	DL	OF	ACC
Mishkin (1957)	2; 2; 4; 2	VL; IL; ML; SL	Lesion (monkey)	Delayed Response; Delayed Alternation	–		✓	X	
Oscar-Berman (1975)	4; 5; 4	DL; VL-O; HA	Lesion (monkey)	Delayed Response	–		✓		
Vérin et al. (1993)	10; 10; 24	DL; PC; HA	Lesion	Delayed Response; Delayed Alternation	–		✓		
Bechara et al. (1998)	9; 10; 21	VM; DL; HA	Lesion	Delayed Response; Delayed Non-Match to Sample	–		✓	✓	✓
Teixeira-Ferreira et al. (1998)	8; 10; 18	DL; TL; HA	Lesion	Delayed Response	–		✓		
D'Esposito and Postle (1999)	7 studies	lateral FL	Meta-analysis	Delayed Response	8, 9, 46		✓		

FP = frontal pole; DL = dorsolateral prefrontal cortex; OF = orbitofrontal cortex; ACC = anterior cingulate cortex; VL = ventral prefrontal cortex; IL = inferior lateral prefrontal cortex; ML = midlateral prefrontal cortex; SL = superior lateral prefrontal cortex; VL-O = ventrolateral-orbital prefrontal cortex; HA = healthy adults; PC = post-central lesion; VM = ventromedial prefrontal cortex; TL = temporal lobe; FL = frontal lobe; ✓ = frontal lobe; ✓ = frontal region damaged and impairment found; X = frontal region damaged but no impairment.

controls have been shown to be impaired with increasing delay, notably when a digit-monitoring task was performed during the delay period (Baldo and Shimamura 2000). As such, in order to discriminate between prefrontal lesion patients and healthy controls, prospective studies may benefit from avoiding interference during the delay period.

Patients with dorsolateral prefrontal lesions have been shown to perform poorly under increasing delays compared to temporal lobe lesion patients and healthy controls across stimulus dimensions (spatial and spatio-temporal; Teixeira-Ferreira et al. 1998). This suggests that, although implicated in target/response delay tasks, the temporal lobe regions may not be necessary or sufficient to cause impairments. Partiot et al. (1996) contrasted the performance of dorsolateral prefrontal lesion patients with subcortical patients including Parkinson's disease and supranuclear palsy on several delay-type tasks. All patient groups exhibited a deficit on the Delayed Response Task and the Delayed Alternation Task administered, committing significantly more errors than healthy controls. However, the type of impairment differed between groups, with dorsolateral prefrontal patients showing perseverative behavior (i.e., the inability to inhibit previous responses and adopt a new response) and subcortical patients showing inattentive behavior (i.e., the inability to maintain response behaviors). Partiot et al. suggested that this result highlights the role of both the dorsolateral prefrontal cortex and subcortical regions such as the striatum in performing target/response delay tasks, and that the functions of the two regions can be dissociated (i.e., learning and inhibition versus maintenance of response programmers).

7.2.3 **Neuroimaging studies**

In rhesus monkeys, cooling[2] of the prefrontal cortex (BAs 9 and 10) has been shown to increase the number of errors on a spatial Delayed Response Task and a color Delayed Match to Sample Task, whereas parietal or no cooling shows no such increase (Bauer and Fuster 1976). Interestingly, specific cells in the dorsolateral prefrontal cortex have been observed to fire in response to cue identity (e.g., color), whereas other cells in the dorsolateral prefrontal cortex (and in the posterior parietal cortex) have been associated with the features of the motor plan (e.g., direction; Niki and Watanabe 1976; Quintana and Fuster 1999). Kojima and Goldman-Rakic (1982) conducted a similar investigation of

---

[2] Cooling is a methodology used to produce 'inactivation' in the regions to which it is applied. Probes are inserted so as to make contact with the surface of the cortex, and rapidly cooled using a thermoelectric reaction. Similar to transcranial magnetic stimulation, the effects of cooling are temporary, making repeated measures designs possible.

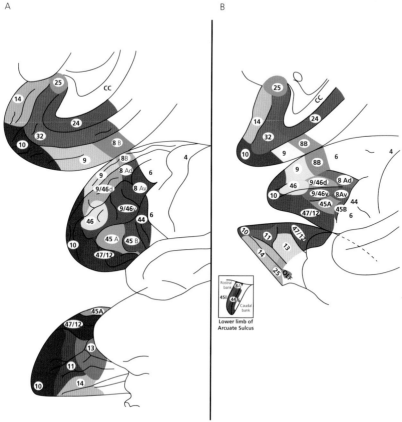

Fig. 1.6 Cytoarchitecture of (A) human and (B) monkey prefrontal cortices. Reprinted from *Cortex*, 48 (1), Michael Petrides, Francesco Tomaiuolo, Edward H. Yeterian, and Deepak N. Pandya, The prefrontal cortex: comparative architectonic organization in the human and the macaque monkey brains, pp. 46–57, Copyright (2012), with permission from Elsevier.

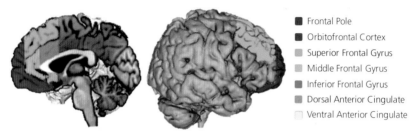

- Frontal Pole
- Orbitofrontal Cortex
- Superior Frontal Gyrus
- Middle Frontal Gyrus
- Inferior Frontal Gyrus
- Dorsal Anterior Cingulate
- Ventral Anterior Cingulate

Fig. 1.7 Subdivision of the frontal lobes.

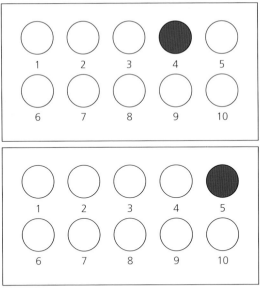

Fig. 2.1 Illustration of a sequential rule ($x + 1$) in the Brixton Spatial Anticipation Test. In this example, the participant sees circle 4 colored blue on the first page (upper) and then has to work out where the colored circle will appear on the next page (lower).

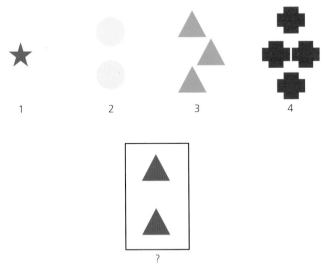

Fig. 4.4 Example of a trial in the Wisconsin Card Sorting Test. Sorted piles of cards are seen along the top, with the new to-be-sorted card at the bottom. The target card can be sorted by shape (pile 3), color (pile 1), or number (pile 2) according to the current sorting rule.

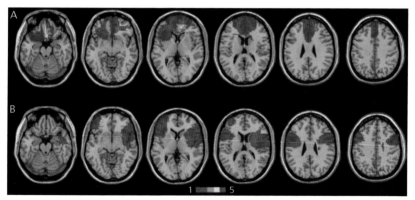

Fig. 8.2 Overlaps of lesions for (A) ventromedial prefrontal group who were impaired on emotion recognition and (B) non-ventromedial prefrontal group who were comparable to controls (Heberlein et al. 2008). Reprinted from Andrea S. Heberlein, Alisa A. Padon, Seth J. Gilihan, et al. Ventromedial frontal lobe plays a critical role in facial emotion recognition, *Journal of Cognitive Neuroscience*, 20(4), pp. 721–733, © 2008 Massachusetts Institute of Technology. Reprinted by permission of MIT Press Journals.

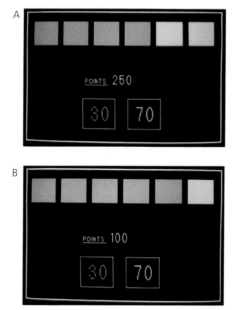

Fig. 9.3 Example of two trials from the Cambridge Gambling Task. Note the difference in probabilities between A (4:2) and B (5:1). Reproduced from Robert D. Rogers, Adrian M. Owen, Hugh C. Middleton, Emma J. Williams, John D. Pickard, Barbara J. Sahakian, and Trevor W. Robbins, Choosing between small, likely rewards and large, unlikely rewards activates inferior and orbital prefrontal cortex, *Journal of Neuroscience*, 20(19), pp. 9029–9038, Figure 1. © 1999, The Society of Neuroscience, with permission.

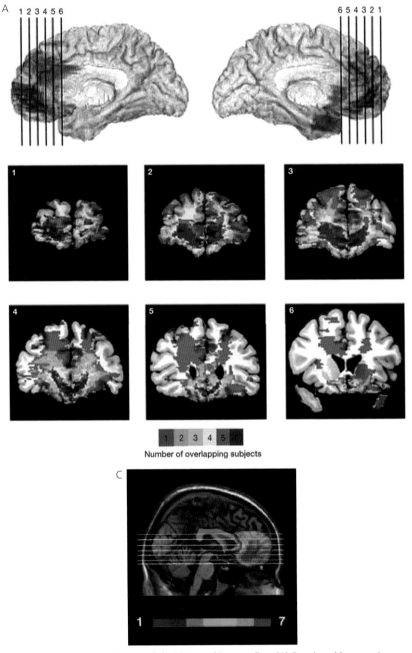

Fig. 9.6 Lesion overlaps in moral decision-making studies. (A) Reprinted by permission from Macmillan Publishers Ltd: *Nature* 446(7138), Michael Koenigs, Liane Young, Ralph Adolphs, Daniel Tranel, Fiery Cushman et al., Damage to the prefrontal cortex increases utilitarian moral judgements, pp. 908–911, Figure 1. Copyright, 2007, Nature Publishing Group. (C) Reproduced from Laura Moretti, Davide Dragone, and Giuseppe de Pellegrino, Reward and social valuation deficits following ventromedial prefrontal damage, *Journal of Cognitive Neuroscience*, 21(1), pp. 128–140. © 2008 by the Massachusetts Institute of Technology. Reprinted by permission of MIT Press Journals.

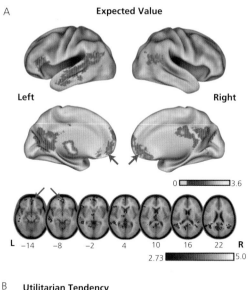

A **Expected Value**

Left   Right

0 ▭▭ 3.6

L −14   −8   −2   4   10   16   22   R

2.73 ▬▬▬ 5.0

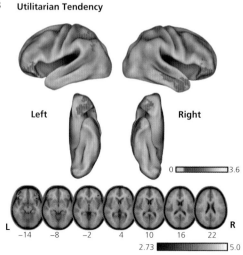

B **Utilitarian Tendency**

Left   Right

0 ▭▭ 3.6

L −14   −8   −2   4   10   16   22   R

2.73 ▬▬▬ 5.0

Fig. 9.7 Utilitarian responses in Moral Decision-Making studies. Top panel: network whose activation increases linearly with value of expected outcome. Ventromedial pre-frontal activation (arrows) sensitive to the "expected moral value" is reported in several studies of economic decision-making. Bottom panel: regions demonstrating increased BOLD activation with increased tendency towards utilitarian responses. Reprinted from Amitai Shenhav and Joshua D. Greene, Moral Judgments Recruit Domain-General Valuation Mechanisms to Integrate Representations of Probvability and Magnitude, pp. 667–77, Figure 3. Copyright (2010), with permission from Elsevier.

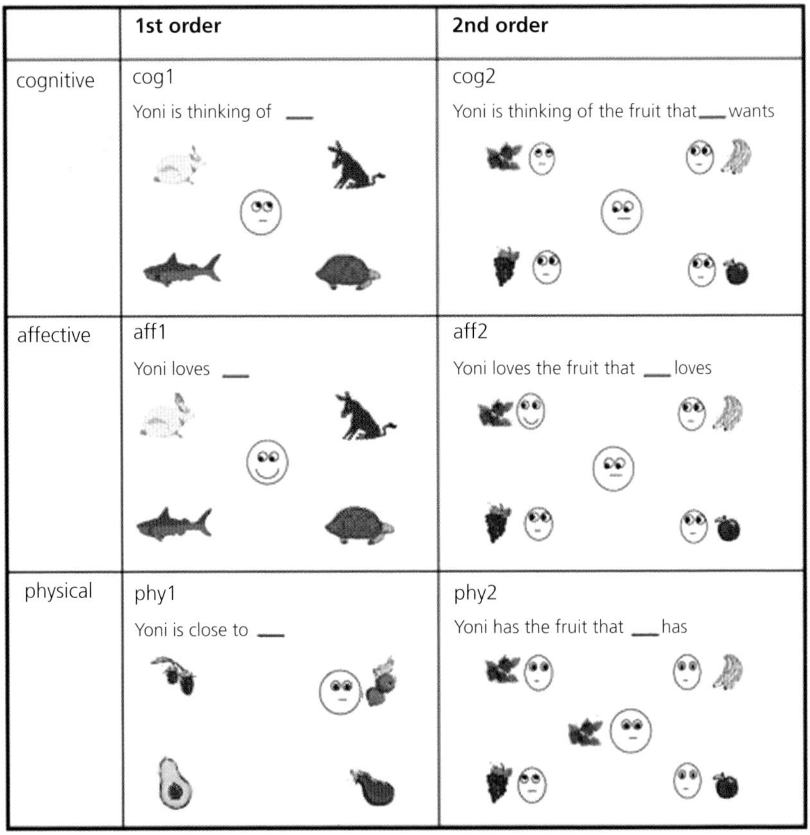

	1st order	2nd order
cognitive	cog1 Yoni is thinking of ___	cog2 Yoni is thinking of the fruit that ___ wants
affective	aff1 Yoni loves ___	aff2 Yoni loves the fruit that ___ loves
physical	phy1 Yoni is close to ___	phy2 Yoni has the fruit that ___ has

Fig. 10.3 Stimuli used in the modified Judgment of Preference Task. Reprinted from *Neuropsychologia* 45 (13), from Elke Kalbe, Marius Schlegel, Alexander T. Sack, Dennis A. Nowak, Manuel Dafotakis, Christopher Bangard, Matthias Brand, Simone Shamay-Tsoory, Oezguer A. Onur, and Josef Kessler, Dissociating cognitive from affective theory of mind: a TMS study, pp. 769–780. Copyright (2010), with permission from Elsevier.

prefrontal neuronal activity in rhesus monkeys, noting phase-locked activity in particular dorsolateral prefrontal neurons where some cells respond specifically to the cue, with the majority of these cells being active during the early part of the delay period (Kojima and Goldman-Rakic 1982). More dorsolateral prefrontal cells modulate their response in line with the delay duration, with longer discharge durations and more negatively skewed discharge profiles as the delay increases (Kojima and Goldman-Rakic 1982). The Delayed Match to Sample Task has also been used to dissociate decision-related responses from motor responses on a neuronal level within both monkey and human brains, with parietal neurons playing a key role during the stages before a response is made (for a review see Freedman and Assad 2011).

In light of non-human primate studies, Goldman-Rakic et al. (1990) have suggested that a distributed network of regions is key to maintaining responses over a delay period. As well as involving the frontal eye fields and premotor cortex, the postulated network also includes the hippocampus and parietal regions, with the dorsolateral prefrontal cortex serving as the hub that links the network together and co-ordinates processing (Goldman-Rakic et al. 1990). Goldman-Rakic et al. suggest that whereas the dorsolateral prefrontal cortex is integral to processing the cue and maintaining a response, when longer delays are encountered, other regions such as the hippocampus act as a longer-term storage buffer. Human neuroimaging studies have lent support to this theory by identifying a fairly widespread network of activation during the Delayed Response Task and other target/response delay tasks (Table 7.5). Using PET, Gold et al. (1996) noted activation in a variety of regions including BAs 6, 8, 9, 10, 46, and 47 after subtracting activation from a no-delay control task using human participants. Activation was most widespread when the task was novel (i.e., the first time participants performed the task); however, performance in this instance was relatively poor (Gold et al. 1996). This pattern of activation suggests that several regions of the prefrontal cortex—including the dorsolateral and ventrolateral prefrontal cortex—may be responsible for performance during the delay period. Also in humans, Goldberg et al. (1996) observed activation in both the dorsolateral prefrontal cortex (BA 46) and ventromedial prefrontal cortex (BA 11), as well as several other regions (e.g., anterior cingulate cortex, parietal lobes, occipital lobes), when subtracting no-delay control task activation from that observed in a spatial Delayed Match to Sample Task (Goldberg et al. 1996; see also Owen et al. 1996b). During a spatial Delayed Response Task, Leung et al. (2002) observed widespread task-related activation in regions such as the middle frontal gyrus (BA 46), inferior frontal gyrus (BA 47), pre-central sulcus, premotor cortex, and lateral occipital cortex. Furthermore, when examining activation during two long-delay conditions

Table 7.5 Target/response delay tasks: Neuroimaging studies

Study	n	Patient/Control Groups	Study type	Task	Brodmann Areas	FP	DL	OF	ACC
Bauer and Fuster (1976)	4	HM	Cooling	Delayed Response; Delayed Match to Sample	—	✓	✓	✓	✓
Niki and Watanabe (1976)	2	HM	Single-unit recording	Delayed Response	—		✓		
Kojima and Goldman-Rakic (1982)	2	HM	Single-unit recording	Delayed Response	—		✓		
Goldman-Rakic et al. (1990)	3 studies	HM	Review (single-unit recording)	Delayed Response	—		✓		
Pascual-Leone and Hallett (1994)	10	HA	rTMS	Delayed Response	—		✓		
Smith et al. (1995)[a]	48	HA	PET	Delayed Match to Sample					
				Location:	6, 32, 46, 47;		✓		✓
				Object:	32, 44		✓		✓
Gold et al. (1996)	18	HA	PET	Delayed Alternation	6, 8, 9, 10, 32, 44, 45, 46, 47	✓	✓	✓	✓
Goldberg et al. (1996)	14	HA	PET	Delayed Match to Sample	6, 11, 44, 46		✓	✓	✓
Owen et al. (1996b)	16	HA	PET	Delayed Match to Sample	6, 9/46		✓		
Bushara et al. (1999)	9	HA	PET	Delayed Match to Sample					
				Auditory:	6, 8/32, 9, 47;		✓	✓	✓
				Visual:	6, 46		✓	✓	✓
Elliott and Dolan (1999)	10	HA	fMRI	Delayed Match to Sample; Delayed Non-Match to Sample					
				Match:	24, 25;		✓		✓
				Non-Match:	6, 11;		✓	✓	✓
				Delay:	44/45		✓		✓

Study	n	Group	Method	Task	BA areas					
Koechlin et al. (1999)	6	HA	fMRI	Delayed Response						
Quintana and Fuster (1999)	2	HM	Single-unit recording	Delayed Response; Delayed Match to Sample Color: Response Direction: Certainty:	 9, 10; 9, 10; 9, 10		✓ ✓ ✓	✓ ✓	✓	✓ ✓
Rypma et al. (1999)	6	HA	fMRI	Delayed Match to Sample Memory load:	6, 24, 44/6; 6, 8, 9, 10, 22/24, 24/32, 44, 45, 46		✓	✓	✓	
Rowe et al. (2000)	6	HA	fMRI	Delayed Response Maintenance: Response Selection:	8; 9/46, 11, 46, 47				✓	
Barrett et al. (2001)	10	HA	PET	Delayed Match to Sample Color: Pattern:	10, 10/46, 11; 11		✓	✓ ✓		
Leung et al. (2002)	30	HA	fMRI	Delayed Response Task: Delay:	6, 6/9/44, 45, 46, 46/9, 46/10, 47; 6, 24/32, 44/6, 46, 46/9		✓	✓		✓
Bunge et al. (2003)	14	HA	fMRI	Delayed Match to Sample; Delayed Non-Match to Sample Delay period:	6, 8, 44					
Curtis et al. (2004)	15	HA	fMRI	Delayed Match to Sample; Delayed Non-Match to Sample Match (Delay): Non-Match (Response):	4, 6, 9, 44, 46, 46/10; 8, 9, 44/45, 46		✓ ✓	✓		✓

Table 7.5 Continued

Study	n	Patient/Control Groups	Study type	Task	Brodmann Areas	FP	DL	OF	ACC
LoPresti et al. (2008)	19	HA	fMRI	Delayed Match to Sample Delay:	6, 8, 10, 46, 47	✓	✓	✓	✓
Schon et al. (2008)	17	HA	fMRI	Delayed Match to Sample Object:	4, 6, 10, 11, 32, 45, 46, 47;	✓	✓	✓	✓
				Location:	6/8, 46			✓	✓
Minzenberg et al. (2009)	5 studies	schiz; HA	Meta-analysis (fMRI)	Delayed Match to Sample	11, 45			✓	
Olsen et al. (2009)	25	HA	fMRI	Delayed Match to Sample					
Robinson et al. (2009)	15	RDep; HA	fMRI	Delayed Non-Match to Sample Familiarity:	6, 9, 10, 13, 32, 46, 47;	✓	✓	✓	✓
				Novelty:	6, 9, 10, 13, 32, 46	✓	✓		✓
Berent-Spillson et al. (2010)	13; 24; 18	CHU; PHU; HA	fMRI	Delayed Match to Sample	13, 32, 45				✓
Yee et al. (2010)	18	HA	fMRI	Delayed Match to Sample					

FP = frontal pole; DL = dorsolateral prefrontal cortex; OF = orbitofrontal cortex; ACC = anterior cingulate cortex; HA = healthy adults; HM = healthy monkeys; rTMS = repetitive transcranial magnetic resonance; PET = positron emission tomography; schiz = schizoprehnic patients; RDep = remitted bipolar patients; CHU = current hormone users; PHU = past hormone users; ✓ = frontal region involved

[a]Combined results from Experiments 1 and 2.

(18 and 24 s) in which behavioral performance was similar, Leung et al. noted that only the middle frontal gyrus (BA 46), but not the inferior frontal gyrus (BA 47), showed sustained activity throughout the delay period in both conditions (Leung et al. 2002).

Event-related neuroimaging studies have also helped to identify distinct phases of activity during performance of target/response delay tasks, with particular prefrontal regions associated with different stages of the task (i.e., decision-related activity and delay-related activity). Curtis et al. (2004) administered both a Delayed Match Task and a Delayed Non-Match to Sample Task to healthy individuals within the fMRI environment, using a 10 s delay period for each task. In the Delayed Match to Sample Task, participants knew the direction of the saccadic eye movement they were cued to make; whereas in the Delayed Non-Match to Sample Task, the direction of saccades was not predictable. Thus, Curtis et al. were able to distinguish the maintenance of motor plans (Delayed Match) from the maintenance of spatial information (Delayed Non-Match). On the Delayed Match Task, frontal eye fields and dorsolateral prefrontal cortex (BAs 9 and 46) exhibited greater delay-related activation early in the delay period (within 3.9 s after the stimulus) when compared to the Delayed Non-Match Task. However, in the latter portion of the delay period (beyond 6.9 s after the stimulus), significantly greater delay-related activation in the inferior parietal sulcus and inferior frontal sulcus was observed in the Delayed Non-Match to Sample Task relative to the Delayed Match to Sample Task (Curtis et al. 2004). Furthermore, activation of the frontal eye fields during the delay period predicted accuracy on each task, with greater activity associated with greater accuracy (Curtis et al. 2004). Support for such a distinction between early and later delay phases has come from electroencephalography investigations which have observed different components across the delay period (e.g., early frontal gamma, later frontal theta; Griesmayr et al. 2010; Kawasaki and Yamaguchi 2013).

One of the ways in which neuroimaging has helped develop our understanding of target/response delay tasks is through the investigation of stimulus type. For example, Bushara et al. (1999) noted modality-specific activation in the Delayed Match to Sample Task. They used an auditory version of the task that was associated with increased activation in the inferior frontal gyrus and medial temporal lobe when compared to a visual version of the same task. Interestingly, the medial prefrontal cortex (BA 6) and inferior parietal and temporal regions were activated during both visual and auditory tasks, suggesting that these areas were associated with task processing, irrespective of modality. In a study conducted by Smith et al. (1995), in which both object- and location-based Delayed Match to Sample Tasks used the same stimuli, a notable difference in recruited regions was observed between the two task conditions. In particular, the location-based task was shown to activate various prefrontal regions (including BAs 46 and 47) whereas the object-based task tapped more temporal and parietal regions (Smith et al. 1995). However, unlike Bushara et al. (1999), Smith et al. (1995) did not directly contrast location-based activation and object-based activation patterns, so they do not give any indication of potential overlap between the two systems. Schon et al. (2008) have also suggested that the pattern of activation during the delay-period of the task differs, with object-based tasks recruiting primarily orbitofrontal regions including BAs 10, 11, and 47 (though also including BA 46 and some anterior cingulate regions), whereas location-based tasks primarily recruit the dorsolateral prefrontal cortex and the frontal eye fields (BAs 6, 8, and 46). Furthermore, familiar objects may rely more heavily on orbitofrontal cortex than other prefrontal regions (Schon et al. 2008). During the delay period of a recognition memory task, the shape-stimulus dimension provokes a pattern of activation in superior frontal, superior parietal, posterior cingulate, and middle occipital gyral regions, whereas the color-stimulus dimension provokes activation of the anterior insula and cuneus (Yee et al. 2010). In a Delayed Match to Sample Task utilizing emotional faces (showing any emotion of either "positive," "neutral," or "negative" valence) as stimuli, LoPresti et al. (2008) noted rather distributed activity across the brain. In the task, participants were required to select a matching probe face to the cue face, based on either the emotion (but not the identity) shown by the face or the identity (but not the emotion) of the face (LoPresti et al. 2008). Activity during a no-delay visuomotor control task (which did not involve Matching to Sample) was then subtracted, leaving significant activation in BAs 6, 8, 10, 19, 28, 40, 46, and 47, amygdala, cerebellum, hippocampus, and insula associated specifically with the phase between cue and probe (LoPresti et al. 2008). Most notably, the face-based Delayed Match to Sample Task (regardless of the match rule—emotion or identity) appears to tap both dorsolateral and ventrolateral prefrontal regions, as well as more posterior regions (LoPresti et al. 2008). Rosenbaum et al. conducted a structural equation modelling investigation of a similar facial Delayed Match to Sample paradigm, where the match was made based on identity of the face (Rosenbaum et al. 2010). By contrast with LoPresti et al. (2008), Rosenbaum et al. (2010) did not describe whether the faces used were emotionally neutral or otherwise. The authors noted that poor performance over the delay was associated with a reduction in prefrontal intraconnectivity, and a strengthening of connectivity between the prefrontal cortex and the amygdala. Such a pattern was particularly prevalent in patients with Alzheimer's disease, and the strengthening of the prefrontal–amygdala network was implicated as a compensatory mechanism for the otherwise disconnected prefrontal regions (Rosenbaum et al. 2010). However, in a visual Delayed Match to Sample Task, PET scanning has implicated similar regions of activation (in both the dorsolateral and ventrolateral prefrontal cortex) during color- and pattern-matching versions (Barrett et al. 2001). Taken together, the above observations suggest dorsolateral prefrontal and parietal involvement in target/response delay tasks across an array of different stimulus types, but with particularly strong associations between dorsolateral prefrontal activation and the delay in location-based visual Delayed Match to Sample Tasks, and ventrolateral prefrontal cortex and amygdala involvement in face-based Delayed Match to Sample Tasks.

However, the involvement of the dorsolateral prefrontal cortex in various target/response delay tasks may be obscured by the effect of working memory load (Rypma et al. 1999). As load increases, so does activation of various frontal regions, including the dorsolateral prefrontal cortex (e.g., BAs 8, 9, 10, 45 and 46; Rypma et al. 1999). Working memory load may therefore explain the differences between those studies implicating the dorsolateral prefrontal cortex in target/response delay tasks and those noting no such involvement. Likewise, the prefrontal cortex is not unique in its involvement in target/response delay tasks, and cells in non-frontal brain regions also differentially respond during the delay period (see Jonides et al. 2005 for a review). Rowe et al. (2000) used an event-related fMRI design to distinguish between phenomena within the delay phase of a spatial Delayed Response Task. Response selection was associated with transient activity in BA 46, but maintenance of spatial working memory was associated with sustained activity of BA 8 during the delay period (Rowe et al. 2000). However, during the "response selection" phase of the task, additional activation was noted in the ventrolateral prefrontal cortex (BAs 11 and 47). No other frontal activation was noted in the "maintenance" phase, suggesting that BA 8 may play a leading role in the maintenance of spatial information in working memory (Rowe et al. 2000). Similarly, Berent-Spillson et al. (2010) noted overall dorsolateral prefrontal (BA 9/46) and anterior cingulate activation (BA 32) in healthy individuals across several delay conditions (0, 1, and 4 s) of a Delayed Match to Sample Task. However, activation in a delay condition of 1 s was not significantly different from the no-delay condition, and a 4 s delay condition differed only in its increasing activation of the hippocampus and medial temporal lobe. This suggests that dorsolateral prefrontal involvement may not scale increasingly in line with delay (Berent-Spillson et al. 2010). Olsen et al. (2009) pointed to the importance of the medial temporal lobe in the Delayed Match to Sample Task, with sustained activation of regions such as the anterior hippocampus being observed during the 30 s delay period. However, activation in the later stages of the delay period was in the posterior hippocampus and parahippocampal cortex, linked to anticipation of the probe onset (Olsen et al. 2009). Robinson et al. (2009) administered a non-verbal Delayed Non-Match to Sample Task to both those patients with remitted bipolar disorder and healthy controls and measured multiple regions of BOLD activation during the task as a whole. Whereas bipolar patients showed increased activation of several prefrontal regions (BAs 6, 9, 10, 11, 24, and 32), healthy controls showed comparatively increased activation in medial temporal regions (BAs 20, 21, and 37). As there was no behavioral difference between the two groups, this points to the importance of a network of several prefrontal and temporal regions in Delayed Non-Match to Sample Task performance (Robinson et al. 2009).

A meta-analysis of schizophrenia studies involving the Delayed Match to Sample Task implicated the activation of different regions for patients with schizophrenia compared to healthy controls (Minzenberg et al. 2009). Of the five studies included in the meta-analysis, four investigated activation differences between schizophrenia and control groups that were not matched for performance (i.e., performance was significantly poorer in schizophrenic individuals versus controls). Although schizophrenic patients exhibited task-related activation of the dorsolateral prefrontal cortex, healthy controls showed no such task-related activation, instead showing activation of the ventrolateral prefrontal cortex (BAs 11 and 45). Furthermore, in an fMRI study conducted by Koechlin et al. (1999), participants performed a delayed choice task that required them to decide whether any two sequentially presented capital letters also appeared sequentially in the word "tablet." Although Koechlin et al. noted general task-related activation in BAs 7, 8, 9, and 40, subtracting the control task from the delayed choice task left no significantly active regions (Koechlin et al. 1999). However, the delay period used by Koechlin et al. was filled with random lower-case letters, which the participants were instructed to ignore. The presence of such distracting stimuli differentiates the paradigm from more common Delayed Response or Delayed Match to Sample studies. The control task itself necessarily loaded upon working memory, as it involved storing both the stimulus previously presented and the current stimulus to decide whether they appeared sequentially within the word "tablet" (similar to an N-Back Task). Therefore, the contrast of the two conditions, instead of revealing delay-related activity, may have instead only tapped distractor-related activation.

Bunge et al. (2003) demonstrated that, whereas dorsolateral prefrontal activation was associated with increasing delay periods, ventrolateral prefrontal cortex (BAs 44, 45, and 47) and frontal pole (BA 10) activation was related to the maintenance and retrieval of the task rules (Bunge et al. 2003). More precisely, rule-guided target/response delay tasks such as the Delayed Match and Delayed Non-Match to Sample Tasks are associated with greater posterior ventrolateral prefrontal activation, but not dorsolateral prefrontal activation, during the delay period. Cue-driven target/response delay tasks, such as the Delayed Response Task, may instead rely on dorsolateral prefrontal activation during the delay period to maintain motor plans (Bunge et al. 2003). Similarly, Elliott and Dolan (1999) directly compared both task-related and delay-related activation in the Delayed Match Task and Delayed Non-Match to Sample Task. Both tasks were associated with activation in the dorsolateral prefrontal cortex, orbitofrontal cortex, and anterior cingulate cortex among others. Although there was some overlap in the patterns of activation, Delayed Match (compared to Delayed Non-Match) performance was associated with the unique activation of BAs 24 and 25, whereas Delayed Non-Match (compared to Delayed Match) performance was associated with activation of BAs 6, 7, and 11 (Elliott and Dolan 1999). The delay-related pattern of activation in each task differed, with Delayed Match to Sample activating the caudate and BA 25 during the delay, and Delayed Non-Match to Sample activating BAs 7 and 32. Therefore, the two tasks appear, to some degree, to tap distinct frontal regions with Delayed Match to Sample uniquely related to medial prefrontal involvement and Delayed Non-Match to Sample uniquely related to more orbital prefrontal regions (Elliott and Dolan 1999).

7.2.4 **Aging studies**

Aging research using animals has helped highlight the role of the prefrontal cortex in maintaining the chosen response over the delay period by protecting against distraction and interference. For example, in one study, aged monkeys were either administered Alpha-2 agonists, which are thought to prevent the depletion of norepinephrine[3] in the prefrontal cortex, or saline prior to performing a spatial Delayed Response Task (Arnsten and Contant 1992). The monkeys receiving the Alpha-2 agonists were less affected by distracting lights or sounds presented during the delay period, in comparison to those control monkeys treated with saline (Arnsten and Contant 1992). Furthermore, overactivity of protein kinase C, which is a method of chemical communication between cells, particularly within the prefrontal cortex, seems to impair

---

[3] Age-related degeneration of structures within the prefrontal cortex that produce catecholamines (such as epinephrine, norepinephrine, and dopamine) has been noted by several early studies (e.g., Bartus et al. 1978; Vijayashankar and Brody 1979). Preventing the depletion of such catecholamines within the prefrontal cortex in older monkeys has been shown to improve working memory functioning (e.g., Arnsten and Goldman-Rakic 1985).

delay-related performance on the Delayed Response Task in non-human primates (Birnbaum et al. 2004).

In humans, the few studies that have investigated the effects of healthy adult aging on Delayed task performance tend to note age-related impairments (Table 7.6). For example, MacPherson et al. (2002) administered a Delayed Response Task to three age groups: a younger group of 30 participants aged 20–38 years, a middle-aged group of 30 participants aged 40–59 years, and an older group of 30 participants aged 61–80 years. On each trial, participants were presented with 12 blue squares and 2–5 of the squares changed color from blue to white simultaneously. A delay followed, during which the screen was blank for 0.5, 30, or 60 s. At the end of the delay, all 12 blue squares reappeared, and participants had to indicate which squares had changed color. MacPherson et al. (2002) found that middle-aged and older adults performed significantly more poorly than the younger participants when there was a 30 s delay, and that the middle-aged group performed significantly more poorly than younger adults when there was a 60 s delay. In an auditory Delayed Match to Sample Task, Chao and Knight (1997) noted that older individuals ($n = 12$, aged 57–71 years) made significantly more errors than younger individuals ($n = 12$, aged 20–22 years). Likewise, they seemed to be more greatly affected by distracting tones. Lamar and Resnick (2004) observed significantly impaired performance on both Delayed Match to Sample Task and Delayed Non-Match

Table 7.6 Target/response delay tasks: Aging studies

Study	n	Participant age groups (years)	Study type	Task	Age effect
Chao and Knight (1997)	12; 12	20–22; 57–71	Cross-sectional (behavioral)	Delayed Match to Sample	✓
Grady et al. (1998)	13; 16	22–28; 62–70	Cross-sectional (neuroimaging)	Delayed Match to Sample	✓
MacPherson et al. (2002)	30; 30; 30	20–38; 40–59; 61–80	Cross-sectional (behavioral)	Delayed Response	✓
Lamar and Resnick (2004)	23; 20	20–40; 60–80	Cross-sectional (behavioral)	Delayed Match to Sample; Delayed Non-Match to Sample	✓ ✓
Lamar et al. (2004)	16; 16	20–40; 60–80	Cross-sectional (neuroimaging)	Delayed Match to Sample; Delayed Non-Match to Sample	✓ ✓

✓ = age effect found; X = age effect not found

to Sample Task in older individuals ($n = 20$, aged 60-80 years) when compared to younger individuals ($n = 23$, aged 20-40 years). Lamar et al. (2004) followed up this observation with an fMRI investigation. Older individuals ($n = 16$, aged 60-80 years) only recruited temporal and parietal regions in the Delayed Match to Sample Task, after subtracting activation from a visuomotor control task, but recruited the dorsolateral prefrontal cortex (BA 9) as well as parietal regions during the Delayed Non-Match to Sample Task. Younger individuals ($n = 16$, aged 20-40 years), meanwhile, showed anterior cingulate (BAs 6 and 24) activation in both tasks, as well as dorsolateral (BA 9) and ventrolateral (BA 47) prefrontal activation specifically during the Delayed Non-Match to Sample Task. When, in each task, the activation of the two age groups was directly contrasted, younger adults exhibited greater dorsolateral prefrontal cortex and anterior cingulate involvement in the Delayed Match to Sample Task than older adults, and greater dorsolateral prefrontal, ventrolateral pre-frontal, and anterior cingulate involvement in the Delayed Non-Match to Sample Task relative to older adults. By contrast, older adults showed greater activation of temporal and occipital regions across both tasks relative to younger adults. Similarly, Grady et al. (1998) found evidence of less ventrolat-eral prefrontal activation yet greater dorsolateral prefrontal activation across all delay conditions (1, 6, 11, and 21 s) within older individuals ($n = 16$, aged 62-70 years) compared to younger individuals ($n = 13$, aged 22-28 years) dur-ing performance of a Delayed Match to Sample Task. However, when exam-ining modulations of activity with increasing delay, increasing prefrontal involvement was only apparent in younger adults. Older adults showed linear changes in activation only in occipital cortex. Furthermore, increased activa-tion of the dorsolateral prefrontal cortex (BAs 9 and 46) and the frontal pole (BA 10) was associated with faster reaction times in younger adults but slower reaction times in older adults. Although older adults responded slower than younger adults in the task overall (across all delay conditions), this age effect did not interact with delay. In light of this relatively intact performance, and subtle differences in the involvement of brain regions between the age groups, Grady et al. suggest that older individuals may use strategies different from those of younger individuals in the attempt to maintain items within memory, and that though these different strategies are successful, they recruit different brain regions.

7.2.5 Summary

There is some suggestion that the dorsolateral prefrontal cortex helps to integrate memory items (including responses) into a plan which details what to do and when to do it (e.g., Goldman-Rakic et al. 1990; Fuster 1999).

The majority of recent human evidence seems to implicate the dorsolateral prefrontal regions in target/response delay tasks, with indications that the Delayed Response Task and Delayed Alternation Task may rely on this region. Whereas target/response delay tasks may in general recruit other prefrontal regions for additional task requirements (such as the ventrolateral prefrontal cortex for rule-guided behavior in Delayed Match Tasks), increasing delay periods in these tasks may be especially useful at tapping the dorsolateral prefrontal cortex (and temporal regions). By subtracting performance in shorter-delay conditions from longer-delay conditions, some marker of dorsolateral prefrontal functioning may be gleaned. However, care must be taken as longer delay periods likely rely more heavily on temporal and subcortical structures such as the hippocampus. Thought must also be paid to the type of stimulus used, with colors, shapes, and faces all involving subtly different patterns of prefrontal involvement, with shapes reportedly providing the most specific dorsolateral prefrontal recruitment. Furthermore, the type of information to be maintained (object identity, spatial location, etc.) also plays a role in the differential recruitment of prefrontal regions, with location-based tasks perhaps being more specific to dorsolateral prefrontal involvement. In terms of aging, older individuals generally perform more poorly on these tasks, and seem to recruit a variety of regions for target/response delay task performance, possibly suggesting a loss of regional specificity if used in aging research.

7.3 **N-Back Task**

7.3.1 **Task description**

The N-Back Task is a widely used task of working memory ability. Participants are presented with a sequence of items (e.g., numbers, letters) one after the other. Each item is followed by a blank delay interval and the participant must decide whether the current item is the same as the one that occurred x items earlier in the sequence (e.g., two items for a 2-back task). For example, in the sequence during 2-back task presentation… D, B, R, B…, participants should respond, "no to the B, no to the R and yes to the B" (see Figure 7.2 for an example). The original N-Back Task was designed by Smith et al. (1996; Experiment 2), and included one 3-back version that tested spatial memory (i.e., the positions of the letters in the display) and one 3-back version that tested verbal memory (i.e., the names of the letters in the display). In the spatial memory 3-back task, participants viewed single letters arranged on the circumference of an invisible circle, and were required to classify whether the letters (irrespective of their identity) had been presented in the same position on the circle three trials prior. For the verbal memory 3-back task, participants were required to

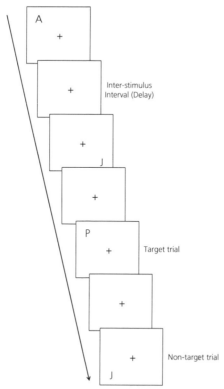

Fig. 7.2 Example of a spatial 2-back task. Each letter is followed by a blank delay interval during which participants should decide whether the letter was the same as the letter presented two items earlier in the sequence.

identify whether the same letters (irrespective of their position) had been presented at any location on the circle three trials prior. One of the unique features of the N-Back Task is that each presented item must be maintained in running, sequential order to enable accurate responding to future probes. Typically, target trials are not cued, so all items are potential targets. The difficulty (or load upon the maintenance system) can be manipulated by increasing the interval between the target and the probe, in terms of interceding stimuli (e.g., one interceding item in a 2-back task versus two interceding items in a 3-back). By doing so, items must be maintained in the face of increasing amounts of interfering stimuli (i.e., the number of intervening trials).

Some researchers use a 0-back task as a baseline condition (e.g., Cohen et al. 1997). The 0-back task requires participants to respond whenever they see a pre-defined stimulus (e.g., the letter H), regardless of its serial position in the sequence. As such, this condition involves no memory recruitment, other than for the identity of the target. By contrast, other researchers have used 1-back conditions (e.g., Carlson et al. 1998) which involve minimal memory recruitment. Since activation is believed to change along with working memory load, it is perhaps more prudent to use a 1-back task as a comparative baseline. Indeed, this would allow researchers to examine scalable increases in executive control-related activity.

7.3.2 Patient and lesion studies

Recent lesion studies have implicated multiple frontal regions—including the lateral and medial prefrontal regions—in the successful performance of the N-Back Task (Table 7.7). For example, Müller et al. (2002) administered two variants of the N-Back Task to a group of four patients with lesions involving the dorsal and ventral regions of the lateral prefrontal cortex (BAs 9, 46, 9/46, 45, and 47), six patients with lesions involving the dorsolateral prefrontal cortex only (BAs 9, 46, and 9/46), five patients with lesions involving the ventromedial prefrontal cortex only (BAs 10, 11, and 12), and 12 healthy controls. In one version of the task, participants had to judge whether the identity of the presented item matched the item presented either one or two items back (i.e., object-based); in the other version of the task, participants had to judge whether the location of the presented item matched the location of the item presented either one or two items back (i.e., spatial-based). Müller et al. (2002) found that only patients with damage involving both the dorsolateral prefrontal cortex and the ventromedial prefrontal cortex exhibited significantly poorer performance than the healthy controls, and that such an impairment was not related to lesion volume. These frontal patients were significantly less accurate than controls on both the 1-back and 2-back versions of the spatial-based task, and on the 2-back but not the 1-back version of the object-based task. In terms of response

Table 7.7 N-Back Task: Patient and lesion studies

Study	n	Patient/ Control Groups	Study type	Stimuli	Brodmann Areas	FP	DL	OF	ACC
Müller et al. (2002)	5; 6; 4; 12	VM; DL; DV; HA	Lesion	Object/ Spatial	9, 10, 11, 12, 45, 46, 47	✓	✓	✓	
Tsuchida and Fellows (2009)	4; 5; 11; 7; 29	lFL, rLF, MFL, VM, HA	Lesion	Letters	–		✓	✓	✓

FP = frontal pole; DL = dorsolateral prefrontal cortex; OF = orbitofrontal cortex; ACC = anterior cingulate cortex; PFC = prefrontal cortex; VM = ventromedial prefrontal cortex; DV = dorsal and ventral prefrontal cortex; HA = healthy adults; lLF = left frontal lobe; rFL = right frontal lobe; MFL = medial prefrontal cortex; ✓ = frontal region damaged and impairment found; X = frontal region damaged but no impairment.

times, these same patients only exhibited significantly slower responses than healthy controls on the low-load condition (regardless of stimulus type). By contrast, patients with more circumscribed damage to either the dorsolateral or the ventromedial prefrontal cortex performed similarly to controls in terms of accuracy and response times. Whereas the results suggest that the dorsolateral and ventromedial prefrontal cortex may play important roles in N-Back performance, each region on its own does not appear to be essential for working memory performance at high loads. However, the lack of a focal ventrolateral, medial, or orbital frontal group and the absence of an analysis accounting for lesion size specifically within the dorsolateral prefrontal and ventromedial prefrontal patient groups may limit any strong conclusions about the localization of the processes associated with N-Back performance from this study.

A later study also examined the involvement of the lateral regions of the prefrontal cortex (including both the dorsolateral and ventrolateral prefrontal cortex) on performance on the N-Back Task under high working memory loads. In this study, Tsuchida and Fellows (2009) found that patients with damage to the dorsolateral prefrontal cortex *and* ventrolateral prefrontal cortex in the left hemisphere showed significantly poorer performance on a letter 2-back task than healthy controls. There were also performance deficits in patients with dorsomedial prefrontal damage (including the dorsal anterior cingulate cortex), suggesting that both the lateral and dorsomedial regions are part of the functional network responsible for N-Back performance. Patients with right lateral prefrontal lesions or lesions in the orbitofrontal cortex were not impaired compared to controls. Tsuchida and Fellows (2009) noted that whereas both left lateral and medial lesion patients were impaired on the N-Back Task, their behavioral impairments were qualitatively different. The lateral frontal patients were less likely to press a button when they were unsure about the probe (i.e., whether it was a target or a non-target), resulting in a lower hit rate than controls, whereas the medial lesion patients were more likely to respond to probes, resulting in a higher false alarm rate than controls. The authors suggest that there are discrete contributions of these two prefrontal regions to N-Back performance, with lateral regions involved in the working memory aspect of the task and medial regions involved in the cognitive control aspect of the task.

7.3.3 Neuroimaging studies

Neuroimaging studies have also suggested that prefrontal regions play a role in N-Back Task performance (Table 7.8). Activation in the dorsolateral prefrontal cortex, as well as the inferior and medial frontal gyri, the medial superior frontal

Table 7.8 N-Back Task: Neuroimaging studies

Study	n	Patient/Control Groups	Study type	Stimuli/task	Brodmann Areas	FP	DL	OF	ACC
Smith et al. (1996)[a]	8	HA	PET	Verbal: Spatial:	9/46, 10/46, 44/45/46/10, 46/9/10; 6, 46/9, 46/10	✓ ✓	✓ ✓		
Cohen et al. (1997)	10	HA	fMRI	N-Back: Load:	4, 6, 8, 9/46, 32, 40, 44; 9		✓ ✓		✓
Carlson et al. (1998)	7	HA	fMRI	2-Back: 1-Back: Load:	6, 6/8, 10, 24/32, 45/47, 46/9; 6/8, 10, 24/32, 45/47; 6, 6/8, 10, 24/32, 45/47, 46/9	✓ ✓ ✓	✓ ✓ ✓		✓ ✓ ✓
D'Esposito et al. (1998)	24	HA	fMRI	Verbal: Spatial:	6, 46; 6, 46	✓ ✓	✓ ✓		
Owen et al. (1998b)	6	HA	fMRI	Spatial: Non-spatial:	6, 6/8, 9, 32/8; 6, 6/8, 9	✓ ✓	✓ ✓		✓
LaBar et al. (1999)	11	HA	fMRI	Letters	6, 44				
Owen et al. (1999)	5	HA	PET	Spatial	6/8, 9/46, 47		✓		
Callicott et al. (2000)	37; 32	schiz, HA	fMRI	Digits	24/32, 47				✓
Jansma et al. (2000)	12	HA	fMRI	Digits	8, 9, 24, 32, 46		✓		✓
Braver et al. (2001b)	28	HA	fMRI	2-Back: Words: Faces:	6, 10, 46/9; 44, 44/45; 6, 10, 44, 44/45, 46/9	✓ ✓	✓ ✓		
Caldú et al. (2007)	75	HA	fMRI	Digits	6, 8, 10, 44, 46/9, 47	✓	✓		

FP = frontal pole; DL = dorsolateral prefrontal cortex; OF = orbitofrontal cortex; ACC = anterior cingulate cortex; HA = healthy adults; PET = positron emission tomography; fMRI = functional magnetic resonance imaging; schiz = schizophrenic patients; ✓ = frontal region involved.

[a]Describes data from Smith et al. (1996) Experiment 2.

gyrus and the anterior cingulate cortex, the parietal cortex, thalamus, caudate nucleus, and putamen (e.g., Cohen et al. 1997; Carlson et al. 1998; Caldú et al. 2007) has been observed in N-Back Tasks with varying memory loads. This suggests that the N-Back Task is not specific in capturing frontal activation.

Instead, manipulating memory and maintenance load within participants may be a more specific method of tapping frontal involvement in the N-Back Task. In one of the earliest investigations, Smith et al. (1996) noted increased dorsolateral prefrontal cortex, ventrolateral prefrontal cortex and frontal pole activation during a 3-back task compared to a simple search task where individuals had to state whether an item's identity or position matched one of three identities or locations established at the beginning of the experiment. Smith et al. suggested that this activation reflected the differing demands placed on the executive mechanisms responsible for updating and shielding the contents of working memory in the face of constant and interfering stimuli.

The effect of load upon activation during the N-Back Task has been further investigated and linked to activation in the dorsolateral prefrontal cortex and parietal regions (Cohen et al. 1997; Jansma et al. 2000; Braver et al. 2001b). Additionally, changes in anterior cingulate activation have been observed both when performing the N-Back Task in general and with increasing memory load (Cohen et al. 1997; Carlson et al. 1998; LaBar et al. 1999). McAllister et al. (1999) administered an auditory N-Back Task to both healthy individuals ($n = 11$) and those with mild traumatic brain injury ($n = 12$) while undergoing fMRI. Strikingly different activation patterns were noted despite similar behavioral performance, and such differences were modulated by working memory load (0-back, 1-back, or 2-back). In healthy individuals, task-general activation was found in BAs 8, 39, 40, and 44 whereas load-specific changes in activation were found in the anterior cingulate cortex (BA 6) and frontal pole (BA 10) regions. By contrast, in the TBI patients, task-general activation was present in the dorsolateral prefrontal cortex (BA 9), frontal pole (BA 10) and parietal (BA 7) regions, with load-specific activation in the anterior cingulate cortex (BA 6), dorsolateral prefrontal cortex (BA 9) and frontal pole (BA 10) regions. It is curious that the load-specific activation pattern observed in the TBI patients resembles that of healthy individuals in other studies (e.g., Smith et al. 1996). The authors suggest that the lack of a deficit in performance despite this different pattern of activation indicates that intact performance during the N-Back Task does not rely on a particular set of regions (especially the dorsolateral prefrontal cortex) but is instead flexible.

Callicott et al. (2000) noted an interesting pattern of performance and fMRI activation between high-performing schizophrenics and healthy individuals. They observed similar behavioral performance on the low-working memory load condition (0-back). However, at higher load conditions (1-back and 2-back), the accuracy of the schizophrenic group declined to a greater degree than the healthy group. Load-related activation differed between the two groups with schizophrenic individuals showing unique dorsolateral prefrontal cortex (BAs 9 and 46), anterior cingulate cortex (BA 32), and frontal pole (BA 10) activation in contrast to the ventromedial prefrontal cortex (BA 47), anterior cingulate cortex (BAs 24 and 32), and parietal (BA 7) activation found in the healthy individuals. Not only does this suggest that schizophrenic patients recruit the dorsolateral prefrontal cortex to a greater degree (which the authors attribute to the functional decline associated with dopaminergic deficits in this prefrontal region) during the N-Back Task, it also suggests that healthy individuals recruit more than just the dorsolateral prefrontal cortex during high-load performance—most notably other prefrontal regions (Callicott et al. 2000).

Whereas most stimulus types share common activation (including the frontal pole, dorsolateral prefrontal cortex and anterior cingulate cortex regions; Smith et al. 1996; D'Esposito et al. 1998), some studies report unique activation patterns for particular stimuli. For example, spatial memory versions of the N-Back Task selectively activate occipital regions BAs 7 and 19 (Smith et al. 1996; Owen et al. 1998b) where non-spatial (e.g., judging identity rather than location) versions of the N-Back Task are slightly less defined, with some studies reporting unique activation in temporal regions (e.g., Owen et al. 1998b) and some reporting unique activation in the dorsolateral prefrontal cortex (e.g., Braver et al. 2001b). This distinction somewhat contradicts the previously discussed conclusions of Müller et al. (2002) who associated widespread lateral prefrontal lesions with particularly prominent spatial N-Back deficits. Furthermore, increasing activation in verbal memory versions of the N-Back Task has been reported in regions widely recognized for their role in language processing (e.g., BAs 44 and 45; Smith et al. 1996; LaBar et al. 1999; Braver et al. 2001b).

The baseline conditions (e.g., 0- or 1-back) with which N-Back manipulations are often compared vary between studies. LaBar et al. (1999) noted that when activation from a 0-back baseline condition was subtracted from the activation during a 2-back condition, no frontal regions remained significantly activated. When the activation associated with a simple working memory span task, in which individuals should hold a sequence of five previously remembered locations (which involves mainly storage abilities rather than more complex working memory processes), was subtracted from a 2-back task, only the dorsolateral prefrontal cortex (BA 46) remained significantly activated (Owen et al. 1999). In another neuroimaging study, with a different baseline condition (i.e., a spatial attention task in which participants must indicate whether a probe item after a delay belonged to the series presented before the delay or was in the same spatial location as a member of the set presented before the delay), activation was noted in the anterior cingulate cortex, Broca's Area, and parietal regions (LaBar et al. 1999). Differences in the baseline conditions adopted by neuroimaging studies may explain the variation in the patterns of activation observed during the N-Back Task.

7.3.4 Aging studies

Healthy aging is associated with poorer performance on the N-Back Task, with reaction times slowing more substantially with increasing memory load than for younger individuals (Kennedy and Raz 2009; Table 7.9). Indeed, age-related differences become more apparent as the memory load increases (Mattay et al. 2006). Furthermore, older individuals especially seem to be affected by lures (i.e., probe stimuli that match a previous stimulus but not the correct number back), with an increased interference effect in terms of both reaction times and accuracy when compared to younger individuals (Schmiedek et al. 2009). An accompanying increased facilitation effect (i.e., faster responses to target probes) led Schmiedek et al. (2009) to suggest a more sensitive "familiarity" mechanism with age, leading to better performance in target trials but an increased susceptibility to non-target trials with previously seen stimuli.

As well as increased right dorsolateral prefrontal cortex activation, older adults exhibit left dorsolateral prefrontal cortex activation—a region not typically recruited by younger individuals (e.g., Mattay et al. 2006). Such bilateral recruitment with age has been observed even in low memory load conditions where accuracy is similar to that of younger individuals (Mattay et al. 2006).

Table 7.9 N-Back Task: Aging studies

Study	n	Participant age groups (years)	Study type	Stimuli/task	Age effect
Dixit et al. (2000)	40	18–48	Cross-sectional (neuroimaging)	Digits	X
Salat et al. (2002)	20; 31	21–43; 72–94	Cross-sectional (neuroimaging)	Letters	✓
Mattay et al. (2006)	10; 12	24–34; 50–74	Cross-sectional (neuroimaging)	Digits	✓
Kennedy and Raz (2009)	52	19–81	Cross-sectional (neuroimaging)	Digits/ Shapes	✓
Schmiedek et al. (2009)	18; 18	20–30; 70–80	Cross-sectional (behavioral)	Spatial	✓

✓ = age effect found; X = age effect not found

Dixit et al. (2000) observed a similar bilateral tendency with increasing age, even in individuals prior to 50 years of age (with an age range of 18–48 years), and associated it with a compensatory mechanism. Those older adults whose performance was poor even on lower memory load conditions did not show such a bilateral pattern of dorsolateral prefrontal cortex activation, instead exhibiting a unilateral pattern similar to that of younger individuals. Moreover, poorer performance with age has been associated with reduced integrity of the white matter tracts associated with frontal subregions (Kennedy and Raz 2009). Since additional right frontal activity is associated with a compensatory mechanism for age-related impairments in verbal working memory (Park and Reuter-Lorenz 2009), reduced connectivity between frontal regions may lead to reduced capacity for such compensation.

Age-related performance on the N-Back Task may also be associated with volumetric changes in the orbital prefrontal cortex. Salat et al. (2002) found that older individuals were both slower and less accurate than younger individuals across all load conditions (0-, 1-, 2-, and 3-back) on the N-back task. Salat et al. also examined the correlations between a composite working memory performance (formed from a battery of tasks including N-Back performance) and orbitofrontal cortex volume. They found that poorer working memory performance was associated with larger orbitofrontal cortex volume, and that both were associated with age (Salat et al. 2002). However, this should be interpreted with caution, as this association may simply represent the relative sparing of the orbitofrontal cortex with age, relative to other prefrontal regions. Indeed, age-related volumetric changes in the frontal lobes are not limited to orbitofrontal cortex areas and often involve reductions in dorsolateral prefrontal cortex volume (e.g., Raz et al. 1999, 2005), non-frontal cortical regions (e.g., Bartzokis et al. 2001; Raz et al. 2005), and white matter (Haug and Eggers 1991; Cook et al. 2007). Such changes in other frontal regions, rather than orbitofrontal cortex volume per se, may well contribute to age-related impairments in N-Back performance.

7.3.5 Summary

Patient and lesion studies have suggested that dorsolateral prefrontal damage is not sufficient to disrupt N-Back performance. Performance is impaired only in patients with more widespread lateral frontal damage involving both the dorsolateral prefrontal cortex and ventrolateral prefrontal cortex. Although dorsomedial lesions also lead to poorer N-Back performance, this is likely to be for reasons qualitatively different from those with lateral prefrontal lesions, with the dorsomedial group finding it more difficult to resist similar lures and the lateral group being poorer at identifying targets. Furthermore, neuroimaging studies have pointed to two networks of regions important for N-Back

Task performance—one involving the dorsolateral prefrontal regions, which are activated across the task, and another involving the anterior cingulate cortex and frontal pole regions, which are activated with increasing memory demands. Although age-related impairments have been noted on the N-Back Task, it has been suggested that, under low memory load conditions, performance can be supplemented by recruiting additional frontal regions. Though it is still unclear why older adults exhibit impaired performance when memory demand is high, recent work has suggested that this is linked to changes in the orbitofrontal cortex.

7.4 **Self-Ordered Pointing Task**

7.4.1 Task description

The Self-Ordered Pointing Task is widely used as a test of response initiation, monitoring, and working memory (Petrides and Milner 1982). Participants are presented with an array of items, such as abstract pictures, everyday objects or words, and are expected to choose any of the items in the array except items they have already chosen. Therefore, when participants are first presented with the array, they are able to select any of the items, but, in the subsequent trials, they should choose any of the items except those that they have already selected in previous trials (see Figure 7.3 for examples of the stimuli). The set size determines the number of selections that participants are required to make. For example, an array of 12 items requires participants to make 12 selections in total. After each selection, the array is rearranged to encourage participants to remember the items they have previously chosen, not simply their locations. In Figure 7.3B, if participants choose the "piano" on the first trial and then "shoes" on the second trial, they should not choose the "piano" or "shoes" on the third trial but should select any of the other 10 items. The difficulty of the task can be manipulated by increasing the size of the array—thus increasing the number of items to be stored within working memory. The number of times a participant makes an error and selects an item that has already been selected is recorded as the primary outcome measure, although reaction times may also be recorded.

Several variations on the original Petrides and Milner (1982) Self-Ordered Pointing Task have been used in the literature. Such variations comprise of the use of different stimuli including numbers, abstract objects, words, etc., as well as encompassing differences in set size varying from eight to 16 items and selection rules (e.g., remembering the specific features of an object versus the location of an object). The stimuli used include "representational drawings" or "object"-based tasks that are intended to manipulate both the array-search strategy and the familiarity or relevance of the items being encoded. By

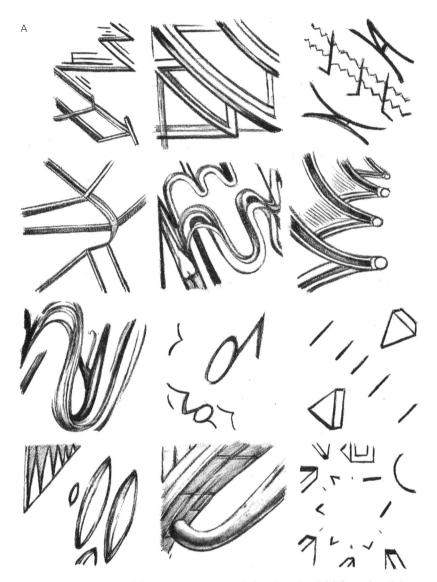

Fig. 7.3 Abstract stimuli (A) and representational-drawing stimuli (B) from the 12-item Self-Ordered Pointing Task. Reprinted from *Neuropsychologia*, 20 (3), Michael Petrides and Brenda Milner, Deficits on subject-ordered tasks after frontal- and temporal-lobe lesions in man, pp. 249–62, figures 4 and 5, Copyright (1982), with permission from Elsevier.

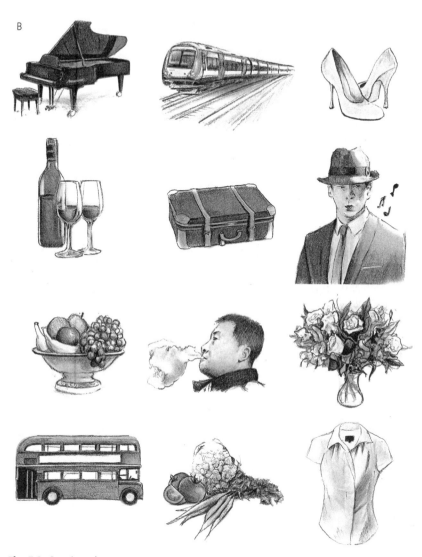

Fig. 7.3 Continued.

comparison, abstract drawings are often used to minimize familiarity effects, and make verbal coding strategies much more difficult to use.

7.4.2 Patient and lesion studies

The Self-Ordered Pointing Task has been developed to assess the ability to arrange, perform, and monitor responses (Petrides and Milner 1982), and performance on the task is reduced following extensive damage to the frontal lobes (Wiegersma et al. 1990; Shallice and Burgess 1991b). Wiegersma et al. (1990) compared the performance of patients with frontal lobe lesions due to tumor excision and healthy controls on a Self-Ordered Pointing Task with numbers as stimuli. Frontal lobe patients committed more repetition selection errors than controls. However, the frontal lesion group included some patients with no prefrontal damage. Furthermore, such general "frontal lobe" patient groups can only reveal so much, and if any frontal subregion is to be implicated in performance, then patients with more specific lesions are required.

A number of studies have examined localization of the processes associated with performance on the Self-Ordered Pointing Task (Table 7.10). Early evidence of specific dorsolateral prefrontal involvement comes from both animal (Petrides 1991, 1995, 2000b) and human (Petrides and Milner 1982; de Zubicaray et al. 1997) lesion studies. Petrides and Milner (1982) investigated performance on four different versions of the Self-Ordered Pointing Task (i.e., two verbal and two non-verbal) in patients with unilateral frontal lobotomy, mostly involving the dorsolateral prefrontal cortex ($n = 23$) or unilateral temporal lobotomy ($n = 56$) as well as in 18 healthy controls. The four tasks differed in the materials used: abstract designs, representational drawings, high-imagery words and low-imagery words. Compared to the controls, the frontal group was impaired on all tasks whereas the temporal group was not impaired on any of the tasks, unless the damage extended to the hippocampus.

Table 7.10 Self-Ordered Pointing Task: Patient and lesion studies

Study	n	Patient/ Control Groups	Study type	Brodmann Areas	FP	DL	OF	ACC
Petrides and Milner (1982)	23; 56; 18	FL; TL; HA	Lesion	–		✓		✓
de Zubicaray et al. (1997)	1; 10	HFI; HA	Lesion	–		✓		
Manes et al. (2002)	5; 4; 5; 5	OF; DL; DM; Mix	Lesion	–		✓		
Berlin et al. (2004)	23; 20	OF; non-OF	Lesion	8, 9, 10, 11, 12, 13, 25, 46	✓	✓		
Chase et al. (2008)	48; 40	FL; HA	Lesion	44, 45				

FP = frontal pole; DL = dorsolateral prefrontal cortex; OF = orbitofrontal cortex; ACC = anterior cingulate cortex; FL = frontal lobe; TL = temporal lobe; HA = healthy adults; HFI = hyperostosis frontalis internal; DM = dorsomedial prefrontal cortex; Mix = dorsal and ventral prefrontal cortex; ✓ = frontal region damaged and impairment found; X = frontal region damaged but no impairment.

De Zubicaray et al. (1997) reported on the case of patient EW who had compression of the dorsolateral prefrontal cortex, resulting from hyperostosis frontalis interna. She was administered three Self-Ordered Pointing Tasks, two spatial and one non-spatial. The spatial tasks included the classic version of Petrides and Milner's Self-Ordered Pointing Task and the Self-Ordered Pointing Task taken from the Cambridge Neuropsychological Test Automated Battery (CANTAB; Sahakian et al. 1988; Owen et al. 1990). The non-spatial task required the generation of letters from the alphabet. Patient EW performed poorly on all three tasks compared to healthy controls, although her impairment was more pronounced for the original task (Petrides and Milner 1982) and the letter generation task. These differing results may relate to the distinct brain regions involved in performing the various versions of the Self-Ordered Pointing Task. Petrides and Milner (1982) found greater impairment in left frontal-damaged patients on the Self-Ordered Pointing Task, and patient EW's frontal lesion was mostly left lateralized. The letter generation task is considered a verbal working memory task and is assumed to depend on intactness of the left hemisphere. Unlike the Petrides and Milner (1982) Self-Ordered Pointing Task, the CANTAB Task requires searching through a series of boxes to find blue tokens and to use them to fill up an empty column on the right side of the screen. Once a token has been found in a box, it will not appear again in that location and participants should avoid returning to that box. This task requires participants to remember the location of the object rather than its specific features (as in Petrides and Milner's version of the task) and it relies on activation of the ventrolateral prefrontal cortex (BA 47), the dorsolateral prefrontal cortex, the frontal pole (BA 10), as well as the anterior cingulate cortex (BA 32) (Owen et al. 1996b). The tokens that are found in the CANTAB Task visibly accumulate, so that the participant is given reward-based feedback that may result in activation in more orbital areas of the prefrontal cortex.

In line with this notion of orbitofrontal involvement on the CANTAB Self-Ordered Pointing Task, patients with orbitofrontal damage have performed poorly on the task compared to non-orbitofrontal patients (Berlin et al. 2004). Two types of errors were investigated: between errors (i.e., how often a box in which a token has already been found is revisited), and within errors (i.e., the number of times a box previously found empty is revisited). Berlin et al. (2004) found that both patient groups performed significantly more poorly than healthy controls, yet their performance was characterized by different types of errors. Non-orbitofrontal patients (most of whom had dorsolateral prefrontal lesions) revisited a box already found empty during the same search more often than orbitofrontal patients. By contrast, orbitofrontal patients were reported to revisit boxes more often where the token was previously found. The authors suggest that the impairment observed in the non-orbitofrontal patients was due primarily to short-term memory deficits, whereas the poor performance reported in the orbitofrontal group was explained as a deficit in learning new reinforcement contingencies (e.g., a token can be found in a box only once). In contradiction to these findings, Manes et al. (2002) compared the performance of patients with discrete orbitofrontal, dorsolateral prefrontal, dorsomedial prefrontal, and large frontal lesions on the CANTAB Self-Ordered Pointing Task and found that the dorsolateral prefrontal group made more errors on the task compared to the orbitofrontal patients, who by contrast performed at the same level as controls. It should be noted that the patients included in the orbitofrontal group in Berlin et al.'s (2004) study had damage to the dorsolateral prefrontal cortex (BAs 9 and 46), whereas damage was restricted to the orbitofrontal area in the patients of Manes et al. (2002).

A contrasting picture is presented by Chase et al. (2008). Here, patients with lesions in the right inferior frontal gyrus (which the study defines as approximately BAs 44 and 45) were compared with non-inferior frontal gyrus lesion patients and healthy controls on a Self-Ordered Search Task taken from the CANTAB. The right inferior frontal gyrus patients made significantly more errors than both the healthy control group and the non-inferior frontal gyrus patients, and suggested that right inferior frontal gyrus patients perform poorly on the task due to poor strategy use. Whereas this seems at odds with the notion that it is primarily the dorsolateral prefrontal cortex that is necessary for successful Self-Ordered Pointing Task performance, it is important to note that the differences in performance between the right inferior frontal gyrus and the non-inferior frontal gyrus patients disappeared when lesion volume was controlled for. Indeed, the lesions categorized as right inferior frontal gyri had larger lesion sizes compared to the non-right inferior frontal gyrus group that perhaps extended into the dorsolateral prefrontal cortex. Moreover, the lesion mapping method adopted by Chase et al. (2008) involved normalizing the lesions to MNI coordinates in order to identify the BAs; thus, the authors are likely to have lost some fidelity, as this method is no longer sympathetic to individual cortical topography.

7.4.3 Neuroimaging studies

Few neuroimaging studies have investigated neural activation during the Self-Ordered Pointing Task, but there appears to be general agreement that the dorsolateral prefrontal cortex is involved in the normal performance of this task (Table 7.11). An early PET study of healthy males found that the mid-dorsolateral prefrontal cortex (BA 46) and the dorsal anterior cingulate cortex (BA 32) were

Table 7.11 Self-Ordered Pointing Task: Neuroimaging studies

Study	n	Patient/ Control Groups	Study type	Brodmann Areas	FP	DL	OF	ACC
Petrides et al. (1993a)	9	HA	PET	9, 32, 46		✓		✓
Petrides et al. (1993b)	10	HA	PET	9, 24, 46		✓		✓
Curtis et al. (2000)	8	HA	PET	6, 9/46, 10/11, 24/32	✓	✓		✓
McLaughlin et al. (2009)	22	psychiatric	MRI	9, 9/46, 46		✓		

FP = frontal pole; DL = dorsolateral prefrontal cortex; OF = orbitofrontal cortex; ACC = anterior cingulate cortex; HA = healthy adults; PET = positron emission tomography; MRI = magnetic resonance imaging; ✓ = frontal region involved.

significantly more activated during the Self-Ordered Pointing Task when compared to a task where pointing to a location was cued by the experimenter (Petrides et al. 1993a, 1993b). Similarly, Curtis et al.'s (2000) PET study reported a significant increase in regional cerebral blood flow in the right dorsolateral prefrontal cortex (BA 9/46) during an object-based Self-Ordered Pointing Task (see Figure 7.4). The task used here differed slightly from the classic Self-Ordered Pointing Task in that it consisted of 11 monochrome 3D shapes which changed position after each selection. The authors attempted to address the problem of participants' perseverative selection of the same location, which takes advantage of the position changes of the stimuli after each selection. By presenting a black square to mask the location of the previous choice, participants were no longer able to exploit this. Unlike the Self-Ordered Pointing Task used by Petrides et al. (1993a), this task elicited additional activations bilaterally in the fronto-marginal gyrus (BA 10/11) and left dorsal anterior cingulate cortex, although only dorsolateral activations correlated strongly with task performance (Curtis et al. 2000).

McLaughlin et al. (2009) took a different approach by examining associations between the brain volumes of frontal regions and Self-Ordered Pointing Task performance among a group of psychiatric outpatients with affective disorders. They found a positive relationship between the volume of both the right and left mid-dorsolateral prefrontal cortex and Self-Ordered Pointing Task scores, and no such relationship for the ventrolateral prefrontal regions of interest. However, with no control group against which to compare the region of interest volumes and cognitive performance, it is unclear whether findings relating to Self-Ordered Pointing Task ability with dorsolateral prefrontal cortex size extend to the healthy population.

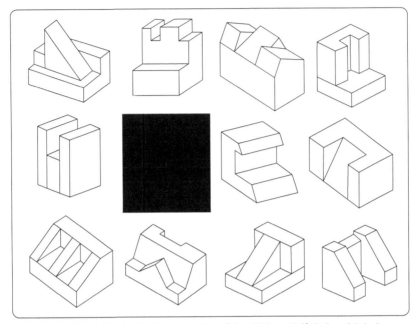

Fig. 7.4 Stimuli used in the "object" version of the 12-item Self-Ordered Pointing task. Reprinted from *Neuropsychologia*, 38 (11), Clayton E Curtis, David H Zald, and José V Pardo, Organization of working memory within the human prefrontal cortex: a PET study of self-ordered object working memory, pp. 1503–10, figures 2 and 3a, Copyright (2000), with permission from Elsevier.

7.4.4 **Aging studies**

Given the dorsolateral prefrontal theory of aging (MacPherson et al. 2002), and the central role that the dorsolateral prefrontal cortex is purported to play in successful Self-Ordered Pointing Task performance, poorer performance would be expected with increasing age; and for the most part the evidence is consistent with this view (Table 7.12). Compared to the performance of younger adults, older participants have been reported to make significantly more Self-Ordered Pointing Task errors (Shimamura and Jurica 1994; Bryan and Luszcz 2001; MacPherson et al. 2002; Salat et al. 2002; Lamar and Resnick 2004). It comes as little surprise that the Self-Ordered Pointing Task has been reported as one of the dorsolateral prefrontal-specific tasks that has the greatest evidence for age effects (MacPherson et al. 2002; Resnick et al. 2007). A detailed study of age effects of the Self-Ordered Pointing Task by Chaytor and Schmitter-Edgecombe (2004) replicated age differences in a cross-sectional study between young and old participants (140 in each group) before demonstrating similar age effects using a longitudinal approach; testing 53 returning members of both groups

Table 7.12 Self-Ordered Pointing Task: Aging studies

Study	n	Participant age groups (years)	Study type	Age effect
Shimamura and Jurica (1994)	41; 17; 11	18–23; 61–70; 71–80	Cross-sectional (behavioral)	✓
West et al. (1998)	40; 40	18–40; 63–78	Cross-sectional (behavioral)	✓
Bryan and Luszcz (2001)	60; 60	17–48; 65–88	Cross-sectional (behavioral)	✓
Garden et al. (2001)	20; 20	30–46; 53–64	Cross-sectional (behavioral)	✓
MacPherson et al. (2002)	30; 30; 30	20–38; 40–59; 61–80	Cross-sectional (behavioral)	✓
Salat et al. (2002)	20; 31	21–43; 72–94	Cross-sectional (neuroimaging)	✓
Chaytor and Schmitter-Edgecombe (2004)	140; 140 53; 53	18–28; 57–93 18–29; 60–85	Cross-sectional (behavioral) Longitudinal	✓ ✓
Lamar and Resnick (2004)	23; 20	20–40; 60–80	Cross-sectional (behavioral)	✓
Resnick et al. (2007)	23; 20	20–40; ≥60	Cross-sectional (neuroimaging)	✓

✓ = age effect found; X = age effect not found

after four years. A significantly impaired performance has also been observed in middle-aged participants when compared to younger participants (Garden et al. 2001). West et al. (1998) suggest that the age-related performance deficit observed on the Self-Ordered Pointing Task may be due to a declining ability to monitor continuously information stored within working memory, rather than simply due to a decrease in working memory span. This may be supported by the observation that a significant proportion of errors committed by older individuals occurs towards the end of a trial as monitoring becomes more difficult.

However, concerns have been raised as to whether these age-related differences are attributable to changes in frontal lobe function. An early study by Shimamura and Jurica (1994) found that, although older individuals performed significantly more poorly than younger individuals, the performance patterns differed between those in their 60s and those in their 70s. Interestingly, those in their 60s performed similarly to healthy controls on the first block of the 16-item version of the Self-Ordered Pointing Task with deficits only showing during a second block of 16 trials. This is compared to the older individuals in their 70s who committed significantly more errors than healthy controls during both blocks of the task. The authors suggest that such a pattern could emerge due to problems suppressing the proactive interference from responses performed during the first block and that this occurs early in the aging process. As age increases, Self-Ordered Pointing Task performance is affected by a more pervasive recognition memory problem rather than a specific working memory decline. Thus, the Self-Ordered Pointing Task likely relies on both working memory components and more general recognition of the abstract patterns or objects. In another study, Bryan and Luszcz (2001) administered executive tasks (e.g., the Wisconsin Card Sorting Test) and processing speed tasks (e.g., Digit–Symbol Substitution), in addition to the Self-Ordered Pointing Task, thus allowing the authors to examine the contribution of each towards age-related differences in Self-Ordered Pointing Task performance. The authors observed that measures of processing speed accounted for the decline in Self-Ordered Pointing Task performance between young and old participants better than executive measures (see also Chaytor and Schmitter-Edgecombe 2004). Thus, the Self-Ordered Pointing Task seems to be sensitive to processing speed changes as well as working memory decline. Whereas this has clear implications for the use of the Self-Ordered Pointing Task in aging research—since a reduction in individual processing speed is one of the major hallmarks of aging (Salthouse 1994; Salthouse and Meinz 1995)—it also suggests that some of the frontal regions implicated by the lesion and neuroimaging data may represent the processing speed demands of the task but not an executive component. However, age-related effects on Self-Ordered Pointing Task performance persist even after controlling for the contribution of processing speed (Chaytor and Schmitter-Edgecombe 2004), thus providing at least some evidence towards the involvement of dorsolateral prefrontal decline.

7.4.5 Summary

Overall, the lesion and patient studies suggest that the dorsolateral prefrontal cortex plays a central role in Self-Ordered Pointing Task performance. However, when tested with different versions of the task (e.g., CANTAB), both dorsolateral prefrontal- and orbitofrontal-damaged patients show impaired performance compared to healthy adults, although their deficits are qualitatively different. That is, the tendency to revisit a box previously found empty is related to working memory deficits and dorsolateral prefrontal damage. By contrast, the tendency to revisit a box where a token had been found previously is related to learning reinforcement contingency deficits and orbitofrontal lesions. The few neuroimaging studies to examine regions of brain activation associated with Self-Ordered Pointing Task performance highlight the importance of the dorsolateral prefrontal cortex, although certain versions of the task might also involve the frontal pole and anterior cingulate cortex. In terms of healthy aging, age effects are consistently reported when older adults perform the Self-Ordered Pointing Task. However, further work is necessary to ascertain whether poor performance on the task is due to an age-related decline in working memory or executive abilities, or to an age-related decline in processing speed.

Chapter 8

Emotional processing

8.1 **Emotion identification**

8.1.1 **Task description**

Different paradigms have been used to investigate the regions of the brain involved in emotion identification. For example, in one such paradigm, participants are shown photographs of faces depicting different emotions (Figure 8.1). Underneath the photographs, adjectives describing different emotions are presented (e.g., happiness, surprise, fear, sadness, disgust, and anger). Participants are asked to decide which adjective best describes the emotion depicted by the face. Other paradigms have asked participants to decide whether the emotion is positive or negative, to rate its intensity, or to make a decision about gender. In vocal versions of the task, participants are presented with emotional sounds (utterances, words, or sentences) and asked to choose a word that best describes the emotion expressed by the sound. Similarly, non-verbal versions of the task often involve identifying emotions from body posture or gait or gestures.

8.1.2 **Patient and lesion studies**

Region-specific evidence for emotion recognition in face-stimuli has been provided by patients with ventromedial prefrontal damage or dysfunction (Beer et al. 2003; Heberlein et al. 2008) (Figure 8.2; Table 8.1). For example, Best et al. (2002) described a facial emotion recognition performance deficit in patients with intermittent explosive disorder. Patients with this condition frequently display impulsive aggressive behaviors, and exhibit significantly less activation of ventromedial prefrontal regions than healthy individuals when viewing certain emotional faces, as well as greater degrees of connectivity between regions such as Brodmann Areas (BAs) 10 and 11 and the amygdala (Coccaro et al. 2007).

However, there is evidence to suggest that ventromedial prefrontal damage may provoke emotion identification deficits that extend to non-visual tasks. For example, Hornak et al. (1996) examined the performance of an array of frontal patients on facial and vocal emotion identification tasks. Those patients with predominantly ventral prefrontal damage—which includes orbital and medial prefrontal areas—performed significantly more poorly on both tasks

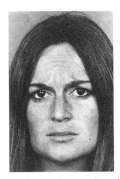

Fig. 8.1 Example of a face portraying sadness taken from the Ekman and Friesen (1976) series. Reproduced from Ekman P. Friesen WV, *Pictures of Facial Affect*. San Francisco, CA: Consulting Psychologists Press © 1976, Consulting Psychologists Press.

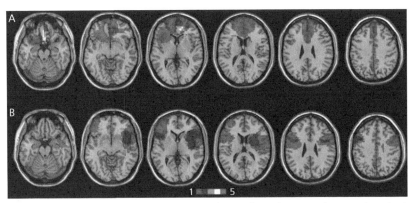

Fig. 8.2 Overlaps of lesions for (A) ventromedial prefrontal group who were impaired on emotion recognition and (B) non-ventromedial prefrontal group who were comparable to controls (Heberlein et al. 2008). Reproduced from Andrea S. Heberlein, Alisa A. Padon, Seth J. Gilihan, et al. Ventromedial frontal lobe plays a critical role in facial emotion recognition, *Journal of Cognitive Neuroscience*, 20(4), pp. 721–733, © 2008, Massachusetts Institute of Technology. Reprinted by permission of MIT Press Journals. Please see color plate section.

when compared to non-ventral frontal patients and healthy controls. This finding was somewhat replicated by Hornak et al.'s (2003) study, which found that ventromedial prefrontal damage may not equally affect visual and verbal emotion identification abilities, and that ventromedial prefrontal lesion patients exhibited varying degrees of impairment on the two tasks. Hornak et al. (2003) also observed that patients with only dorsolateral prefrontal lesions performed well on the facial and the vocal emotion identification tasks. By

Table 8.1 Emotion identification: Patient and lesion studies

Study	n	Patient/Control Groups	Study type	Task	Brodmann Areas	FP	DL	OF	ACC
Beer et al. (2003)	5; 5	OF; HA	Lesion	Faces					✓
Blair and Cipolotti (2000)	1; 1; 5; 5	OF; Dysex; Psych; HA	Lesion (single case)	Faces				✓	
Coccaro et al. (2007)	10; 10	IED patients; HA	Patient (neuroimaging)	Faces	10, 11	✓		✓	
Heberlein et al. (2008)	7; 8; 16	VM; DL; HA	Lesion	Faces		✓		✓	✓
Hornak et al. (1996)	12; 11	VM; non-VM	Lesion	Faces; Vocal				✓	✓
Hornak et al. (2003)	11; 6; 6; 4; 8	DL/OM; bOF; uOF; BA 9/ ACC; BA 9/ACC+OF	Lesion	Faces/Vocal	8, 9, 10, 11, 12, 25, 46	✓		✓	✓
Mah et al. (2005)	20; 9; 23	VM; DL; HA		TSI Expressions	6, 8, 9, 10, 11, 12, 13, 14, 24, 32, 44, 45, 46, 47	✓		✓	✓
Shamay-Tsoory et al. (2003)	12; 6; 17; 19	VM; DL; PC; HA		Faces, Vocal					

FP = frontal pole; DL = dorsolateral prefrontal cortex; OF = orbitofrontal cortex; ACC = anterior cingulate cortex; HA = healthy adults; Dysex = dysexecutive syndrome; Psych = psychomathic inmates; VM = ventromedial prefrontal cortex; OM = orbitomedial; bOF = bilateral orbitofrontal; uOF = unilateral orbitofrontal; TSI = tests of social intelligence; PC = posterior cortex; ✓ = frontal region damaged and impairment found; X = frontal region damaged but no impairment.

contrast, patients within the ventromedial prefrontal group who showed performance deficits had lesions encompassing BAs 11 and 12, as well as parts of the anterior cingulate cortex. Keane et al. (2001) noted similar findings from patients with frontal-variant frontotemporal dementia (fvFTD), with impaired performance observed both in facial and vocal emotion identification tasks. The authors also observed a significant correlation between facial and vocal task performance, and suggested that a single functional deficit—emotion identification—underlies the poor performance of fvFTD patients, rather than two domain-specific deficits. Mah et al. (2005) further suggest that the emotion recognition deficits exhibited by ventromedial prefrontal lesion patients extend beyond facial and verbal stimuli. Indeed, ventromedial prefrontal patients seem also to perform poorly when required to identify an emotion from a non-verbal stimulus such as a gesture or body posture (Mah et al. 2005).

However, the recognition of certain emotions may be impaired to a greater degree than others. For example, Fernandez-Duque and Black (2005) note that frontotemporal dementia patients are impaired at recognizing negative emotions from facial stimuli, but perform normally with more positive emotions. Blair and Cipolotti (2000) described the case of patient JS who developed sociopathy after damage to the ventromedial prefrontal regions of the brain bilaterally. Compared to the performance of dysexecutive syndrome patients (i.e., those with more dorsolateral prefrontal involvement), patient JS had problems recognizing emotions from facial expressions—especially fear and disgust. Similar deficits regarding identifying anger, disgust, and surprise were observed within intermittent explosive disorder patients, with especially poor performance on facial emotion identification compared to healthy controls (Best et al. 2002). By contrast, Beer et al. (2003) observed that the impairment in identifying emotions found in patients with orbitofrontal lesions was limited to faces showing embarrassment or shame, with the recognition performance of other emotions such as fear and happiness similar to healthy controls.

Furthermore, not all such studies have observed an emotional identification deficit that is specific to ventromedial prefrontal patients. Most notably, a study conducted by Shamay-Tsoory et al. (2003) found that ventromedial and dorsolateral prefrontal lesion patient groups did not significantly differ in their performance on both facial and vocal emotion recognition tasks, though these groups did perform more poorly than healthy control participants. Instead, the authors suggest a right-sided hemispheric bias in that damage to the right frontal lobe was associated with a greater number of errors on both tasks. Having said this, the majority of patient and lesion study evidence does seem to suggest varying degrees of emotional identification deficits among ventromedial prefrontal lesion patients. Whether this deficit is specific to ventromedial prefrontal damage remains somewhat unclear, as patients with dorsolateral prefrontal damage seem also to show recognition-based deficits, though this is likely attributable to problems with more executive task demands (Shamay-Tsoory et al. 2003). It also remains to be seen whether ventromedial prefrontal damage produces problems recognizing particular emotions or whether the consequences of damage are more widespread (Heberlein et al. 2008).

8.1.3 Neuroimaging studies

Some neuroimaging studies also support the central role played by the ventromedial prefrontal cortex in emotion identification (Lange et al. 1993; Morris et al. 1998; Blair et al. 1999; Nakamura et al. 1999; Narumoto et al. 2000; Gorno-Tempini et al. 2001; Iidaka et al. 2001; Keightley et al. 2003) (Table 8.2). In a PET study, Nakamura et al. (1999) measured regional cerebral blood flow in healthy adults while they were presented with images of faces whose emotions were categorized as calm, happy, sad, angry, surprised, and disgusted. They were asked to assess each face as positive (e.g., happy), neutral (e.g., calm), or negative (e.g., sad, angry). Greater activity was evident in the inferior frontal cortex and the ventromedial prefrontal cortex, specifically the orbitofrontal cortex. Lange et al. (1993) scanned nine participants with functional magnetic resonance imaging (fMRI) while performing three different tasks with photographs depicting happiness (considered neutral) and fear (Ekman and Friesen 1976): passive view, gender decision, and emotion judgment, which required participants to decide whether the emotion depicted was more or less emotional than the previous expression. Results showed that emotion decision specifically activated the ventromedial prefrontal cortex. There is also evidence that ventromedial prefrontal activation relates to specific emotions. In a PET investigation, Blair et al. (1999) scanned healthy adults performing a task that required gender discrimination of faces depicting various degrees of sadness and anger. The ventromedial prefrontal cortex responded to anger but not to sadness, indicating that different networks underlie different emotions.

The main role of the ventromedial prefrontal cortex in emotion recognition has also been supported by electrophysiological investigations. Streit et al. (2003) investigated the temporal and spatial characteristics of the neural representation of facial emotion recognition by means of magnetoencephalography in 12 healthy adults. Materials consisted of 30 Ekman and Friesen (1976) photographs of faces depicting the six basic emotions (happiness, anger, fear, surprise, disgust, and sadness), neutral faces and photographs of objects. They found stronger responses to emotional faces at short latencies (within 180 ms from the stimulus onset) in the orbitofrontal cortex, the amygdala, the

Table 8.2 Emotion identification: Neuroimaging studies

Study	n	Patient/ Control Groups	Study type	Task	Brodmann Areas	FP	DL	OF	ACC
George et al. (1993)	9	HA	PET	Faces	9, 10, 24	✓	✓		✓
Lange et al. (1993)	9	HA	fMRI	Faces	47		✓		
Imaizumi et al. (1997)	6	HA	PET	Vocal	–		✓		
Phillips et al. (1997)	7	HA	fMRI	Faces	32, 46		✓		✓
Sprengelmeyer et al. (1998)	6	HA	fMRI	Faces	46, 47		✓	✓	
Morris et al. (1998)	5	HA	PET	Faces	–				✓
Blair et al. (1999)	13	HA	PET	Faces	32, 47				✓
Nakamura et al. (1999)	7	HA	PET	Faces	–			✓	
Narumoto et al. (2000)	8	HA	fMRI	Faces: delayed matching	47			✓	
Gorno-Tempini et al. (2001)	10	HA	fMRI	Faces	11/47			✓	
Harmer et al. (2001)	7	HA	rTMS	Faces	32/24				✓
Iidaka et al. (2001)	12	HA	fMRI	Faces	11			✓	
Keightley et al. (2003)	10	HA	fMRI	Faces: Implicit	10, 24, 32, 46, 47	✓	✓	✓	✓
				Explicit	9, 32		✓		✓
Streit et al. (2003)	4	HA	MEG	Faces	–			✓	✓
Wildgruber et al. (2005)	10	HA	fMRI	Vocal	47			✓	
Britton et al. (2006)	12	HA	fMRI	Faces	–			✓	✓
Ethofer et al. (2006)	24	HA	fMRI	Vocal	45/46		✓		

FP = frontal pole; DL = dorsolateral prefrontal cortex; OF = orbitofrontal cortex; ACC = anterior cingulate cortex; HA = healthy adults; PET = positron emission tomography; fMRI = functional magnetic resonance imaging; rTMS = repetitive transcranial magnetic stimulation; MEG = magnetoencephalography; ✓ = frontal region involved.

posterior fusiform cortex and the occipital cortex, and between 200 and 360 ms in the orbitofrontal cortex, the inferior frontal cortex, and the anterior cingulate cortex. The activation of some areas only at later stages has led authors to suggest that activation of these areas represent a deeper social evaluation of the stimuli, whereas earlier activation corresponds to a quicker evaluation of the emotional significance of the stimulus.

Despite these results, other studies reported activation in both the ventromedial prefrontal cortex and the dorsolateral prefrontal cortex during emotion tasks (George et al. 1993; Phillips et al. 1997; Sprengelmeyer et al. 1998; Keightley et al. 2003; Britton et al. 2006). A recent meta-analysis of 100 neuroimaging studies involving facial emotional processing revealed that both medial and inferior-lateral areas of the prefrontal cortex were activated (Sabatinelli et al. 2011). Emotion recognition studies typically ask participants to decide whether the emotion depicted is positive or negative. Activation of the dorsolateral prefrontal cortex seems to relate to the specific type of emotion presented, in that negative emotions, such as disgust and fear, have been related to dorsolateral prefrontal activation. In an fMRI study, Phillips et al. (1997) investigated brain activation during the presentation of faces depicting fear and disgust, and found that disgust activated the dorsolateral prefrontal cortex (BA 46). In a similar paradigm, Sprengelmeyer et al. (1998) assessed facial emotion recognition in healthy subjects during a gender discrimination task on images of faces portraying disgust, fear, anger, and neutral expressions. Although all emotions activated the ventromedial prefrontal cortex, there was also specific emotion-related brain activity: fear was associated with activation of the dorsolateral prefrontal cortex: disgust and anger showed additional activation in the insula and the temporal lobe, respectively, suggesting that different emotions are processed by different neural substrates. These results suggest that negative emotions, such as disgust and fear, may involve activation of the dorsolateral prefrontal cortex (Phillips et al. 1997; Sprengelmeyer et al. 1998).

The dorsal activation also relates to specific task demands. Narumoto et al. (2000) investigated emotion recognition in eight healthy participants. The task consists of the presentation of a sample stimulus (a face or a word depicting an emotion, e.g., sadness), followed after a delay of 400 ms, by the presentation of two choice stimuli (always photographs of faces). The aim of the task was to match the emotion depicted by the first stimulus with the emotion depicted by one of the two subsequent faces. Compared to a rest condition, the emotional tasks activated both the ventromedial and the dorsolateral prefrontal cortex. Although the results support involvement of both ventromedial and dorsolateral prefrontal cortex, the activation of these brain regions may relate not only to emotion processing, but also to the working memory component of the task.

When brain activity common to emotion and working memory processes was controlled by comparing the emotional task with a gender-matching control task, the neural activity for emotion processing was restricted to the ventromedial prefrontal cortex.

Whereas most neuroimaging studies have focused on emotion identification of static faces, a few studies have examined the neural correlates of dynamic expression identification. For example, in a PET study, Kilts et al. (2003) required participants to make explicit static and dynamic emotion intensity judgments about angry and happy faces, as well as to perform a control face-processing task in which they should judge the direction of a face. Separate conjunction analyses were conducted for each emotion to identify the common activation for static and dynamic faces. For angry faces, activation was revealed in the bilateral medial (BAs 6 and 8), bilateral superior (BAs 6, 8 and 10), right middle (BAs 8 and 10), and left inferior (BA 45) frontal regions. Similar brain regions were associated with the recognition of happy static and dynamic faces (i.e., bilateral medial, BAs 6 and 8, bilateral superior, BAs 6 and 8, right middle, BA 9 and left inferior, BA 45/47 frontal regions, as well as the posterior cingulate, BA 23, and left central gyrus, BA 4). This work suggests that both static and dynamic emotional expressions activate approximately the same frontal regions. However, other studies have demonstrated additional frontal activation associated with emotion identification from dynamic faces. In an fMRI study involving 10 participants, LaBar et al. (2003) morphed prototypical facial expressions with neutral expressions to create dynamic expressions of fear and anger. When the dynamic expressions were contrasted against the static ones, LaBar et al. (2003) reported bilateral activation in the ventrolateral prefrontal cortex (BAs 45 and 47) and dorsomedial prefrontal cortex (BA 32) as well as the substantia innominata, amygdala, parahippocampal gyrus (BA 28/36), fusiform gyrus (BA 19/37), and the left precentral sulcus (BA 6). In another fMRI study of 22 healthy participants in which morphed dynamic stimuli of happy and fearful faces were contrasted with static faces, Sato et al. (2004) reported activation in the right inferior frontal gyrus (BA 44) as well as the inferior and middle occipital gyri (BAs 19 and 37), the inferior and middle temporal gyri (BAs 21 and 37), and the fusiform gyrus (BA 37). These latter two studies suggest the involvement of both medial and lateral prefrontal regions in the identification of dynamic facial expressions. Of course, as these dynamic stimuli are often morphs, these findings may not reflect the processing of natural facial motion.

Other studies also suggest that specific brain activation relates to task demands (Gorno-Tempini et al. 2001; Keightley et al. 2003). Keightley et al. (2003)

compared emotion-related activity during implicit and explicit processing. Their participants were presented with emotional faces taken from a magazine and asked to decide about the gender of the person (implicit condition) or the emotional valence (explicit condition). The implicit condition activated an extensive network of brain areas that included the ventromedial and dorsolateral prefrontal cortex, whereas the explicit judgment of the emotional valence activated the dorsolateral prefrontal cortex, suggesting that activation depends on the task demands with the explicit judgment involving mainly dorsal frontal activation.

Emotion recognition has also been related to activation of the anterior cingulate cortex. Harmer et al. (2001) applied repetitive transcranial magnetic stimulation (rTMS) over the anterior cingulate cortex (BA 32/24) to healthy participants during discrimination of angry and happy faces. rTMS impaired recognition of anger but not of happiness. Activation of the anterior cingulate cortex has been reported in other studies, and it has been suggested that the anterior cingulate cortex is involved especially in processing anger, sadness, disgust, and fear (Blair et al. 1999; Phillips et al. 1997; Morris et al. 1998).

Both ventromedial and dorsolateral prefrontal activity is associated with vocal versions of emotion recognition tasks (Imaizumi et al. 1997; Wildgruber et al. 2005). In an fMRI investigation, Ethofer et al. (2006) scanned their participants while they were listening to adjectives pronounced with different intonations: happiness, anger, or neutral. Recognition of the speech intonation was associated with activity in the bilateral inferior and middle frontal gyrus (BA 45/46).

8.1.4 **Aging studies**

The current literature suggests that aging may well be accompanied by an impaired ability to identify certain emotions (Table 8.3). Across various types of visual or auditory stimuli, older participants have been reported to be less accurate and slower than their younger counterparts at identifying depicted emotions (Oscar-Berman et al. 1990; Gunning-Dixon et al. 2003). There also appears to be some evidence for a different blood oxygen level-dependent response between old and young groups during performance of this type of task; older individuals have been reported to exhibit activations confined to the ventromedial prefrontal cortex, whereas a younger group activated a more distributed network including both the ventromedial and lateral frontal areas for happy faces, though there was no age effect in identifying this emotion (Keightley et al. 2007). Conversely, Gunning-Dixon et al. (2003) found additional activation of the anterior cingulate (BA 32) and bilateral lateral prefrontal cortex (BAs 9/46 and 47) during emotional discrimination in contrast to right-sided activation of BAs 9/46 and 44 in the younger group. However, there is a large degree of inconsistency surrounding the precise emotions affected, both across modalities and

Table 8.3 Emotion identification: Aging studies

Study	n	Participant age groups (years)	Study type	Task	Age effect
Malatesta et al. (1987)	30	25–40; 45–60; 65–80	Cross-sectional (behavioral)	Video clips	✓
Oscar-Berman et al. (1990)	12; 15	23–49; 51–70	Cross-sectional (behavioral)	Faces Voices	✓ ✓
Brosgole and Weisman (1995)	155; 28	Younger, mean = 27.5 Older, mean = 75.2	Cross-sectional (behavioral)	Faces (cartoon animals)	✓
Montepare et al. (1999)	20; 21	18–22; 65–81	Cross-sectional (behavioral)	Video clips	✓
MacPherson et al. (2002)	30; 30; 30	20–38; 40–59; 61–80	Cross-sectional (behavioral)	Faces	✓
Phillips et al. (2002a)	30; 30	20–40; 60–80	Cross-sectional (behavioral)	Faces	✓
Calder et al. (2003, Study 1)	24; 24	18–30; 58–70	Cross-sectional (behavioral)	Faces	✓
Calder et al. (2003, Study 2a)	73; 32; 29; 35; 58	17–30, 31–40, 41–50, 51–60, 61–70	Cross-sectional (behavioral)	Faces	✓
Calder et al. (2003, Study 2b)	28; 23; 29; 22; 23	18–30, 31–40,41–50, 51–60, 61–75	Cross-sectional (behavioral)	Faces	✓
Gunning-Dixon et al. (2003)	8; 8	19–29; 57–79	Cross-sectional (behavioral)	Faces	✓
Sullivan and Ruffman (2004a)	24; 24	20–46; 60–82	Cross-sectional (behavioral)	Faces	✓
Sullivan and Ruffman (2004b, Study 1)	31; 30	20–38; 60–84	Cross-sectional (behavioral)	Faces	✓
Sullivan and Ruffman (2004b, Study 2)	28; 28	18–29; 63–79	Cross-sectional (behavioral)	Faces	✓
	28; 28	18–29; 63–79	Cross-sectional (behavioral)	Voices	✓
Wong et al. (2005)	20; 20	Younger, mean = 19.2 Older, mean = 69.5	Cross-sectional (behavioral)	Faces	✓
Keightly et al. (2006)	30; 30	Younger M = 25.7 Older M = 72.5	Cross-sectional (neuroimaging)	Faces	✓

(continued)

Table 8.3 Continued

Study	n	Participant age groups (years)	Study type	Task	Age effect
MacPherson et al. (2006)	29; 29	20–38; 61–80	Cross-sectional (behavioral)	Faces	✓
Isaacowitz et al (2007)	189; 90; 78	18–39; 40–59; 60–85	Cross-sectional (behavioral)	Lexical	✓
Keightly et al. (2007)	10; 11	Younger, mean = 27.2 Older, mean = 69.6	Cross-sectional (neuroimaging)	Faces	✓
Suzuki et al. (2007)	34; 34	18–25; 62–81	Cross-sectional (behavioral)	Faces	✓
Baena et al. (2010)	39; 39	18–35; 60–90	Cross-sectional (behavioral)	Faces	✓
Mill et al. (2009)	147; 208; 93; 71; 50; 34	18–20; 21–30; 31–40; 41–50; 51–60; 61–84	Cross-sectional (behavioral)	Faces Voices	✓ ✓
Hunter et al. (2010, Study 1)	25; 25	19–40; 60–80	Cross-sectional (behavioral)	Faces Voices	✓ ✓
Hunter et al. (2010, Study 2)	20; 20	18–23; 63–78	Cross-sectional (behavioral)	Faces Voices	✓ ✓

✓ = age effect found; X = age effect not found

between investigations of the same modality. Given that the recognition of distinct emotions involves different brain regions (for a review see Ruffman et al. 2008), the pattern of age-related impairment in detecting specific emotions is useful when considering the regional specificity of this task.

Some studies have reported age-related decrements in identifying only one emotion, such as anger (faces: Baena et al. 2010; video: Montepare et al. 1999) or sadness (MacPherson et al. 2002; Moreno et al. 1993; MacPherson et al. 2006; Suzuki et al. 2007) with no effect on any other emotion tested. However, several studies report effects of age on the detection accuracy of both anger and sadness in cartoon animal faces (Brosgole and Weisman 1995), static human faces (Phillips et al. 2002a; Mill et al. 2009) as well as moving images and emotional vocalizations (Sullivan and Ruffman 2004a). Even the same method from the same research group yields variable results, initially reporting age effects on fear and sadness labelling (Keightley et al. 2006), and then sadness, anger and disgust (Keightley et al. 2007).

Other data suggest a combination of fear and anger (Calder et al. 2003) which may not be impaired in the auditory domain (Wong et al. 2005), whereas others have also reported impairments in mainly negative emotion identification in various permutations (anger and disgust, Sullivan and Ruffman 2004b; sadness, anger, and fear in faces, Orgeta and Phillips 2008, or in video, Malatesta et al. 1987; anger, sadness, surprise, and fear, Hunter et al. 2010; anger, disgust, fear, and happiness, Isaacowitz et al. 2007). Further still, Allen and Brosgole (1993) reported that no impairment on any emotion recognition from faces accompanies old age (which has since been reported elsewhere; Borod et al. 2004), but their older participants did show an impairment in detecting emotion from auditory stimuli, although they did not specifically test hearing acuity. More recently, a meta-analysis attempted to identify clarity among this apparent inconsistency (Ruffman et al. 2008). The authors included 24 data sets, comprising 962 young and 705 old participants over multiple modalities, and reported that age is accompanied by impairments in detecting anger and sadness, with a trend towards superior sensitivity to disgust. Moreover, when congruent emotional information is presented through multiple modalities (e.g., faces and voices), older adults' ability to identify emotion improves (Hunter et al. 2010; Lambrecht et al. 2012).

In the context of age-related cognitive decline, we would not expect to see impairment in the ability to identify emotions whose detection is mediated by the ventromedial prefrontal cortex. This would include the identification of emotions such as anger and sadness, which have been shown to activate the anterior cingulate and orbitofrontal cortex in the case of anger (Sprengelmeyer et al. 1998; Blair et al. 1999; Blair and Cipolotti 2000; Fine and Blair 2000; Iidaka et al. 2001; Murphy et al. 2003) and the anterior cingulate (Blair et al. 1999; Phan et al. 2002; Murphy et al. 2003; Killgore and Yurgelun-Todd 2004; Lennox et al. 2004; Salloum et al. 2007) and the dorsomedial prefrontal cortex (Murphy et al. 2003) in sadness. Yet, older adults are found to be poorer than younger adults at correctly recognizing these emotions (e.g., Moreno et al. 1993; Phillips et al. 2002a; MacPherson et al. 2006; Suzuki et al. 2007; Mill et al. 2009; Baena et al. 2010).

The reported pattern of impairment in identifying anger and sadness with aging appears to contradict the expected pattern of performance, as detection of these emotions involves ventromedial rather than dorsolateral prefrontal regions. Further, the literature suggests that this trend cannot be explained by the age of the faces that participants are being asked to rate (Borod et al. 2004; Ebner and Johnson 2009), or by their ethnicity (MacPherson et al. 2006). One explanation for this pattern is that connectivity between the frontal lobes and other parts of a distributed network that aid emotion detection may be affected, rather than the ventromedial or dorsolateral prefrontal cortex per se

(Ruffman et al. 2008). On the other hand, it has been suggested that perceptual and attentional difficulties may offer some explanation. As observed by Calder et al. (2000), the identification of fear, anger, and sadness in faces relies on the examination of the upper half of the face. Evidence from Wong et al. (2005) reports a tendency in older adults to fixate predominantly on the lower half, thus putting themselves at a perceptual disadvantage. Indeed, fewer fixations on the top half of the face were associated with poorer performance on identification of fear, anger, and sadness. Therefore, it could be that attentional differences may be a root cause for the pattern of behavior seen with age, which has been postulated to relate to changes in the integrity of the frontal eye field and other more anterior portions of the dorsolateral prefrontal cortex (Wong et al. 2005).

8.1.5 **Summary**

Evidence from patient studies, neuroimaging and aging suggests that emotional processing requires integration of higher-order processing from a variety of frontal lobe regions. Emotion identification deficits are most consistently reported among those with ventromedial prefrontal lesions or patients with ventromedial-related pathology. Functional imaging also frequently identifies ventromedial prefrontal activation associated with the recognition of emotion. However, the specificity of ventromedial prefrontal involvement remains unclear, as dorsolateral prefrontal lesion patients also show recognition-based deficits, and the activity of other lateral and medial frontal regions has been reported during emotion identification tasks. It has been suggested that deficits due to non-ventromedial prefrontal lesions or additional non-ventromedial prefrontal activity may be due to the disruption of other processes necessary for task performance that do not necessarily relate to the integration of visceral information (e.g., the dorsolateral prefrontal cortex and possible attentional/executive processes). This hypothesis may also explain apparent age effects on the identification of specific emotions (fear, anger and sadness); accurate recognition of these emotions relies on attending to cues present in the upper half of the face, otherwise relevant information will not be available to process their actual emotional valence correctly. Thus, although it has been postulated that the ventromedial prefrontal regions are less susceptible to the effects of age-related decline than dorsolateral prefrontal regions, age effects on emotion recognition may be due to altered attentional guidance rather than visceral integration per se. A competing explanation is that other non-frontal regions also undergo age-related changes such that emotion identification is disrupted, but there are currently insufficient data to reliably parse these competing accounts.

Chapter 9

Social decision-making

9.1 Implicit Association Task

9.1.1 Task description

The Implicit Association Task (IAT) was designed to assess access to attitudes, stereotypes and self-concepts that unconsciously influence our behavior (Greenwald and Banaji 1995). The logic underlying the Implicit Association Task is that judgments that are congruent with an individual's implicit pre-existing association between a target category (e.g., insects) and an evaluative category (e.g., unpleasant words) should be performed more accurately and faster than judgments that are incongruent with a pre-existing association (e.g., insects and pleasant words; see Figure 9.1). The strength of the implicit association is the difference in the time taken to make these congruent and incongruent judgments (Hummert et al. 2002). The Implicit Association Task has been used to assess automatic associations between target concepts such as race (e.g., black versus white names/photographs: Greenwald et al. 1998), gender/career (e.g., male versus female; Rudman et al. 2001), smoking (e.g., Andrews et al. 2010), and positive and negative evaluative attributes. Since task performance does not often correlate with an individual's explicit attitudes, the Implicit Association Task has been interpreted as a measure of implicit or unconscious beliefs or attitudes (Greenwald et al. 1998).

The Implicit Association Task typically consists of five steps (see Table 9.1). In the first step, the individuals are asked to discriminate between two targets (e.g., flower and insects) and to respond to one category of targets (e.g., flowers: orchid) by pressing a button on the keyboard with their left hand, and to the other category (e.g., insects: ant) by pressing a button on the keyboard with their right hand. In the second step, individuals respond to a positive word (e.g., heaven) by pressing the response key (e.g., left) previously associated with flowers, and to negative words (e.g., vomit) with the response key (e.g., right) previously associated with insects. In the third step (i.e., congruent condition), the first and the second tasks are combined. Individuals are instructed to respond with their left hand to both flowers and positive words, and with their right hand to both insects and negative words. In the fourth step, the task is similar to step 2 but with the target response keys reversed. For example, individuals should

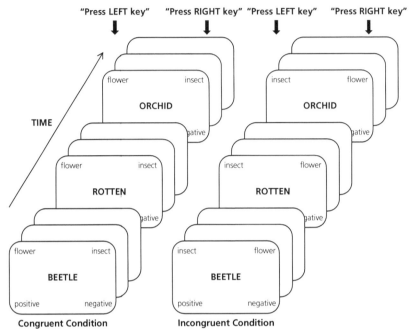

"Press LEFT key"   "Press RIGHT key" "Press LEFT key"   "Press RIGHT key"

Congruent Condition   **Incongruent Condition**

Fig. 9.1 Example of the flowers and insects version of the Implicit Association Task. Individuals are asked to categorize words presented in the middle of the computer screen. In the congruent condition, individuals should press the same left-hand response button to categorize words as *flowers* or *positive* and the same right-hand response button to categorize words as *insects* or *negative*. In the incongruent condition, the flowers and insects switch sides, so that individuals should now categorize the words as *flowers* or *negative* by pressing the left button or *insects* or *positive* by pressing the right button. The difference in response latencies between the congruent and incongruent conditions provides a measure of implicit attitudes towards flowers and insects (i.e., the "IAT effect"). Adapted from *Neuropsychologia*, 47 (10), Marta Gozzi, Vanessa Raymont, Jeffrey Solomon, Michael Koenigs, and Jordan Grafman, Dissociable effects of prefrontal and anterior temporal cortical lesions on stereotypical gender attitudes, pp.2125–2132, Figure 1, Copyright (2009), with permission from Elsevier.

respond to flowers with their right hand and to insects with their left hand. Finally, in the fifth step (i.e., incongruent condition), the reversed target discrimination task from step 4 is combined with the associated attribute discrimination task from step 2. As such, the final step resembles the task in step 3, but with the category responses reversed. The main outcome (the IAT effect) is the difference in time taken to respond to the third and the fifth steps. This provides a measure of the strength of the implicit association, so that a larger IAT effect reflects stronger implicit associations. Healthy individuals typically show faster

Table 9.1 Schematic description of Implicit Association Task[a]

Task description	Condition				
	1 Target discrimination	**2** Associated attribute discrimination	**3** Congruent condition	**4** Reversed target discrimination	**5** Incongruent condition
Task instructions	< FLOWER INSECT >	< positive negative >	< FLOWER < positive INSECT > negative >	FLOWER > < INSECT	FLOWER > < positive < INSECT negative >
Sample stimuli	ANT > < ORCHID < DAISY BEE > < TULIP BEETLE > WASP > < LILY	< lucky < heaven stink > vomit > < peace evil > < cheer rotten >	< ORCHID < peace BEE > evil > WASP > < lucky < DAISY rotten >	< BEE < WASP DAISY > < BEETLE ORCHID > LILY > < ANT TULIP >	< heaven TULIP > Stink > < ANT < Cheer LILY > vomit > < BEETLE

< = left response key, > = right response key

[a]Reproduced from Anthony G. Greenwald, Debbie E. McGhee, and Jordan L. K. Schwartz, Measuring individual differences in implicit cognition: the Implicit Association Test, *Journal of Personality and Social Psychology* 74(6), pp. 1464–1480, Figure 1. © 1998, American Psychological Association.

responses for compatible concepts mapped on to a single response key (flowers + positive words compared to flower + negative words; Greenwald et al. 1998).

9.1.2 Patient and lesion studies

Few studies have explored the effects of focal frontal brain damage on Implicit Association Task performance, but there is evidence to suggest that the ventral areas of the prefrontal cortex play a role when accessing automatic associations (Table 9.2). Forbes et al. (2012) investigated performance on an Implicit Association Task that measured the strength of gender associations in a group of traumatic brain injury (TBI) patients and healthy controls. Response times (RTs) were slower in the TBI group compared to healthy controls when the patients made congruent judgments (e.g., male/strong or female/weak) but not incongruent judgments (e.g., male/weak or female/strong). However, the slower RTs on both the congruent and incongruent blocks were correlated with volume loss in the ventromedial prefrontal cortex, suggesting that this prefrontal area is involved in making automatic associative judgments.

Milne and Grafman (2001) compared the performance of seven patients with ventromedial prefrontal lesions, three patients with dorsolateral prefrontal damage and 15 healthy controls on a gender Implicit Association Task. Patients with ventromedial prefrontal damage showed a significantly smaller IAT effect when congruent RTs were subtracted from incongruent RTs compared to the dorsolateral prefrontal lesion patients, although the ventromedial patients only showed a trend for a smaller IAT effect than healthy controls. Whereas the dorsolateral prefrontal lesion group produced a higher IAT effect than healthy controls, the difference was not significant; that is, both groups showed faster RTs during the congruent than the incongruent conditions. This

Table 9.2 Implicit Association Task: Patient and lesion studies

Study	*n*	Patient/ Control Groups	Study type	Task	Brodmann Areas	FP	DL	OF	ACC
Milne and Grafman (2001)	7; 3; 15	VM; DL; HA	Lesion	Gender	11, 12, 13, 14, 47			✓	
Gozzi et al. (2009)	18; 15; 43	VM; VL; HA	Lesion	Gender	–			✓	✓
Forbes et al. (2012)	177; 49	TBI; HA	VBLSM	Gender	–		✓		✓

FP = frontal pole; DL = dorsolateral; OF = orbitofrontal cortex; ACC = anterior cingulate cortex; VM = ventromedial prefrontal cortex; HA = healthy adults; VL = ventrolateral prefrontal cortex; TBI = traumatic brain injury; VBLSM = voxel based symptom mapping; ✓ = frontal region damaged and impairment found; X = frontal region damaged but no impairment.

finding indicates that patients with dorsolateral prefrontal lesions and healthy controls both show a strong association between target and evaluative categories, whereas ventromedial prefrontal lesions result in a deficit in the ability to access these associations automatically.

A more recent lesion study conducted by the same research group reported that medial and lateral areas of the ventral prefrontal cortex play a different role in Implicit Association Task performance (Gozzi et al. 2009). The performance of a subgroup of 18 patients with ventromedial prefrontal lesions was compared with that of a subgroup of 15 patients with ventrolateral prefrontal lesions from a sample of 154 penetrating head-injured patients on a gender Implicit Association Task. Ventromedial prefrontal lesions were associated with a larger IAT effect (i.e., stronger implicit associations) compared to healthy control participants, whereas ventrolateral prefrontal damage was associated with a smaller IAT effect (i.e., weaker implicit associations). Damage to the dorsolateral prefrontal cortex did not predict Implicit Association Task performance. The authors suggest that the ventromedial prefrontal cortex may be associated with the ability to overcome unacceptable social behavior (e.g., stereotypical attitudes), whereas the ventrolateral prefrontal cortex may play a role in the executive elements of the Implicit Association Task, including inhibition.

9.1.3 Neuroimaging studies

Neuroimaging studies exploring the neural correlates of Implicit Association Task performance have shown that specific brain areas are activated during the congruent and incongruent blocks (Table 9.3). The lateral prefrontal cortex is thought to be associated with response inhibition during incongruent trials (Chee et al. 2000; Phelps et al. 2000; Knutson et al. 2006, 2007; Luo et al. 2006; Krendl et al. 2012). For example, Luo et al. (2006) investigated the neural correlates of implicit moral attitudes using functional magnetic resonance imaging (fMRI) and observed activation of the ventrolateral prefrontal cortex during task performance. The IAT effect (i.e., increased RTs to incongruent trials in step 5) was associated with greater activation of the premotor cortex, the anterior cingulate cortex, and the ventrolateral prefrontal cortex (Brodmann Area (BA) 47) compared to the congruent trials (in step 3). As ventrolateral prefrontal activation has emerged during the performance of tasks that require individuals to withhold or to change a motor response (e.g., Go/No-Go task, response reversal), the researchers interpreted the ventrolateral prefrontal activation as reflecting the processing of response conflict.

Other imaging studies have found that the dorsolateral prefrontal cortex also plays a central role in inhibiting automatic responses when making incongruent

Table 9.3 Implicit Association Task: Neuroimaging studies

Study	n	Patient/ Control Groups	Study type	Task		Brodmann Areas	FP	DL	OF	ACC
Chee et al. (2000)	8	HA	fMRI	Flowers/ insects		–		✓	✓	✓
Phelps et al. (2000)	14	HA	fMRI	Race		–				✓
Richeson et al. (2003)	15	HA	fMRI	Race		6, 9, 10, 24, 32, 46	✓	✓		✓
Knutson et al. (2006)	24	HA	fMRI	Politics Congruent:		6, 9, 10, 32, 45, 46, 47;	✓	✓		✓
				Incongruent:	6, 9, 32, 47		✓			✓
Luo et al. (2006)	20	HA	fMRI	Moral attitudes		6, 13, 24, 25, 47				✓
Beer et al. (2008)	16	HA	fMRI	Race		11/25, 44	✓			✓
Knutson et al. (2007)	20	HA	fMRI	Race/gender Congruent:		8, 9, 10	✓			✓
				Incongruent:	8, 9, 46		✓			
Quadflieg et al. (2009)	20	HA	fMRI	Gender		10	✓			
Cattaneo et al. (2011)	36	HA	rTMS	Gender		–		✓		
Krendl et al. (2012)	20	HA	fMRI	Stigma		9, 10, 32, 47	✓	✓		✓

FP = frontal pole; OF = orbitofrontal; DL = dorsolateral; ACC = anterior cingulate cortex; HA = healthy adults; fMRI = functional magnetic resonance imaging; rTMS = repetitive transcranial magnetic stimulation; tDCS = transcranial direct current stimulation; ✓ = frontal region involved.

judgments (Chee et al. 2000; Richeson et al. 2003). For example, Chee et al. (2000) scanned individuals using fMRI while they were performing the flowers/insects version of the Implicit Association Task. Prefrontal activation (BAs 9 and 47) was associated with the incongruent condition (step 5) relative to the congruent condition (step 3), with the dorsolateral prefrontal cortex being activated to a greater extent than the ventrolateral prefrontal cortex. Further support to the view that the dorsolateral prefrontal cortex is involved in inhibiting habitual responses comes from Richeson et al. (2003), who investigated the correlation between the performance of white individuals on a racial Judgment variant of the Implicit Association Task and performance on the Stroop Task, a measure of inhibition. Those individuals who demonstrated the greatest racial bias performed the most poorly on the Stroop Task. In a separate session in the fMRI scanner, participants were instructed to indicate whether black and white faces appeared on the right or the left of the screen. Blood oxygen level-dependent (BOLD) responses were significantly greater for black faces compared to white faces in the dorsolateral prefrontal cortex (BA 9) and the anterior cingulate cortex (BA 32). Therefore, the brain regions often shown to be important for inhibition were activated significantly more when making decisions about faces that were incongruent rather than congruent with the participants' own ethnicity. As racial bias only predicted activation in the dorsolateral prefrontal cortex when exposed to black faces, Richeson et al. (2003) suggested that this dorsolateral activation was specifically related to the cognitive effort needed to control racial thoughts and behaviors.

The central role played by the dorsolateral prefrontal cortex in inhibiting stereotypical responses in the Implicit Association Task is further supported by a recent transcranial magnetic stimulation investigation (Cattaneo et al. 2011). Temporary disruption of the dorsolateral prefrontal cortex during the performance of a gender variant of the Implicit Association Task (e.g., male/female and strong/weak attributes) increased the participants' gender bias compared to the control condition (i.e., stimulation of the vertex). In particular, the authors noted an increased error rate during incongruent trials (e.g., male/weakness). Whereas the dorsolateral prefrontal cortex is mainly associated with response inhibition (i.e., the incongruent condition), the ventromedial prefrontal cortex is involved in accessing previously acquired social knowledge and processing emotional information necessary to make judgments (i.e., the congruent condition; Knutson et al. 2006, 2007; Quadflieg et al. 2009). For example, Knutson et al. (2006) scanned participants during a version of the Implicit Association Task that required individuals to categorize Republican or Democratic US politicians. The authors included two post-scan measures: the valence strength (i.e., positive or negative feelings towards each politician) and the affiliation strength (i.e., how likely they were to vote for the politician). fMRI showed that performance on the congruent condition was associated with a distributed brain network, which included BA 47 (relative to the incongruent condition) and left BA 9 (relative to the control condition). The incongruent condition was instead associated with activation of BA 10 (relative to the congruent condition) and bilateral dorsolateral prefrontal cortex (BA 9 and 46) and BA 47 (relative to the control condition). The bilateral activation of the dorsolateral prefrontal cortex during the incongruent versus congruent conditions suggests that this area of the prefrontal cortex is mainly recruited when the task requires unusual (i.e., not habitual) responses. Further analysis showed that frontal pole (BA 10) activity correlated with valence strength, whereas lateral prefrontal activity correlated instead with affiliation strength. These results were interpreted in terms of two networks involved in Implicit Association Task performance, one associated with knowledge of stereotypes and emotional processing, the second to deliberative and factual knowledge. This notion of dual networks contributing to Implicit Association Task performance is not dissimilar to the dual-process theory of moral judgments (Greene et al. 2001), whereby both emotional and controlled cognition guide moral reasoning and decision-making (see Section 9.3).

In a second fMRI study, Knutson et al. (2007) found that accessing automatic social beliefs (i.e., the congruent condition) involved activation of the medial frontal gyrus (BAs 10 and 13) and the superior frontal gyrus (BA 8 extending to BA 9), whereas the suppression of automatic association (i.e., the incongruent condition) was associated with activation of the dorsolateral prefrontal cortex only (BAs 9 and 46). Similar results emerged in an fMRI study exploring the separate contributions of automatic and controlled components to brain activation during Implicit Association Task performance (Beer et al. 2008). In this study, the researchers computed two parameters based on the Implicit Association Task error rate: the activation parameter, which refers to the degree to which associations are automatically activated (e.g., white/pleasant), and the detection parameter, which reflects the detection of incongruent responses (e.g., white/unpleasant). fMRI showed that the activation parameter was associated with activation of BA 11 and 47. By contrast, the detection parameter was associated with activity in BA 46. Together these findings indicate that the response suppression component of the Implicit Association Task mainly relies on lateral prefrontal activity (dorsolateral and ventrolateral prefrontal cortex), whereas accessing social information involves the medial (BAs 10 and 13) and lateral (BAs 9 and 47) regions of the prefrontal cortex.

9.1.4 Aging studies

Studies have explored the effect of age on Implicit Association Task performance (Table 9.4). These aging studies have generally shown a larger IAT effect in older compared to younger adults on versions of the task measuring implicit attitudes towards flowers/insects, younger/older adults, race, as well as gender in relation to science/art and career/family (Hummert et al. 2002; Nosek et al. 2002). Some researchers have pointed out that the age effect on Implicit Association Task performance reflects a general slowing associated with aging in addition to older adults' access to implicit attitudes. For example, Hummert et al. (2002) investigated the IAT effect for the target category age in a group of 36 younger (mean age = 21.9 years), a group of 38 young-old (mean

Table 9.4 Implicit Association Task: Aging studies

Study	n	Participant age groups (years)	Study type	Task	Age effect
Hummert et al. (2002)	36; 38; 40	18–29; 55–74; 75–93	Cross-sectional (behavioral)	Age	✓
Nosek et al. (2002)	28, 108–160, 857	< 23; 23–50; ≥50	Cross-sectional (behavioral)	Web IAT	✓
Roefs and Jansen (2002)	30; 31	Obese, mean = 46.3 Normal, mean = 40.5	Cross-sectional (behavioral)	Diet	✓
Gonsalkorale et al. (2009)	15, 752	11–15; 16–20; 21–30; 31–40; 41–50; 51–60; 61–70; ≥71	Cross-sectional (behavioral)	Race	✓
Stewart et al. (2009)	112	40–91	Cross-sectional (behavioral)	Race	✓

IAT, Implicit Association Task; ✓ = age effect found; X = age effect not found.

age = 69.4 years), and a group of 40 old-old (mean age = 80.4 years) adults. They reported that the old-old adults demonstrated more positive attitudes towards the young and negative attitudes towards the old than younger adults. However, when the Implicit Association Task data were z-score-transformed to adjust the response latencies for an individual's mean response time and standard deviation, there was no significant difference in the implicit attitudes between younger and older adults. These results suggest that age differences in Implicit Association Task performance may emerge as a consequence of the effect of age on processing speed.

Other studies have not reported age effects on Implicit Association Task performance. For example, in a much larger-scale web-based study involving thousands of participants, all age groups demonstrated a negative bias in implicit attitudes towards older adults (Nosek et al. 2002). By contrast, when a gender/science version of the Implicit Association Task was performed online in the same study, an implicit association between men and science and women and liberal arts was increasingly reported as adults aged from 50 years onwards. It is difficult to parse to what degree the shift toward this greater implicit association is related to age-related brain changes versus an artefact of age-related cultural differences. Thus, these data cannot easily be used to aid with the functional localization of Implicit Association Task performance within the frontal lobes.

Some studies have investigated whether age differences in performance on the Implicit Association Task are accounted for by differences in the strength of the automatic associations or by a decline in inhibitory skills with age

(Gonsalkorale et al. 2009; Stewart et al. 2009). Gonsalkorale et al. (2009) modelled the responses on the racial Implicit Association Task according to the quadruple process model. This model assumes that four processes are responsible for the performance on tasks measuring implicit biases: the *activation of association*, which refers to the activation of automatic associations; the *detection process*, which refers to the discrimination between appropriate and non-appropriate responses (i.e., incongruent trials); the *overcoming bias*, which refers to the ability to overcome automatic associations during incongruent conditions; and the *guessing parameter*, which refers to the tendency to provide general responses when individuals do not have an association that guides their behavior. Gonsalkorale et al. administered the racial Implicit Association Task to a group of participants aged 11–94 years who were subdivided into the following age groups: 11–15, 16–20, 21–30, 31–40, 41–50, 51–60, 61–70, ≥71 years. The IAT effect increased with increasing age, indicating that older participants had stronger racial associations compared to younger adults. The *overcoming bias* estimated parameter declined with age, suggesting that older participants were less able to inhibit their automatic associations than younger adults rather than having difficulty in regulating automatically activated associations.

Other studies support the view that the age effect on inhibitory processes moderates the larger IAT effect in older individuals (Roefs et al. 2002; Stewart et al. 2009). For example, Stewart et al. (2009) administered the racial Implicit Association Task to a group of participants aged 40–91 years, finding a larger IAT effect in older than in middle-aged participants. Separate automatic and controlled components of the Implicit Association Task were derived from errors on the task using the process-dissociation procedure (Jacoby 1991). Regression analysis indicated that this increase in the IAT effect with age was explained by age-related losses in the control component of the Implicit Association Task (i.e., inhibition) but not automatic processes.

9.1.5 Summary

Overall, the Implicit Association Task studies discussed above indicate that both automatic and controlled processes play a role in Implicit Association Task performance. Whereas the medial prefrontal cortex is thought to be involved in the automatic processing of social emotional information (i.e., the congruent trials), the lateral prefrontal cortex is mainly recruited during the inhibition of strong habitual responses (i.e., the incongruent trials). Age effects observed on the Implicit Association Task are thought to reflect decline in inhibitory functioning, rather than the automatic processing of social and emotional information.

9.2 **Iowa Gambling Task**

9.2.1 **Task description**

The Iowa Gambling Task is a common[1] and clinically recognized method of assessment designed to tap impairments in decision-making associated with ventromedial prefrontal lesions (Bechara et al. 1994). In the Iowa Gambling Task, participants are initially given a fake amount of $2000 or £2000 (depending on whether the task is administered in the USA or UK) and are requested to pick a card from one of four decks of cards laid before them (see Figure 9.2).

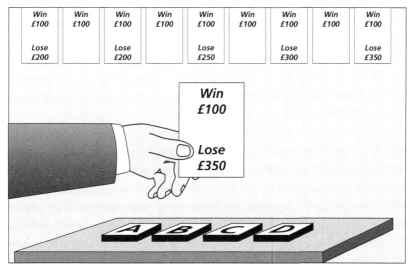

Fig. 9.2 The version of the Iowa Gambling Task in pounds sterling used by MacPherson et al. (2009). Participants choose one card at a time from decks A, B, C, or D, changing deck when they so wish. Each card has a reward associated with it but some cards also have a penalty, which is transacted in fake money. The run of cards at the top of Figure 9.2 denotes the rewards and punishments if participants were to choose from deck A, a high-risk deck. Selecting cards predominantly from decks A and B will eventually result in a loss, whereas selecting cards from decks C and D will result in gains. Reproduced from Iowa Gambling Task Impairment Is Not Specific To Ventromedial Prefrontal Lesions, Sarah E. MacPherson, Louise H. Phillips, Sergio Della Sala et al., *The Clinical Neuropsychologist*, © 2009, Taylor & Francis Ltd. http://www.tandf.co.uk/journals.

---

[1] Other common gambling tasks are also discussed briefly below, where relevant. However, as the Iowa Gambling Task is prevalent both in clinical use and in research attempting to localize frontal functions, it will be the focus of this review.

Table 9.5 Iowa Gambling Task contingencies for each deck over 10 card selections, and the net yield after 10 selections from a given deck

Deck	Average reward value	Reward frequency	Average punishment value	Punishment frequency	Net yield
A	$100	10/10	$250	5/10	−$250
B	$100	10/10	$1250	1/10	−$250
C	$50	10/10	$50	5/10	+$250
D	$50	10/10	$250	1/10	+$250

Note that each card has both a reward and a punishment.

Participants are asked to earn as much money as possible from choosing the cards. Typically, they should make 100 card selections in total, although they are not made aware of this. Decks A, B, C, and D have different properties, each with different rates of winning and losing. Both the magnitude and the frequency of rewards and punishments differ between the decks (see Table 9.5). Cards from decks A and B result in the same high win, but deck A also involves frequent low losses whereas deck B results in infrequent high losses. Cards from decks C and D result in the same lower win, but deck C involves frequent low losses whereas deck D involves infrequent high losses. Participants should learn to choose cards from decks C and D rather than decks A and B, as selecting more cards from the former results in losing less money overall.

A similar task is the Cambridge Gambling Task (Rogers et al. 1999) in which participants are asked to decide whether a target (a token) is hidden beneath a blue or a red box, and how much money to bet their decision on (see Figure 9.3). However, ten blue and red boxes are shown at the same time and in different proportions (e.g., four blue and six red boxes), hence the participant is provided with an indication of the probability of the accuracy of their choice (e.g., 60% chance that the target is in a red box). From this probability, participants can decide how much money to bet on their decision according to their confidence, with more biased proportions (e.g., 9:1) tending to provoke higher-value bets. As will be discussed in this section, there is some indication that the Iowa Gambling Task and the Cambridge Gambling Task differ in terms of regional recruitment of prefrontal regions (see Clark et al. 2003). Performance on both of these gambling tasks can be measured in terms of a net score (in the case of the Iowa Gambling Task this is the number of choices from good decks minus the number of choices from bad decks; in the case of the Cambridge Gambling Task, this is the number of choices from the high-proportion color of boxes), or in the amount of money earned at the end of the task.

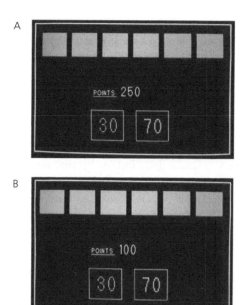

Fig. 9.3 Example of two trials from the Cambridge Gambling Task. Note the difference in probabilities between A (4:2) and B (5:1). Reproduced from Robert D. Rogers, Adrian M. Owen, Hugh C. Middleton, Emma J. Williams, John D. Pickard, Barbara J. Sahakian, and Trevor W. Robbins, Choosing between small, likely rewards and large, unlikely rewards activates inferior and orbital prefrontal cortex, *Journal of Neuroscience*, 20(19), pp. 9029–9038, Figure 1. © 1999, The Society of Neuroscience, with permission. Please see color plate section.

Bechara et al. suggest that cognitive processes alone are insufficient to make the decisions that result in the best overall outcome on the Iowa Gambling Task. The Somatic Marker Hypothesis (Damasio et al. 1991; Bechara et al. 1996) asserts that bioregulatory and emotional signals (i.e., somatic markers) help to bias decisions towards the best outcome. In particular, the presence of such biasing signals has been measured through skin conductance responses (SCRs), which are observed before individuals are consciously aware of the best choice to make (Bechara et al. 1997). Turnbull et al. (2003) developed a task in which participants evaluated the diary events of trainee firefighters in a format similar to the Iowa Gambling Task, so that instead of monetary rewards and punishments (direct reinforcement), the participants received indirect emotional reinforcement in the form of "good" and "bad" diary events (Turnbull et al. 2003). This meant that participants received rewards and punishments indirectly through the consequences of others' rather than their own actions and so they could not rely on somatic markers to guide their decision-making.

Interestingly, whereas healthy participants on the Iowa Gambling Task show gradual learning over sub-blocks (i.e., a shift towards selections from "good" decks), no such learning behavior was observed in the Firefighter Task with an equal number of selections from "bad" diaries compared to "good" diaries (Turnbull et al. 2003). This suggests that gambling tasks such as the Iowa Gambling Task require direct emotional reinforcement to generate the appropriate somatic markers used to guide decision-making.

Lin et al. (2007) showed that, in healthy participants, the deck preference tends to lie with deck C rather than deck A, because deck C has fewer losses than a higher value outcome overall. In a modified Iowa Gambling Task, Chiu and Lin (2007) nearly doubled the gain–loss amounts in each trial to ensure that the losses in deck C were noticeable, but kept the frequency of rewards and punishments, as well as the net outcome, the same for each of the decks. Instead of choosing the deck with the best outcome (deck C), participants choose from both decks equally, suggesting that participants may be tracking and using the reward frequency, rather than magnitude, as a simple and immediate strategy (but not the optimum strategy) for successful performance (Chiu and Lin 2007). There has been some indication of a "Prominent Deck B" phenomenon whereby healthy participants show a preference for deck B despite it being a "bad" deck (Dunn et al. 2006). This preference has been explained in terms of both reward-value (both rewards and losses are high) and gain–loss frequency (gains are frequent and losses are rare), in that participants tend to choose the high-value frequent-gain deck B, despite its large loss (Lin et al. 2007). Lin et al. administered a simplified two-phase version of the Iowa Gambling Task in which "good" and "bad" decks were equated for their gain–loss frequency (i.e., AACC and BBDD versions of the Iowa Gambling Task). For example, deck A contained five losses and five gains (of 10 cards) that would result in a net loss of $250, whereas deck C also contained five losses and five gains but resulted in a net profit of $250. By contrast, decks B and D both contained nine gains and only one loss, but in the case of deck B this was large ($1250), resulting in a net loss. In the A–C deck version, participants picked more cards from deck C (the optimum deck) and developed this preference early in the task. However, in the B–D deck version, participants picked equally from both decks and performance did not shift over time, suggesting that long-term outcome was not used by participants to guide their decisions (Lin et al. 2007). Furthermore, van den Bos et al. (2006) identified that whereas in the original Iowa Gambling Task "bad" decks (A and B) rewarded $100 and "good" decks (C and D) rewarded only $50, resulting in a 2:1 ratio of reward magnitude, manipulating this amount can influence the decision-making strategy used. The authors administered versions of the Iowa Gambling Task in which the ratio of the reward between "bad" decks and "good" decks ranged from 1:1 (i.e., all decks rewarded $50 per selection) to 6:1 (i.e., "bad" decks rewarded $300 and "good" decks rewarded $50 per selection). Importantly, the magnitude of the punishments for each deck was also manipulated to preserve the original net gains and losses. In the 1:1 condition, in which "bad" and "good" decks rewarded the same amount per card selection, the performance of healthy individuals was significantly better both in terms of "good" card selections and in net gain relative to the original (2:1) task. Increasing the bad:good bias (e.g., 4:1 or 6:1) resulted in impaired performance relative to the original task, with healthy participants picking more "bad" cards and earning less money overall (van den Bos et al. 2006).

Although the administration of the Iowa Gambling Task differs between studies in various ways, there appears to be little difference in terms of performance when the task is presented on a computer rather than a paper-and-pencil version, or when a delay between card selections is enforced (Bowman et al. 2005). Moreover, performance in terms of learning the optimum strategy and picking cards from "good" decks does not appear to differ between real and fake (as in the original Bechara et al. task) monetary reward conditions (Bowman and Turnbull 2003). However, there is some indication that real monetary conditions lead to bias towards high-risk but high-reward decks in the middle of the task. Later in the task, as high-value punishments are encountered, decisions are biased away from these decks (Bowman and Turnbull 2003). Bowman and Turnbull suggest that this represents the generation of stronger somatic marker signals when real monetary rewards are used, though it may also indicate that the more direct experience afforded by monetary reinforcements was necessary to motivate participants to perform well. Finally, the range of scores obtained from healthy control performance in fake monetary conditions is larger than in real monetary conditions (Bowman and Turnbull 2003). As such, clinical studies using a fake monetary Iowa Gambling Task may inadvertently increase the chance of detecting no deficit in a particular patient (i.e., a false rejection), as extremely poor performance can also be observed in the healthy population (Bowman and Turnbull 2003).

Brand et al. distinguished between decision-making under ambiguity and decision-making under risky conditions (Brand et al. 2006). In particular, as the Iowa Gambling Task involves decisions based on no prior or explicit knowledge of the value or frequency of rewards from any given deck, participants must rely on emotion-based "gut" feelings (ambiguity). By contrast, gambling tasks such as the Game of Dice task provide explicit probabilities and control over the magnitude of the reward or punishment (Brand et al. 2006). In the Game of Dice task, participants are asked to choose a single number

(1 to 6) or a combination of several numbers before throwing a single die (e.g., Brand et al. 2005a). The monetary gain or loss per dice roll is determined by the choice of numbers, with a single digit bringing the biggest reward but also the biggest penalty if wrong, and increasing combinations of numbers bringing reduced values of reinforcement (two-numbers > three-numbers > four numbers). The more numbers in the combination, the less risky the decision, since the better the chance of one of the numbers being rolled. Thus, participants are provided with an explicit indication of the probability of the accuracy of their choice and thus the risk associated with their decision (fewer numbers yield a smaller chance of a reward).

Given the association between gambling disorders and impaired performance on the Iowa Gambling Task, there may be some indirect evidence of ecological validity (e.g., Brand et al. 2005b; Linnet et al. 2010). Similarly, the construct validity is relatively good—there is some evidence to suggest that ambiguous decision-making abilities may be tapped by early blocks of the Iowa Gambling Task but that risky decision-making abilities may be tapped in latter blocks, since participants are often aware of the probabilities associated with each deck (see Buelow and Suhr 2009 for a review). Significant correlations between Iowa Gambling Task performance and performance on other executive tasks—even those which do not involve emotional processing—suggest that cognitive factors (as well as emotional factors) play a role in decision-making during the Iowa Gambling Task (Buelow and Suhr 2009). Specifically, performance on the Iowa Gambling Task and the Game of Dice Task correlates with Modified Card Sorting Task (a test of inhibitory control and problem-solving) and Trail-Making Task (a test of set-shifting) performance (Brand et al. 2005a, 2005b; Barry and Petry 2008).

9.2.2 Patient and lesion studies

Research has provided evidence of localization of the processes associated with performing the Iowa Gambling Task (Table 9.6). Bechara et al. (1994) observed that individuals with ventromedial prefrontal lesions performed significantly more poorly than healthy controls, and seemed to choose mainly from decks A and B. Therefore, Bechara et al. (1994) concluded that such patients seemed to pay little attention to any potential loss, and focused on those decks with high win values even if they resulted in a net loss (see Figure 9.4). Furthermore, Bechara et al. (1998) found that patients with anterior ventromedial prefrontal lesions performed significantly more poorly than healthy controls on the Iowa Gambling Task, but not on a task designed to test working memory (a Delayed Response Task). By contrast, those with dorsolateral prefrontal lesions performed significantly more poorly on a delay-based working memory task, but

Table **9.6** Iowa Gambling Task and similar tasks: Patient and lesion studies

Study	*n*	Patient/Control Groups	Study type	Task	Brodmann Areas	FP	DL	OF	ACC
Bechara et al. (1994)	7; 44	VM; HA	Lesion	IGT	–			✓	✓
Bechara et al. (1996)	7; 12	VM; HA	Lesion (SCR)	IGT	–			✓	✓
Bechara et al. (1997)	6; 10	VM; HA	Lesion (SCR)	IGT	–			✓	✓
Bechara et al. (1998)	9; 10; 21	VM; DL; HA	Lesion	IGT	–			✓	✓
Bechara et al. (1999)	5; 5; 13	VM; AM; HA	Lesion (SCR)	IGT	–			✓	✓
Rahman et al. (1999)	8; 8	fvFTD; HA	Patient	CGT	–				
Manes et al. (2002)	5; 4; 5; 5; 13	VM; DL; DM; Mix; HA	Lesion	IGT CGT Risk task	–		✓ X X	X X X	X X X
Tranel et al. (2002)	3; 4	Left VM; right VM	Lesion Left: Right:	IGT	–			✓	✓
Clark et al. (2003)	24; 22; 21	Left FL; Right FL; HA	Lesion	IGT CGT Risk task	–		✓	X	X
Fellows and Farah (2005b)	9; 11; 17; 14	VM; DL; HA1; HA2	Lesion	IGT	–		✓	✓	
Torralva et al. (2007)	20; 10	fvFTD; HA	Patient	IGT	–				
MacPherson et al. (2009)	14; 6; 24	VM; non-VM; HA	Lesion	IGT	10, 11, 12, 13, 14, 47	✓	✓	✓	✓
Roca et al. (2010)	21; 25	FL; HA	Lesion	IGT	–			X	X

FP = frontal pole; DL = dorsolateral prefrontal cortex; OF = orbitofrontal cortex; ACC = anterior cingulate cortex; VM = ventromedial prefrontal cortex; HA = healthy adults; IGT = Iowa Gambling Task; SCR = skin conductance responses; AM = amygdala; fvFTD = frontal variant frontotemporal dementia; CGT = Cambridge Gambling Task; DM = dorsomedial prefrontal cortex; Mix = dorsal and ventral prefrontal cortex; FL = frontal lobe; ✓ = frontal region damaged and impairment found; X = frontal region damaged but no impairment.

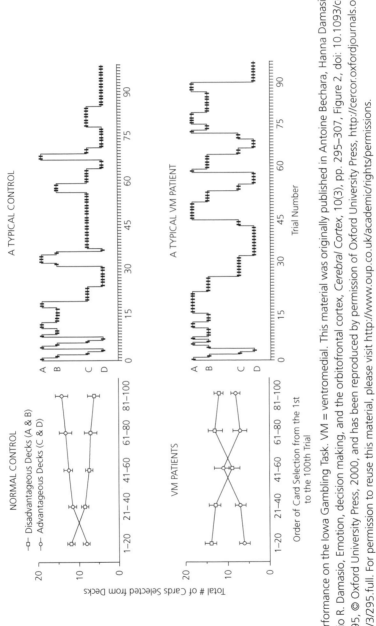

Fig. 9.4 Performance on the Iowa Gambling Task. VM = ventromedial. This material was originally published in Antoine Bechara, Hanna Damasio, and Antonio R. Damasio, Emotion, decision making, and the orbitofrontal cortex, *Cerebral Cortex*, 10(3), pp. 295–307, Figure 2, doi: 10.1093/cercor/10.3.295, © Oxford University Press, 2000, and has been reproduced by permission of Oxford University Press, http://cercor.oxfordjournals.org/content/10/3/295.full. For permission to reuse this material, please visit http://www.oup.co.uk/academic/rights/permissions.

not on the Iowa Gambling Task. Those patients with posterior ventromedial prefrontal lesions were impaired on both tasks, suggesting that such lesions affected both decision-making and working memory (Bechara et al. 1998). Patients with frontal variant frontotemporal dementia (fvFTD; involving primarily ventromedial prefrontal cortex), however, are able to make correct decisions based on probability, but take longer to make such decisions and risk more money regardless of the likelihood of the outcome (Rahman et al. 1999; see also Torralva et al. 2007).

Furthermore, whereas patients with primarily ventromedial prefrontal damage and healthy controls show changes in SCRs after choosing a card (regardless of a win or a loss), only healthy controls develop a modified, anticipatory SCR before choosing a card from a disadvantageous deck (Bechara et al. 1996). Such SCR changes are thought to reflect somatic markers that are present in emotional responses—and their emergence during the decision-making process is thought to represent the involvement of shared mechanisms between the decision-making process and the emotion associated with that decision (Bechara et al. 2000). Healthy controls unconsciously use such an anticipatory SCR to guide their decision-making, even before becoming aware of the optimum behavioral strategy for maximizing wins (i.e., choosing only from decks C and D; Bechara et al. 1997). As such, the anticipatory SCR indicates some level of emotional response to the predicted outcome of a given action, and this marker can be used to inform or direct decisions before the conscious use of strategies (Bechara et al. 2000). There is also some suggestion that both markers of decision-making deficits (performance and anticipatory SCRs) are significantly reduced in right ventromedial prefrontal lesion patients, more so than in left ventromedial prefrontal lesion patients (Tranel et al. 2002). Right ventromedial prefrontal lesion patients have been shown to exhibit greater social and emotional dysfunction than left ventromedial prefrontal lesion patients, suggesting a right-sided asymmetry in both decision-making and social and emotional abilities (Tranel et al. 2002).

Interestingly, the integrity of the amygdala appears to play a part in Iowa Gambling Task performance, with amygdala lesion patients also showing both behavioral impairments (picking more cards from "bad" decks) and a lack of a modified anticipatory SCR relative to healthy controls when performing the Iowa Gambling Task (Bechara et al. 1999). However, Bechara et al. have suggested distinguishable roles for the amygdala and the ventromedial prefrontal cortex, with damage to the former also impairing the reactionary SCR (when receiving a reward or punishment), but damage to the latter leaving the reactionary SCRs relatively intact (Bechara et al. 1999).

Research has shown that healthy participants are often explicitly aware of the best strategy to adopt in order to perform successfully on the Iowa Gambling

Task as well as the relative values of each deck (Maia and McClelland 2004). Decisions made during Iowa Gambling Task performance are not only guided by the non-conscious emotion-guided signals proposed by the 'somatic marker hypothesis', but also conscious knowledge. Maia and McClelland also note that, since the "bad" decks initially present large rewards in the deck, ventromedial prefrontal patients may simply be failing the Iowa Gambling Task because they are unable to reverse their behavioral response when the card selections associated with the "bad" decks start punishing participants (i.e., a reversal learning deficit rather than an insensitivity to the negative consequences of their actions; Maia and McClelland 2004). In response to Maia and McClelland, Bechara et al. suggest that the deficit exhibited by ventromedial prefrontal patients in terms of reversal learning can also be accounted for by the somatic marker hypothesis (Bechara et al. 2005). They suggest that the same emotional processes that inform the patients' decisions also contribute to the "stop" signal necessary for preventing perseveration (Bechara et al. 2005). Furthermore, even with knowledge of contingencies, ventromedial prefrontal patients (for whom the emotional signals are not present) still fail the task, suggesting that cognitive processes in the absence of emotion are not adequate for successful performance (Bechara et al. 2005).

However, some investigations into Iowa Gambling Task performance have been less supportive for the necessary involvement of the ventromedial prefrontal cortex. For example, Clark et al. (2003) found that although some frontal lesion patients (particularly those with right frontal lesions) did pick significantly more cards from the disadvantageous decks, performance was correlated with the volume of the lesion outside the ventromedial prefrontal cortex in more lateral areas such as the inferior frontal gyrus, the medial frontal gyrus, and the superior frontal gyrus (Clark et al. 2003). Clark et al. also noted that right frontal lesion patients, but not left frontal patients, bet more money per bet than healthy controls did on the Cambridge Gambling Task. However, such performance was not significantly correlated with lesion volume in any prefrontal region (including the ventromedial prefrontal cortex). Interestingly, Manes et al. (2002) found that patients with ventromedial prefrontal lesions performed similarly to normal controls on several decision-making tasks (including versions of the Iowa Gambling Task). The only resemblance to a deficit observed in such patients was a significantly longer thinking time before they made a choice. By contrast, patients with dorsolateral prefrontal lesions performed significantly more poorly on the Iowa Gambling Task as well as the spatial working memory task from the Cambridge Neuropsychological Test Automated Battery (CANTAB; Manes et al. 2002). Patients with diffuse lesions to the frontal lobes also performed more poorly on the Iowa Gambling

Task, showing particularly risky decision-making behavior. Manes et al. (2002) conclude that in decision-making tasks such as the Iowa Gambling Task, it is the interplay between dorsolateral and ventromedial prefrontal areas that is necessary for successful performance, not the ventromedial prefrontal cortex alone. Similarly, MacPherson et al. (2009) observed that both ventromedial prefrontal and non-ventromedial frontal lesion patients chose significantly more "bad" cards than healthy controls, with no difference between the performance of the two frontal patient groups (see Figure 9.5). Fellows and Farah (2005b) observed a similar result, but found that when ventromedial prefrontal and dorsolateral prefrontal patients performed a task similar to the Iowa Gambling Task in which the decks were re-ordered so that the "loss" cards were presented first, the ventromedial prefrontal patients performed as well as controls whereas the dorsolateral prefrontal patients were impaired compared to

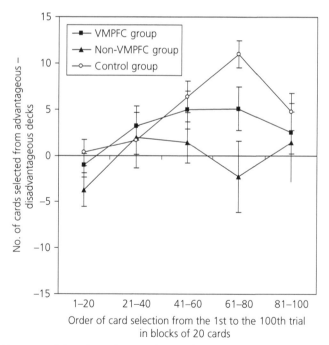

Fig. 9.5 Ventromedial prefrontal cortex (VMPFC) versus non-VMPFC patients on Iowa Gambling Task. Reproduced from Iowa Gambling Task Impairment Is Not Specific To Ventromedial Prefrontal Lesions, Sarah E. MacPherson, Louise H. Phillips, Sergio Della Sala et al., *The Clinical Neuropsychologist*, © 2009, Taylor & Francis Ltd. http://www.tandf.co.uk/journals.

both ventromedial prefrontal patients and healthy controls (Fellows and Farah 2005b). By rearranging the decks in this manner, Fellows and Farah removed the "reversal learning" component of the Iowa Gambling Task, hence participants did not have to alter an already established stimulus–reward association and adapt their responses accordingly. Thus, the tendency of patients with ventromedial prefrontal lesions to underperform on the Iowa Gambling Task is likely due to deficits in dealing with switches of reward contingencies rather than decision-making per se. Similarly, Roca et al. (2010) noted that those patients with inferior medial prefrontal lesions performed similarly to patients with other frontal lesions, and that the differences in terms of final outcome on the Iowa Gambling Task between patients and healthy controls disappeared after controlling for IQ.

Despite a weight of evidence suggesting that ventromedial prefrontal lesion patients fail the Iowa Gambling Task, the fact that other patient groups, including those with dorsolateral prefrontal damage, also fail the task raises concerns over its specificity. However, some analysis of the pattern of performance may improve the Iowa Gambling Task's utility as different patient groups appear to fail for different reasons. In particular, using both reversal- and no-reversal-learning conditions of the Iowa Gambling Task may help to distinguish between ventromedial prefrontal and dorsolateral prefrontal involvement.

9.2.3 Neuroimaging studies

Several neuroimaging studies have examined the regions within the frontal lobes that are activated when healthy participants perform the Iowa Gambling Task inside the scanner (Table 9.7). Lawrence et al. used an event-related fMRI paradigm to examine regional activation associated with particular events within the Iowa Gambling Task—such as choosing from a bad deck, or receiving a reward (Lawrence et al. 2009). The researchers noted overall task-related activation (after subtracting activation from a non-decision-making control task in which participants were instructed which deck to choose from) in the ventromedial prefrontal cortex (BA 11) and anterior cingulate cortex (BAs 6, 24, and 32). Card selections from "bad" decks (i.e., decks A and B) provoked activation in the dorsolateral prefrontal cortex (BA 9), ventrolateral prefrontal cortex (BAs 10 and 47), and anterior cingulate cortex (BAs 24 and 32) and "wins" (i.e., positive rewards regardless of deck) provoked primarily thalamic and striatal activation. Activation during the selection of cards from "bad" decks was positively correlated with task performance (Lawrence et al. 2009). Similarly, Rogers et al. (1999) found significantly increased positron emission tomography activation within the ventrolateral and ventromedial prefrontal

Table 9.7 Iowa Gambling Task and similar tasks: Neuroimaging studies

Study	n	Patient/Control Groups	Study type	Task	Brodmann Areas	FP	DL	OF	ACC
Elliott et al. (1997)	6	HA	PET	Guessing task	11, 47			✓	
Rogers et al. (1999)	8	HA	PET	CGT	4, 10, 10/11, 11, 47			✓	
Bolla et al. (2004)	10; 10	HW; HM	PET	IGT Men: Women:	9, 10, 11, 47; 11		✓	✓ ✓	
Fukui et al. (2005)	14	HA	fMRI		9, 10, 11		✓	✓	
Northoff et al. (2006)	14	HA	fMRI	Unexpected affective judgment: Expected affective judgment:	10, 46; 8, 10	✓ ✓	✓		
Lin et al. (2008)	24	HA	fMRI	IGT Anticipation: Feedback:	–				✓
Lawrence et al. (2009)	17	HA	fMRI	Task: Risky decisions: Wins:	4, 6, 11, 24, 32; 6, 8, 9, 10, 32, 47; 6, 24	✓	✓	✓ ✓	✓ ✓ ✓
Li et al. (2010)	10	HA	fMRI		–		✓	✓	✓
Stern et al. (2010)	20	HA	fMRI	Uncertainty during feedback: Uncertainty during decisions:	4, 24, 32; 6, 8, 9, 10, 11, 32, 44, 45, 46, 47	✓	✓	✓	✓ ✓
Suhr and Hammers (2010)	58	HA	NIrS		–		✓		

FP = frontal pole; DL = dorsolateral prefrontal cortex; OF = orbitofrontal cortex; ACC = anterior cingulate cortex; HA = healthy adults; PET = positron emission tomography; CGT = Cambridge Gambling task; HW = healthy women; HM = healthy men; IGT = Iowa Gambling Task; fMRI = functional magnetic resonance imaging; NIrS = near-infrared spectroscopy; ✓ = frontal region involved.

regions (BAs 10, 11, and 47) during the Cambridge Gambling Task, regardless of whether the boxes were 4:2 or 5:1 in terms of color. By contrast, subtracting the 5:1 (low risk) from the 4:2 (high risk) condition revealed significant activation only in the ventrolateral prefrontal cortex (BA 11) and anterior cingulate cortex (BAs 6 and 24). Rogers et al. suggested that whereas the ventrolateral and ventromedial prefrontal cortex may be involved in decision-making, a separate network of ventrolateral prefrontal and anterior cingulate regions helps to track changes in reinforcement and risk (Rogers et al. 1999).

In addition to ventromedial prefrontal activation, recent neuroimaging studies have yielded evidence of dorsolateral prefrontal activation in healthy individuals performing the Iowa Gambling Task, particularly within BA 9 (Clark et al. 2003; Fukui et al. 2005; Suhr and Hammers 2010). As the reversal of learned associations is likely to be underpinned by ventromedial prefrontal functions (see Fellows and Farah 2003, 2005b), it might be that the decision-making component of the Iowa Gambling Task is supported by dorsolateral prefrontal functions. Even if this is not the case, the results of three neuroimaging studies suggest that successful Iowa Gambling Task performance may rely on both ventromedial prefrontal and dorsolateral prefrontal functions (Clark et al. 2003; Fukui et al. 2005; Suhr and Hammers 2010). Li et al. (2010) noted a wider pattern of activation during the entire Iowa Gambling Task including the ventromedial prefrontal cortex, dorsolateral prefrontal cortex, ventrolateral prefrontal cortex, anterior cingulate cortex, striatum and insula. Furthermore, using event-related fMRI, Lin et al. (2008) demonstrated that ventromedial prefrontal activation was specifically related to the phase after a decision was made, but only when large losses were incurred, suggesting an error-monitoring role. By contrast, only the basal ganglia and the insula were associated with decision-making per se, showing activation during the phase immediately before the card selection. However, using event-related fMRI methods, subtracting "safe" card selections (from decks C and D) from "risky" selections (from decks A and B) leads to significant activation only in the ventromedial prefrontal cortex (BA 10), suggesting that the ventromedial prefrontal cortex may be involved in decisions where the potential risks are high and can be anticipated (Fukui et al. 2005).

Bolla et al. (2004) noted gender differences in brain activation when performing the Iowa Gambling Task. Bolla et al. observed that the activation pattern shown throughout the whole task by men was more right-sided and ventrolateral (BAs 10 and 47), whereas women's activation was more focused on the left dorsolateral prefrontal cortex (BA 9). Interestingly, this difference in the pattern of activation was associated with a difference in performance, with men performing better overall and appearing to improve their Iowa

Gambling Task performance faster than women (Bolla et al. 2004). Although this study is limited by the small sample size (men: $n = 10$; women: $n = 10$), it does suggest that consideration should be taken when assessing brain activation in male and female participants using the Iowa Gambling Task, as they may differ at least in the strategies which they adopt to perform the task, and the regions which they recruit during performance. Interestingly, gender differences in terms of behavioral performance may be attenuated by requiring participants to contemplate personal moral dilemmas between sub-blocks of the Iowa Gambling Task (Overman et al. 2006). The researchers suggest that by encouraging participants to think critically but emotionally, the decisions made by both men and women become more influenced by somatic markers. However, it is unclear whether such a method could also reduce gender differences in terms of brain activation.

In a review of ambiguous decision tasks, such as the Iowa Gambling Task, and risky decision tasks, such as the Game of Dice Task, Brand et al. (2006) implicate distinguishable brain networks associated with performance on each. In particular, while fronto-limbic networks are involved in both tasks and thought to support the representation of somatic markers as well as the self-monitoring process in terms of certainty, the fronto-striatal networks are implicated only in risky decision-making, and are thought to represent anticipation of a given reward (Brand et al. 2006). Similarly, the ventrolateral prefrontal cortex has been associated with the use of reward-based decision-making under ambiguity, with anterior portions (BAs 10 and 11) helping to inhibit previously rewarded (but now punished) decisions and posterior portions (BA 47), upregulating processing during risky decisions (Elliott et al. 2000). Indeed, when ambiguity is absolute (i.e., the reinforced stimulus is randomly selected on each trial), the ventromedial prefrontal cortex appears to play a role in tracking feedback across trials (Elliott et al. 1997). Stern et al. (2010) suggest a similar role for the ventromedial prefrontal cortex in evaluating evidence and tracking certainty, allowing for "safer" decisions to be made when the outcome of the decision is uncertain. Ventromedial prefrontal activation during unexpected affective judgments correlates positively with healthy adults' performance on the Iowa Gambling Task, suggesting that the greater the recruitment of such regions in emotional decisions, the better the decision-making under ambiguity (Northoff et al. 2006).

In summary, neuroimaging studies have helped to clarify the conditions under which the ventromedial prefrontal cortex is involved in Iowa Gambling Task performance. Ventromedial prefrontal regions appear to be consistently activated in studies requiring decisions to be made based under ambiguous risk. Similarly, both the ventromedial prefrontal cortex and the anterior cingulate cortex operate in unison to track and adapt to changing reward contingencies.

Hence, closer analysis of Iowa Gambling Task performance, particularly in risky card selections or after high losses, could help to distinguish ventromedial prefrontal involvement from the more dorsolateral prefrontal involvement also prevalent during task performance.

9.2.4 Aging studies

Studies examining the effects of healthy adult aging on Iowa Gambling Task performance have yielded conflicting results (Table 9.8). MacPherson et al. (2002) administered the Iowa Gambling Task to younger (n = 30, aged 20–28 years), middle-aged (n = 30, aged 40–59 years), and older (n = 30, aged 61–80 years) individuals. No significant age-related impairment in Iowa Gambling Task performance, in terms of card selections, was observed, with older and middle-aged adults performing as well as their younger counterparts. Similarly, Denburg et al. (2005) noted that only a subset of older individuals (n = 14, aged 56–85 years) showed an impairment on the Iowa Gambling Task. This impaired subgroup (n = 14) was similar to the unimpaired older adult group in terms of demographic characteristics such as age, education, and health status, as well as in terms of performance on other cognitive tests such as the Wisconsin Card Sorting Test and verbal fluency. However, whereas the performance of the unimpaired older adults optimized over time (i.e., by selecting more cards from good decks), the impaired older adults selected from bad decks consistently over the course of the task. Wood et al. found that older individuals (n = 67, aged 65–88 years) performed similarly to younger individuals (n = 88, aged 18–34 years) both in terms of overall "good" card selections and in terms of learning over the five sub-blocks (Wood et al. 2005). However, there was some indication that the two age groups performed the

Table 9.8 Iowa Gambling Task and similar tasks: Aging studies

Study	n	Participant age groups (years)	Study type	Task	Age effect
MacPherson et al. (2002)	30; 30; 30	20–28; 40–59; 61–80	Cross-sectional (behavioural)	IGT	X
Deakin et al. (2004)	41; 46; 45; 45	17–27; 28–40; 41–52; 53–79	Cross-sectional (behavioural)	CGT	✓
Denburg et al. (2005)	51; 29	26–55; 56–85	Cross-sectional (behavioural)	IGT	✓
Wood et al. (2005)	88; 67	18–34; 65–88	Cross-sectional (behavioural)	IGT	X

IGT = Iowa Gambling Task; CGT = Cambridge Gambling task; ✓ = age effect found; X = age effect not found.

Iowa Gambling Task in different ways. By fitting models to each of the age groups that account for the speed of learning, the weight given to rewards, and the sensitivity of the decision to probabilities, Wood et al. were able directly to contrast the strategy of younger and older participants. Age effects were noted on all three model parameters. Older individuals learned from relatively short-term representations of reward, showing a strong influence from recent decisions, particularly those that were rewarded, but quickly rejecting any influence from past decisions (i.e., forgetting past large-value punishments). By contrast, younger individuals appeared to use all past decisions and reinforcements to inform their decisions, and placed particular importance on negatively reinforced decisions. This explains the similar performance between the age groups in the initial stages of the Iowa Gambling Task (where there are no past decisions to influence behavior), but the eventual divergence in terms of "good" deck selections as time goes on (Wood et al. 2005). Given the various observations of working memory impairments with age noted elsewhere (e.g., MacPherson et al. 2002; Park et al. 2002; Bopp and Verhaeghen 2005), it could be that older adults are forced to rely on a short-term strategy to reduce the working memory load and the need for working memory resources.

In the Cambridge Gambling Task, Deakin et al. (2004) noted that, in a large group of adults from across the lifespan ($n = 177$, mean age = 41 years), older individuals risked fewer points per bet than younger individuals, and that older adults showed an attenuated modulation of betting behavior in response to the probability of success (i.e., a smaller increase in bet value when viewing high proportions). Similarly, older individuals took longer to make decisions than younger individuals regardless of the probability of the outcome (Deakin et al. 2004). This echoes earlier suggestions in the literature of a reduction in gambling and risk-taking behaviors with age (Mok and Hraba 1991). However, within older individuals, the degree of decision-making impairment does not appear to be associated with age directly, suggesting that some other factors, such as general slowed learning, explain the poorer performance observed in some older individuals (Denburg et al. 2005), though this has yet to be investigated.

Older adults may differ from younger adults on the Iowa Gambling Task, at least in the manner in which they perform the task. Due to decrements in working memory abilities, older adults may be using short-term strategies to track reward contingencies, thus leading to more conservative gambling behavior than their younger counterparts.

9.2.5 Summary

There appears to be fairly consistent evidence from both lesion and neuroimaging studies to suggest that the ventromedial prefrontal cortex is involved in

Iowa Gambling Task performance. However, other regions such as the dorsolateral prefrontal cortex have also been associated with performance. It is possible that the recruitment of these regions represents differential functions within the Iowa Gambling Task itself, with the ventromedial prefrontal cortex responsible for tracking reward contingencies and the dorsolateral prefrontal cortex involved in the actual decision-making. This broadly fits with the suggestion of both emotional and cognitive biasing signals informing decisions (see Bechara et al. 2000). Moreover, although decisions on the Iowa Gambling Task can be made using a mixture of both types of signal, those patients with damage to the ventromedial prefrontal cortex show an impaired pattern of behavior consistent with dysfunction of the emotional signals (i.e., somatic markers). Whereas damage to other regions beyond the frontal lobes appears also to impair decision-making, the pattern of performance (in terms of selecting cards from "good" decks) is usually distinct from those ventromedial prefrontal patients. However, the Iowa Gambling Task is complex, and its administration differs between research groups in terms of factors such as reward contingencies and type of reward or punishment. Thus, interpretation of the overall support for the involvement of specific prefrontal regions in Iowa Gambling Task performance is difficult. Finally, there appears to be little evidence for specific decision-making impairments with age, as older adults either perform as well as younger adults on the Iowa Gambling Task, or fail for other reasons such as memory.

9.3 **Moral Decision-Making Task**

9.3.1 **Task description**

The Moral Decision-Making Task was initially developed to investigate the contributions of emotional and "controlled" cognition to moral reasoning and decision-making. In its original form, the participant is presented with a series of 60 dilemmas (Greene et al. 2001). A question follows each one, asking the participant whether they would endorse a suggested course of action, in order to resolve the dilemma, by simply answering yes or no. The scenarios typically fall into two categories: moral and non-moral. The action required to achieve the suggested resolution in moral scenarios varies in its severity, but will often require the participant to contravene personal moral boundaries (i.e., doing harm to other people). The value of the outcome is also manipulated (e.g., thousands of lives will be saved), providing various levels of conflict between the desire to observe personal moral boundaries, and to benefit the greater good. By contrast, non-moral scenarios contain no moral content, but rather present participants with both actions and outcomes that have low moral or emotive benefit or value.[2] In healthy participants, levels of endorsement typically decrease with the extremity of the personal moral violation required. Likewise, the response time taken to arrive at a decision increases with the level of conflict elicited between (i) the severity of the course of action required and (ii) the moral value of the potential outcome.

A further degree of distinction can be made within the moral category, whereby the type of action required is manipulated as either personal (e.g., causing direct physical harm to someone) or impersonal (e.g., pressing a switch or throwing a lever). However, studies vary in the way that they differentiate the various moral dilemma scenarios. Stories can be categorized in terms of high and low conflict based on reaction times (e.g., Greene et al. 2001), based on independent ratings of emotional salience (e.g., Koenigs et al. 2007), or in terms of the type of moral conflict induced (e.g., Kahane and Shackel 2008). Further variants include visual representations (Harrison et al. 2008), or short sentences or scenarios in which one must simply judge whether a moral violation has occurred (e.g., Moll et al. 2002a).

Example of a moral dilemma (low conflict) taken from the supplementary material of Koenigs et al. (2007):

> *You are visiting the sculpture garden of a wealthy art collector. The garden overlooks a valley containing a set of train tracks. A railway workman is working on the tracks, and an empty runaway trolley is heading down the tracks toward the workman. The only way to save the workman's life is to push one of the art collector's prized sculptures down into the valley so that it will roll onto the tracks and blocks the trolley's passage. Doing this will destroy the sculpture.*
>
> *Is it appropriate for you to destroy the sculpture in order to save this workman's life?*

Example moral dilemma (high conflict) taken from the supplementary material of Koenigs et al. (2007):

> *Enemy soldiers have taken over your village. They have orders to kill all remaining civilians. You and some of your townspeople have sought refuge in the cellar of a large house. Outside you hear the voices of the soldiers who have come to search the house for valuables. Your baby begins to cry loudly. You cover his mouth to block the sound. If you remove your hand from his mouth, his crying will summon the attention of the soldiers who will kill you, your child and the others hiding out in the cellar. To save yourself and the others, you must smother your child to death.*
>
> *Is it appropriate for you to smother your child in order to save yourself and the other townspeople?*

---

[2] Although responses to non-moral scenarios are not central to the frontal regional specificity of this test, it is important to note that some of the non-moral decisions are arguably not dilemmas at all (Kahane & Shackel 2008).

9.3.2 **Patient and lesion studies**

Lesion studies provide evidence to support the role of the ventromedial pre-frontal cortex in moral cognition (Ciaramelli et al. 2007; Koenigs et al. 2007; Moretti et al. 2009) (Table 9.9). In each study, groups with lesions primarily overlapping on the subgenual anterior cingulate cortex (BAs 24 and 32) and BAs 10, 11 and 12 were significantly more likely to endorse a utilitarian solu-tion to high-conflict moral dilemmas than were controls (Figure 9.6). In the Koenigs et al. (2007) paper, performance was compared to an additional brain-damaged control group comprising three with lateral prefrontal damage, one with dorsomedial prefrontal damage, and a further eight with non-frontal pathology (M. Koenigs, personal communication) whose scores did not differ from controls. However, neither of the other studies contained a control group that had lesions to other frontal lobe regions. A more recent study (Young et al. 2010) compared a ventromedial prefrontal lesion group with brain-damaged and healthy controls on a different task (in which participants had to judge the permissibility of an action, given the presence or absence of a protagonist's intention to do harm, and a harmful or neutral outcome). In direct contrast to the harsh judgment passed on protagonists who intended to cause harm by the control groups, the ventromedial prefrontal lesion group appeared to judge the moral permissibility of the scenario on the outcome, irrespective of the initial intention. Though the lesion control group had lesions outside the ven-tromedial prefrontal cortex, amygdala, insula and right somatosensory cortex,

Table 9.9 Moral Decision-Making: Patient and lesion studies

Study	n	Patient/ Control Groups	Study type	Task	Brodmann Areas	FP	DL	OF	ACC
Ciaramelli et al. (2007)	7; 12	VM[a]; HA	Lesion	Dilemmas	10, 12, 24, 32	✓		✓	✓
Koenigs et al. (2007)	6; 12; 12	VM[a]; BDC; HA	Lesion	Dilemmas	–		✓	✓	✓
Moretto et al. (2009)	8; 7; 18	VM[a]; BDC; HA	Lesion	Dilemmas	10, 11, 24, 32	✓		✓	✓
Grossman et al. (2010)	19; 19	fvFTD; HA	Patient (fMRI)	Social decisions	11			✓	
Young et al. (2010)	9; 7; 8	VM[a]; BDC; HA	Lesion	Judgments	–			✓	✓

FP = frontal pole; DL = dorsolateral prefrontal cortex; OF = orbitofrontal cortex; ACC = anterior cingulate cortex; VM = ventromedial prefrontal cortex; HA = healthy adults; BDC = brain damaged controls; fvFTD = frontal variant frontotemporal dementia; ✓ = frontal region damaged and impairment found; X = frontal region damaged but no impairment.

[a]Lesion predominantly involves medial OF and ventral ACC.

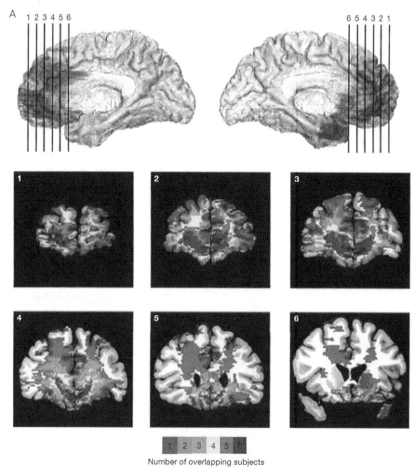

Fig. 9.6 Lesion overlaps in moral decision-making studies. (A) Reprinted by permission from Macmillan Publishers Ltd: *Nature* 446(7138), Michael Koenigs, Liane Young, Ralph Adolphs, Daniel Tranel, Fiery Cushman et al., Damage to the prefrontal cortex increases utilitarian moral judgements, pp. 908–911, Figure 1, Copyright, 2007, Nature Publishing Group. Please see color plate section. (B) This material was originally published in Elisa Ciaramelli, Michela Muccioli, Elisabetta Làdavas, and Giuseppe di Pellegrino, Selective deficit in personal moral judgment following damage to ventromedial prefrontal cortex, *Social Cognitive and Affective Neuroscience*, 2(2), pp. 84–92, Figure 1, doi: 10.1093/scan/nsm001, © 2007, Oxford University Press, and has been reproduced by permission of Oxford University Press. http://scan.oxfordjournals.org/content/2/2/84.full. For permission to reuse this material, please visit http://www.oup.co.uk/academic/rights/permissions. (C) Reproduced from Laura Moretti, Davide Dragone, and Giuseppe de Pellegrino, Reward and social valuation deficits following ventromedical prefontal damage, *Journal of Cognitive Neuroscience*, 21(1), pp. 128–140, Figure 1, © 2008 by the Massachusetts Institute of Technology. Reprinted by permission of MIT Press Journals. Please see color plate section.

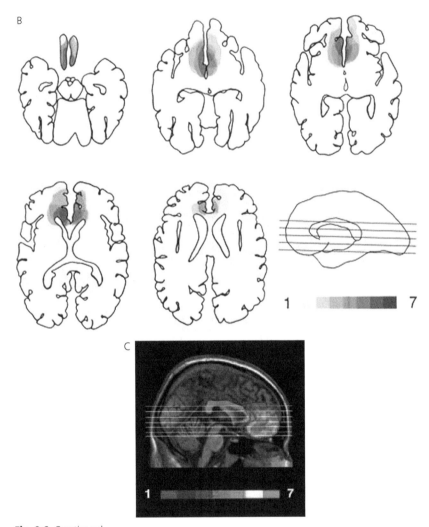

Fig. 9.6 Continued

there was no explicit dorsolateral prefrontal comparison group. Therefore, whereas there is replicated evidence from different research groups that lesions to the ventromedial prefrontal cortex disrupt the normal pattern of moral decision-making compared to healthy participants, evidence is still lacking regarding the specificity of the ventromedial prefrontal cortex as the only frontal region to yield this pattern of behavior. Therefore, replication of the data from Koenigs et al. showing patterns of performance related to dorsolateral prefrontal dysfunction is merited.

Further evidence to implicate the ventromedial prefrontal cortex in accurate moral judgment comes from patients with frontal variant frontotemporal dementia (fvFTD; Grossman et al. 2010). Participants were presented with brief social scenarios such as running a red light at 02:00 when either (i) driving a sick child to hospital or (ii) being observed by a police car. When compared to controls, the fvFTD group endorsed moral rule violations with a negatively valenced feature or outcome significantly more than controls, and showed atrophy in the ventromedial prefrontal regions that were activated when healthy participants performed the task.

The performance of clinical populations has also been examined using this paradigm. A recent study examined the neural correlates of moral decision-making in a group of 17 psychopaths of varying severity (Glenn et al. 2009). They found that individuals who were rated particularly highly on the interpersonal factor of psychopathy (i.e., callous and manipulative) exhibited a reduction in activation in the ventromedial prefrontal cortex during the moral decision-making scenarios developed by Greene et al. However, the absence of a control group makes it hard to generalize these neural correlates to a normal population. Moreover, the moral decisions made by the participants are not reported (and would be of little use without a control group for comparison), preventing interpretation of these findings in the context of behavior. In fact, another study comparing the pattern of responses in moral decision-making between psychopaths and controls reported that there was no difference in their moral judgments (Cima et al. 2010). Whereas this may suggest that emotional processes are not causal agents for normal performance on such tests, the functional differences reported by Glenn et al. may reflect the motivational state of participants (i.e., seeking to deceive versus giving honest responses) and the fact that controls and psychopaths may have been attempting explicitly to do different things, rather than reflecting an implicit difference in processing during moral decision-making.

9.3.3 Neuroimaging studies

Neuroimaging studies suggest that both the dorsolateral and ventromedial prefrontal cortices play a role in moral decision-making (Table 9.10). Greene et al. (2001) developed the original set of 60 moral reasoning scenarios in order to investigate their dual-process theory of moral judgments, whereby both emotional and controlled cognition are synthesized to guide moral reasoning and decision-making. Using fMRI in normal healthy participants, the authors reported the increased engagement of the medial prefrontal cortex (BA 9/10) and decreased activity of BA 46 during decision-making for moral–personal tasks when compared to moral–impersonal and non-moral conditions. This finding has been subsequently replicated (Greene et al. 2004). An increase in reaction times was also reported between judgments approving of personal harm to others compared to judgments that disapproved these actions, but a subsequent

Table 9.10 Moral Decision-Making: Neuroimaging studies

Study	n	Patient/ Control Groups	Study type	Task	Brodmann Areas	FP	DL	OF	ACC
Greene et al. (2001)	9	HA	fMRI	Dilemmas	9, 10				
Moll et al. (2002a)	7	HA	fMRI	Judgments	10, 11			✓	
Moll et al. (2002b)	7	HA	fMRI	Moral emotions	10, 11			✓	
Greene et al. (2004)	41	HA	fMRI	Dilemmas	9/10, 24				✓
Borg et al. (2006)	24	HA	fMRI	Dilemmas	10, 9/46	✓	✓		
Harenski and Hamann (2006)	10	HA	fMRI	Moral emotions	6, 9/10				
Pérez-Alvarez et al. (2006)	15	Adolescents	fMRI	Cartoons	10/11, 24/25/32			✓	✓
Young et al. (2007)		HA	fMRI	Moral per-missibility of scenarios	–			✓	✓
Harrison et al. (2008)	22	HA	fMRI	Cartoons	–			✓	✓
Prehn et al. (2008)	23	HA	fMRI	Judgments	10/11, 11/47			✓	
Pujol et al. (2008)	10	Adolescents	fMRI	Cartoons	9/10, 32				✓
Young and Saxe (2008a)	17	HA	fMRI	Moral per-missibility of scenarios	–			✓	✓
Young and Saxe (2008b)	14	HA	fMRI	Moral per-missibility of scenarios	–			✓	✓

FP = frontal pole; DL = dorsolateral prefrontal cortex; OF = orbitofrontal cortex; ACC = anterior cingulate cortex; HA = healthy adults; fMRI = functional magnetic resonance imaging; ✓ = frontal region involved.

re-analysis of the data suggests that this was primarily driven by very fast disapproval reaction times on a select few dilemmas (McGuire et al. 2009). Using moral dilemmas slightly different from those developed by Greene et al., Borg et al. (2006) have reported further replication of evidence suggesting two complementary moral decision networks. They compared moral dilemmas that were presented in either dramatic or muted languages, but were still based on standard philosophical scenarios, and non-moral scenarios that involved destruction of personal objects rather than non-moral unpleasant stimuli or semantic improprieties (Borg et al. 2006). The authors reported that the ventromedial prefrontal regions were more active during elevated moral content, whereas dorsolateral prefrontal regions were preferentially recruited for non-moral decisions. In addition, they observed that whereas the dorsolateral prefrontal cortex was more active during moral scenarios where individuals had to process the numerical consequences of their actions, the orbitofrontal cortex was activated when processing the intention of doing harm to others, along with the right middle frontal gyrus (BA 8). Similarly, Moll et al. (2002a) reported that the ventromedial prefrontal cortex was also activated during the judgment of emotionally charged moral sentences, whereas only the lateral orbitofrontal cortex was recruited during evocative non-moral scenarios. This region has also been implicated in processing morally salient images (Moll et al. 2002b; Harenski and Hamann 2006).

Greene et al. (2004) reported activation of the anterior cingulate cortex (BA 32) during decision-making in higher-conflict scenarios. A large body of evidence suggests a role for the anterior cingulate cortex in conflict processing. Its connections with both the dorsolateral prefrontal cortex and orbitofrontal cortex (e.g., Beckmann et al. 2009), and its involvement in sensitivity to social pain (Etkin et al. 2006) are consonant with the dual process theory of moral decision-making, whereby cingulate activity reflects the high conflict between dorsal and orbital processing of information in a given scenario. Two more recent studies developed cartoons based on the original scenarios, reporting that the ventromedial prefrontal area (including the ventral anterior cingulate cortex) was significantly more active while judging emotional situations when compared to non-emotional situations; this contrasted with increased dorsolateral prefrontal activation in the non-emotional condition (Perez-Alvarez et al. 2006; Pujol et al. 2008).[3] Another study which involved judging vignettes based on difficult/personal moral dilemmas also reported significant ventromedial prefrontal activation (including the ventral anterior cingulate cortex), although the activations were compared with a resting state rather than with impersonal or non-moral stories (Harrison et al. 2008).

Using a slightly different task, in which participants had to judge whether or not a social norm had been violated based on a two-sentence passage, the involvement of both the dorsolateral and ventromedial prefrontal cortex in moral decision-making was replicated (Prehn et al. 2008). The authors

---

[3] It is important to note that both of these studies were examining activations in adolescents, and therefore may not be fully representative of adult neural responses.

reported that higher dorsolateral prefrontal recruitment was associated with poorer accuracy in identifying social violations. However, they also reported that over-recruitment of the left ventromedial prefrontal cortex tended to be associated with lower moral judgment competence, which is at odds with the previously reported data.

The consistent reporting of involvement of the ventromedial prefrontal cortex in moral decision-making has been explored in further detail, by manipulating when and how key details of the scenario are presented to participants (Young et al. 2007; Young and Saxe 2008a, 2008b). During this task, participants are presented with scenarios in which an ambiguous moral action is described in segments (background; the neutral or negative intention of the protagonist; outcome describing a neutral or negative result). The participant is then asked to rate the moral permissibility of the protagonist's behavior. Thus, this task requires participants to integrate information about the intentions of others (i.e., theory of mind) with the factual background and outcome to arrive at a moral judgment. Whereas other non-frontal regions (i.e., the temporo-parietal junction and precuneus) were activated during the integration of relevant factual, theory of mind, and moral information, the ventromedial prefrontal cortex was significantly more active when the morally relevant feature of the suggested action was displayed.

Thus, most of the published functional imaging literature appears to support the idea of two cognitive streams occupying mutually competing roles in our moral decision-making. Whereas the dorsolateral prefrontal cortex's contribution to moral decision-making represents the exertion of controlled cognitive processes, the ventromedial prefrontal processes more implicit emotional responses. This dual contribution is ostensibly supported by the findings that increased cognitive load exerts a selective interference effect by increasing utilitarian-style decision-making (Greene et al. 2008). However, in apparent contradiction, Shenhav and Greene (2010) report that participants exhibiting a more utilitarian profile are associated with *increased* activation in the orbitofrontal cortex, specifically in lateral areas (Figure 9.7). As the authors note, this contradiction may be reconciled by the differences between the experimental tasks, as well as the way the data are analyzed: whereas in previous studies, participants are required to make a concrete yes/no judgment about the acceptability of a suggested action, Shenhav and Greene's study was designed to examine the economics of moral decisions by systematically varying the moral value of action/inaction in the context of variable probabilities of risk. They suggest that this could reflect differences in the way the scenario variables are manipulated, therefore representing a different task demand.

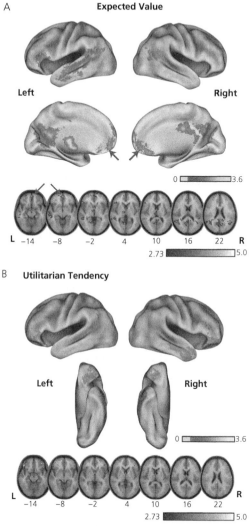

Fig. 9.7 Utilitarian responses in Moral Decision-Making studies. Top panel: network whose activation increases linearly with value of expected outcome. Ventromedial prefrontal activation (arrows) sensitive to the "expected moral value" is reported in several studies of economic decision-making. Bottom panel: regions demonstrating increased BOLD activation with increased tendency towards utilitarian responses. Reprinted from *Neuron*, 67 (4), Amitai Shenhav and Joshua D. Greene, Moral Judgments Recruit Domain-General Valuation Mechanisms to Integrate Representations of Probability and Magnitude, pp. 667–77, Figure 3, Copyright (2010), with permission from Elsevier. Please see color plate section.

Table 9.11 Moral Decision-Making: Aging studies

Study	n	Participant age groups (years)	Study type	Task	Age effect
Moran et al. (2012)	31; 17	Younger, mean = 23.0 Older, mean = 71.8	Cross-sectional (neuroimaging)	Moral permissibility of scenarios	✓

✓ = age effect found; X = age effect not found

9.3.4 Aging studies

To our knowledge, there are no studies that have directly assessed the effects of age on the moral decision-making task (Greene et al. 2001). However, Moran et al. (2012) administered a moral judgment task (Young et al. 2007 described above) to 31 younger and 17 older adults while inside the fMRI scanner. Older adults' ratings of action permissibility appeared to use less information about the actors' intentions than younger adults' ratings. In other words, older adults were less inclined to blame actors for their negative intentions if the outcome was neutral, and more likely to blame actors for a negative outcome if their intentions were neutral when compared to their younger counterparts. The authors then examined participants' BOLD responses, contrasting activity when judging scenarios with neutral intention and negative outcome against activity when judging scenarios with neutral intention/neutral outcome. Older adults showed significantly reduced activation in the ventromedial prefrontal cortex (mainly ventral anterior cingulate cortex) and medial frontopolar cortex than the younger group (Table 9.11).

9.3.5 Summary

The extant data on this task appear supportive of the dual process theory of moral decision-making, whereby both dorsolateral and ventromedial prefrontal regions make discrete processing contributions. Functional neuroimaging indicates that ventromedial prefrontal activity is related to the emotional valence of actions related to harming others, whereas dorsolateral prefrontal activity is related to dilemmas that place importance on numerical and rule-based information. Conflict between these mutually competing cognitive streams is thought to be instantiated in the anterior cingulate cortex, consistent with its hypothesized role in conflict processing from this and other experimental paradigms. Lesion studies are also generally supportive of this view, with damage to the orbital and ventral cingulate regions resulting in more utilitarian decision-making. It would follow that dorsolateral prefrontal lesions would result in the converse pattern of decisions, yet there is a distinct absence of large, well-characterized dorsolateral lesion groups. Hence, this task has potential sensitivity to frontal pathology through divergent profiles of moral decision-making, but further empirical research is fundamentally required. Moreover, it remains unclear to what extent lesions to the ventral anterior cingulate cortex and orbitofrontal cortex differentially affect moral decision-making performance, and future studies should examine the performance of patients with clearly localized lesions in these brain areas. It may also well be the case that reciprocal ventral anterior cingulate-orbitofrontal cortex reciprocal connectivity must remain intact, but identifying a suitably well-powered sample to test this directly would be highly challenging. Age effects on this specific task are lacking, though there appear to be age-related effects on the more complex Young et al. (2007) task, suggesting subtle alterations in the way that factual, moral, and theory of mind information are integrated, which is reflected in a reduced task-related ventromedial prefrontal BOLD response in older adults.

9.4 **Ultimatum Game**

9.4.1 **Task description**

The Ultimatum Game is a task widely used as a measure of economic decision-making. Participants are told that a proposer will share a certain amount of money with them (e.g., £10) and that they can choose either to accept or reject the offer. If the respondent accepts the offer (e.g., £8 to the proposer: £2 to the respondent), the money will be divided as proposed. If, instead, the respondent rejects the offer, neither player will receive anything (Figure 9.8).

Economically rational performance on the task predicts that even when the proposer offers the smallest amount of money, the respondent should accept it. However, research has shown that offers to the respondent that are <20–30% of the total amount are often rejected, and that rejection rates increase as offers become more "unfair" (Guth et al. 1982; Bolton and Zwick 1995; Nowak et al.

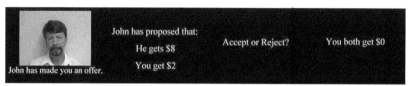

Fig. 9.8 Schematic representation of the Ultimatum Game. Reprinted from Michael Koenigs and Daniel Tranel, Irrational economic decision-making after ventromedial prefrontal damage: evidence from the Ultimatum Game, *The Journal of Neuroscience*: the official journal of the Society for Neuroscience, 27(4), pp. 951–956. doi: 10.1523/JNEUROSCI.4606-06.2007. © 2007, The Society for Neuroscience.

2000). Participants are thought to reject offers due to the negative emotions elicited by unfair offers, and, by rejecting these unfair offers, participants seem to believe that they are punishing the proposer (Blount et al. 1995; Pillutla et al. 1996; Bosman et al. 2001).

9.4.2 Patient and lesion studies

Neuropsychological research has examined localization within the frontal lobes of the processes associated with performing the Ultimatum Game (Table 9.12). Koenigs and Tranel (2007) assessed the performance of patients with ventromedial prefrontal lesions, patients with non-ventromedial prefrontal lesions, and healthy controls performing the Ultimatum Game. The non-ventromedial prefrontal group included patients with lesions in the dorsolateral prefrontal cortex, superior mesial prefrontal cortex, lateral temporal, or thalamic regions. No significant difference was found between the patient and control groups in terms of their acceptance of fair offers. However, ventromedial prefrontal patients accepted a smaller proportion of unfair offers compared to the non-ventromedial prefrontal and healthy control groups. The authors suggest that the higher rejection of unfair offers is due to the ventromedial prefrontal patients' inability to modulate their anger when such offers are presented. However, Koenigs and Tranel (2007) did not directly investigate their participants' emotional responses to the offers.

An alternative explanation for the higher rejection rate for unfair offers is reduced sensitivity to the financial benefit of the offer regardless of the amount, in line with previous studies indicating the role played by the

Table 9.12 Ultimatum Game: Patient and lesion studies

Study	n	Patient/ Control Groups	Study type	Condition	Brodmann Areas	FP	DL	OF	ACC
Koenigs and Tranel (2007)	7; 14; 14	VM; non-VM; HA	Lesion	Unfair offers:	10, 11, 25, 32	✓		✓	✓
Krajbich et al. (2009)	6; 20; 16	VM; non-VM; HA	Lesion		10, 11, 25, 32	✓		✓	✓
Moretti et al. (2009)	7; 6; 14	VM; non-frontal; HA	Lesion	Unfair offers, no cash:	10, 11, 12, 24, 32	✓		✓	✓
				Unfair offers, with cash:		✓		✓	✓

FP = frontal pole; DL = dorsolateral prefrontal cortex; OF = orbitofrontal cortex; ACC = anterior cingulate cortex; ✓ = frontal region damaged and impairment found; X = frontal region damaged but no impairment.

ventromedial prefrontal cortex in the representation of rewards (O'Doherty et al. 2001). Moretti et al. (2009) compared the performance of patients with ventromedial prefrontal damage, patients with damage outside the frontal cortex, and healthy controls on three versions of the Ultimatum Game in which offers were made by a human partner (human opponent with no cash), a computer (computer opponent), or by a human partner who offered actual cash (human opponent with cash). In line with the results reported by Koenings et al. (2007), the ventromedial prefrontal patients accepted fewer offers than the non-ventromedial prefrontal and healthy control groups in both the human opponent with no cash and computer opponent conditions. Within the ventromedial prefrontal group, patients were more likely to accept an unfair offer in the human opponent with cash condition than in the human opponent with no cash condition. No significant difference in the acceptance rate emerged between the human opponent with no cash and the computer opponent condition. By contrast, the healthy controls accepted more offers in the computer opponent condition than the human opponent without cash condition, but there was no difference between the acceptance of human opponent with and without cash unfair offers. There were no significant differences in the acceptance rates of the three conditions in the non-ventromedial prefrontal group. This difference in rejection rates for offers made by a human and a computer in healthy individuals has been interpreted as a reaction to social unfairness from human partners (Blount 1995; Sanfey et al. 2003; Rilling et al. 2004). This does not occur in ventromedial prefrontal patients, as they do not differ in their acceptance rates in the human and computer opponent conditions. Furthermore, the subjective judgments of anger and fairness of the ventromedial prefrontal group in relation to each offer did not differ from those of healthy controls and non-ventromedial prefrontal groups: this speaks against the view that ventromedial prefrontal patients reject more offers because they feel angrier when presented with unfair offers. The stronger skin conductance responses to unfair offers compared to fair offers in healthy adults contrasted with the similar responses to fair and unfair offers in ventromedial prefrontal patients, and confirms that these patients do not overreact to unfairness. The finding that ventromedial prefrontal patients accepted more offers when real money was used further suggests that ventromedial prefrontal patients do not overreact to unfair offers; rather their rejection depended on whether the offer was visible and immediately attainable. Taken as a whole, it seems that control individuals' motivation is related to the intentionality of the opponent (i.e., unfair offers intentionally made by humans). By contrast, ventromedial prefrontal patients instead seem to rely more on immediate gains and losses.

Ventromedial prefrontal damage has also been related to impaired processing of social emotions, such as guilt. Krajbich et al. (2009) used a version of the Ultimatum Game that instructed participants to play a one-shot version of the task where they had to divide 50 points. They played the game twice, once as the proposer and once as the respondent. As the proposer, participants were asked how much they would offer: offering more than zero would be interpreted as a consequence of guilt. As the responder, participants were asked to indicate the minimum amount they would demand in order to accept the offer. A feeling of guilt would emerge if there were a tendency to offer more than they would be expected to be offered themselves. The ventromedial prefrontal group did not offer less or demand more than the controls. However, whereas controls showed that they would offer more than their minimum acceptable offer, ventromedial prefrontal lesion patients did not offer more than they demanded themselves. These results have been interpreted as a reduction in the feeling of guilt in the ventromedial prefrontal patients, which leads them to offer no more than what they would demand.

Further support for the involvement of the ventromedial prefrontal cortex in the acceptance of unfair offers comes from a study investigating performance on the Ultimatum Game in a group of psychopaths (Koenigs et al. 2010). The authors proposed that primary psychopathy emerges due to a deficit in affective and attentional processing that may also underlie the deficit in ventromedial prefrontal functioning (Barrash et al. 2000; Anderson et al. 2006). The results of this study revealed that primary psychopaths accepted fewer unfair offers than healthy controls. When the patients' performance was compared with previously published data (Koenigs and Tranel 2007; Krajbich et al. 2009), it appeared that primary psychopaths performed similarly to ventromedial prefrontal patients on the Ultimatum Game, supporting the view that damage to the ventromedial prefrontal cortex reduces the acceptance rate of unfair offers.

9.4.3 Neuroimaging studies

Neuroimaging studies have reported activation of both the ventromedial and dorsolateral prefrontal cortex during Ultimatum Game performance (Table 9.13). In one such study, Tabibnia et al. (2008) conducted an fMRI study of healthy participants playing a stake version of the Ultimatum Game. The possible outcome for the participant was the same in fair and unfair conditions, but the total amount available to the proposer was varied to seem more fair (e.g., seven out of 15 offered) versus more unfair (e.g., seven out of 23 offered). The fMRI results showed greater ventromedial prefrontal activity associated with offers perceived as more fair compared to more unfair. Greater

Table 9.13 Ultimatum Game: Neuroimaging studies

Study	n	Patient/ Control Groups	Study type	Condition	Brodmann Areas	FP	DL	OF	ACC
Sanfey et al. (2003)	19	HA	fMRI	Unfair offers:	–		✓		✓
Rilling et al. (2004)	19	HA	fMRI		8, 9, 32				✓
van't Wout et al. (2005)	7	HA	rTMS	Unfair offers:	–		✓		
Knoch et al. (2006)	52	HA	rTMS	Unfair offers:	–		✓		
Tabibnia et al. (2008)	12	HA	fMRI	Fair offers:	–	✓		✓	
Harlé and Sanfey (2012)	18; 20	YA; OA	fMRI	Unfair offers:	–		✓		

FP = frontal pole; DL = dorsolateral prefrontal cortex; OF = orbitofrontal cortex; ACC = anterior cingulate cortex; HA = healthy adults; fMRI = functional magnetic resonance imaging; rTMS = repetitive transcranial magnetic stimulation; YO = younger adults; OA = older adults; ✓ = frontal region involved.

ventrolateral prefrontal activation accompanied by reduced activation of the anterior insula was also observed when accepting an unfair offer, suggesting that the ventrolateral prefrontal cortex modulates the negative emotions elicited by unfair offers, leading to acceptance of the offer.

Unfair offers have also been associated with greater activation in the dorsolateral prefrontal cortex in healthy younger (Sanfey et al. 2003; Rilling et al. 2004) as well as older adults (Harlé and Sanfey 2012). In Sanfey et al. (2003), 19 healthy adults underwent fMRI while they performed the Ultimatum Game against a human partner or with a computer. In line with previous studies, participants accepted all fair offers and the rejection rate of low offers increased as the offers became more unfair. Moreover, the rejection of unfair offers was higher for offers made by the human than by the computer opponent, indicating that participants had a stronger emotional response to unfairness when they played with a human than with a computer partner. In terms of the neuroimaging results, increased activation of the dorsolateral prefrontal cortex and the insula was reported for unfair compared to fair offers. However, whereas the strength of activation in the insula correlated with the rejection rate of unfair offers, the dorsolateral prefrontal activation was constant across all unfair offers. Dorsolateral prefrontal activation has also been associated with the maintenance of the cognitive goals of a given task (see Section 4.1, Goal

Neglect), in this case accepting as much money as possible. Activation of the insula, instead, was related to the negative emotions elicited by the unfair offer, a notion consistent with previous studies that have shown activation of the insula during the evaluation and representation of negative emotions (Calder et al. 2001). Insula activation increased as offers became more unfair, and participants with stronger activation of the anterior insula rejected a higher proportion of unfair offers. These results indicate that the final decision on whether to accept an offer depends on the relative activation of both the dorsolateral prefrontal cortex and the anterior insula, with greater insula activation over the dorsolateral prefrontal cortex leading to the rejection of an unfair offer, whereas greater dorsolateral prefrontal activity over the insula results in the acceptance of an unfair offer. Tabibnia et al. (2008) showed a similar relationship between the lateral prefrontal areas and the insula during Ultimatum Game performance. However, unlike Sanfey et al. (2003), Tabibnia et al. (2008) found greater ventrolateral prefrontal activation when accepting unfair offers. This result suggests that the dorsolateral and the ventrolateral prefrontal cortex play different roles when individuals are presented with unfair offers: the dorsolateral prefrontal cortex may be involved in maintaining the task goal (i.e., earning as much money as possible); the ventrolateral prefrontal cortex is thought to be involved in moderating the negative emotion elicited by unfair offers.

The central role for the dorsolateral prefrontal cortex in the Ultimatum Game has also been demonstrated in studies showing that Ultimatum Game performance is affected by the temporary disruption of the dorsolateral prefrontal cortex (van't Wout et al. 2005; Knoch et al. 2006). For example, Knoch et al. (2006) found that, following repetitive transcranial magnetic stimulation (rTMS) application over the right dorsolateral prefrontal cortex, participants accepted a greater proportion of unfair offers. Despite these behavioral results, the subjective judgments of fairness for each offer did not change after rTMS compared to sham conditions, suggesting that the dorsolateral prefrontal cortex is involved in the ability to implement fair behavior, and that after its disruption, the decision is guided by the goal of accepting as much money as possible.

9.4.4 Aging studies

At present, only a few studies have investigated the effect of age on the Ultimatum Game and the results are contradictory (Table 9.14). Some studies found that the rejection of low offers increases as people become older (Beadle 2009; Harlé and Sanfey 2012; Roalf et al. 2012) and show that the final decision to accept or reject an offer might depend on the ability to empathize. For example,

Table 9.14 Ultimatum Game: Aging studies

Study	*n*	Participant age groups (years)	Study type	Age effect
Nguyen et al. (2011)	129	26–88	Cross-sectional (behavioral)	X
Beadle et al. (2012)	40; 40	24–45; 55–81	Cross-sectional (behavioral)	✓
Harlé and Sanfey (2012)	18; 20	18–27; 55–78	Cross-sectional (neuroimaging)	✓
Roalf et al. (2012)	29; 30	21–45; 65–85	Cross-sectional (behavioral)	✓
Bailey et al. (2013)	35; 37	18–33; 65–92	Cross-sectional (behavioral)	✓

✓ = age effect found; X = age effect not found

Beadle et al. (2012) found that older adults with a high level of empathy were more likely than young participants with high empathy to reject unfair offers. The researchers suggest that the effect of empathy on behavior depends on different motivations. For example, empathy in economic decision-making might be used to benefit either the self or others: in this study, older participants with high empathy would maximize their own benefit by rejecting unfair offers. By contrast, high empathy in younger participants would enhance their prosocial behavior towards others (Beadle et al. 2012). A recent fMRI study showed that older adults accepted fewer low offers of $3 out of $10 than younger adults, whereas no age differences emerged on the acceptance of equal division of money ($5) and low offers of $2 and $1 (Harlé and Sanfey 2012). These findings indicate that age affects the acceptance of the intermediate offers, thought to be moderately unfair, whereas no age effect emerged for the most unfair offers. The behavioral performance was accompanied by greater dorsolateral prefrontal activation for all unfair offers in older adults compared to young participants, suggesting that older participants rely more than younger adults on the cognitive processes associated with decision-making (e.g., goal maintenance, the processing of game rules) to compensate for the cognitive decline that occurs as people age.

Other researchers explain the age effect on the Ultimatum Game in terms of emotion regulation. For example, Bailey et al. (2012) administered the Ultimatum Game to a group of younger and older adults. In this task, the age of the proposers was also manipulated. At the end of the task, the participants rated their anger in relation to each offer made. Both younger and older felt angrier to low offers made by a younger than by an older proposer. Yet, only young participants rejected more unfair offers made by a young person. This result suggests that the ability to regulate negative emotions (as those elicited by unfair offers) is enhanced as people become older. A final aging study using the classic Ultimatum Game, however, showed that age did not affect the acceptance rate of fair and unfair offers (Nguyen et al. 2011).

These contradictory results might be explained in terms of the different methodologies employed. For example, the participants in Bailey et al. (2012) were first instructed to make offers to future participants. Participants were told that if their offers were included in a future study and were accepted, they would be paid accordingly. As noted by the researchers, the type of offers made (e.g., fair or unfair) might have affected the willingness to accept monetary divisions in the role of respondents. Beadle (2009) and Beadle et al. (2012) employed the Repeated Fixed Opponent Ultimatum Game. In this task, participants play against the same opponent across all trials, whereas, in the classic Ultimatum Game, the opponents change from trial to trial. It has been claimed that when participants interact with the same player, it is necessary to show that they will not accept low offers (Nowak 2000). Therefore, the higher rejection of low offers in the older group might be due to older adults being more inclined than younger participants to make it clear that they will not accept unfair treatment. Finally, Nguyen et al. (2011) found that personality-related factors (e.g., Big Five) but not cognitive (e.g., intelligence) and demographic (e.g., age, education) variables discriminated between the performance of rational and irrational participants (e.g., accepting any type of offer or rejecting low unfair offers, respectively) on the classic Ultimatum Game. The researcher, however, did not compare the performance of younger and older participants.

9.4.5 Summary

Lesion and neuroimaging studies have shown that both the ventromedial prefrontal cortex and the dorsolateral prefrontal cortex are involved in Ultimatum Game performance. The dorsolateral prefrontal cortex is related to the ability to implement a sense of fairness, expressed by the higher rejection of unfair offers. The ventromedial prefrontal cortex, however, is involved in representing the value of the reward, and damage to this region is associated with reduced sensitivity to the value of the reward.

Chapter 10

Theory of mind

10.1 Animations Task

10.1.1 Task description

The Animations Task is a computer-based task that assesses an individual's ability to attribute mental states to moving geometric shapes (e.g., a large red triangle and a small blue triangle moving around a white background) based on their silent interaction (see Figure 10.1; Abell et al. 2000; Castelli et al. 2000, 2002). The task is based on the early work of Heider and Simmel (1944), which demonstrated that the movement of simple shapes was sufficient to allow individuals to attribute complex mental states such as intentions and beliefs. It is the movement and the interaction between the stimuli rather than the stimuli themselves that are central to the ability to make these complex attributions (Berry et al. 1992; Berry and Springer 1993). Each animation involves either a complex theory of mind interaction, in which one shape reacts to another shape's mental state (e.g., teasing, coaxing), a simpler goal-directed interaction that does not require "mind reading" (e.g., dancing together, chasing one another) or random actions in which the two shapes do not interact (e.g., floating around). In the theory of mind interaction, participants are told that the shapes refer to people (e.g., grandmother and grandson); in the goal-directed interaction, participants are told that the shapes refer to animals (e.g., mother duck and duckling); and in the random actions, the shapes are simply referred to as shapes (e.g., triangles). The animations last between 34 and 45 s, and, after each one, participants have to provide an explanation of what is happening in the interaction (verbal descriptions) or choose the correct description from a possible four descriptions that best describes the shapes' movement (multiple choice; see Box 10.1 for examples). The detailed scoring criteria for verbal descriptions are provided in Abell et al. (2000), and examples of the animations can be viewed online at https://sites.google.com/site/utafrith/research#TOC-Tasks-to-probe-intuitive-mentalisin. The verbal descriptions do not require participants to provide complex narratives in order to achieve high scores on the task (Castelli et al. 2002).

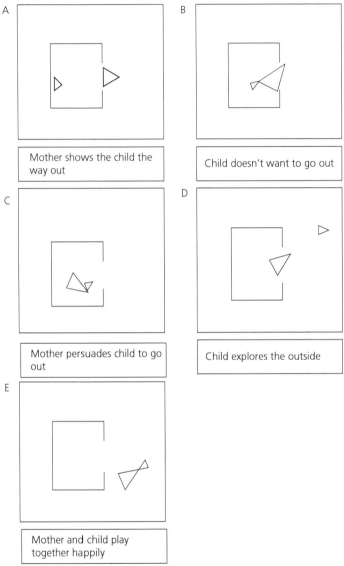

Fig. 10.1 Example of a theory of mind animation in which the big triangle is coaxing the little triangle to come out of a pen. The captions are not presented during the actual task. Reprinted from *NeuroImage*, 12 (3), Fulvia Castelli, Francesca Happé, Uta Frith, and Chris Frith, Movement and Mind: A Functional Imaging Study of Perception and Interpretation of Complex Intentional Movement Patterns, pp. 314–325, Appendix 3 Copyright (2000), with permission from Elsevier.

Box 10.1 Examples of the correct and lure descriptions for a theory of mind animation and a goal-directed animation

Theory of mind animation

Correct: Red encourages Blue to go out (theory of mind description)
Lure 1: Red barges Blue out (goal-directed description)
Lure 2: Blue skips out past Red (goal-directed description)
Lure 3: Red and Blue are moving around aimlessly (random movement description)

Goal-directed animation

Correct: Red and Blue are fighting (goal-directed description)
Lure 1: Blue is offended by Red (theory of mind description)
Lure 2: Blue is chasing Red (goal-directed description)
Lure 3: Red and Blue are moving around aimlessly (random movement description)

Data from Chris M. Bird, Fulvia Castelli, Omar Malik, Uta Frith, and Masud Husain, The impact of extensive medial frontal lobe damage on "Theory of Mind" and cognition, *Brain*, 127(4), pp. 914–928, doi:10.1093/brain/awh108, 2004.

10.1.2 Patient and lesion studies

Much of the literature examining the localization of the processes associated with performing the Animations Task has involved neuroimaging. The only lesion study to examine performance on the Animations Task is that of Bird et al. (2004) (Table 10.1). The authors administered a range of theory of mind tests to patient GT, who had a lesion involving the orbital and medial frontal regions due to a bilateral infarction in the anterior cerebral artery. When GT performed the multiple choice version of the Animations Task, she was not impaired compared to healthy controls at identifying the theory of mind or the goal-directed animations. However, as GT's lesion did not involve the entire ventromedial prefrontal cortex and her performance was not compared to brain damaged controls, this study on its own is not adequate to conclude that the ventromedial prefrontal cortex is not necessary for successful performance on the Animations Task, nor whether other frontal regions might be necessary. Further neuropsychological work is needed.

10.1.3 Neuroimaging studies

By contrast with the lesion studies, several neuroimaging studies have examined the neural correlates of the Animations Task (Table 10.2). One of the first

Table 10.1 Animations Task: Patient and lesion studies

Study	n	Patient/ Control Groups	Study type	Brodmann Areas	FP	DL	OF	ACC
Bird et al. (2004)	1	ACA	Lesion (single case)	–			X	X

FP = frontal pole; DL = dorsolateral prefrontal cortex; OF = orbitofrontal cortex; ACC = anterior cingulate cortex; ACA = anterior cerebral artery infarct; ✓ = frontal region damaged and impairment found; X = frontal region damaged but no impairment.

Table 10.2 Animations Task: Neuroimaging studies

Study	n	Patient/ Control Groups	Study type	Brodmann Areas	FP	DL	OF	ACC
Castelli et al. (2000)	6	HA	PET	9				
Gobbini et al. (2007)	12	HA	fMRI	8, 9, 45				
Castelli et al. (2002)	10; 10	Autistic; HA	PET	9				
Martin and Weisberg (2003)	12	HA	fMRI	–			✓	✓
Kana et al. (2009)	12; 12	Autistic; HA	fMRI	8, 9, 13, 45			✓	

FP = frontal pole; DL = dorsolateral prefrontal cortex; OF = orbitofrontal cortex; ACC = anterior cingulate cortex; HA = healthy adults; PET = positron emission tomography; fMRI = functional magnetic resonance imaging; ✓ = frontal region involved.

studies was a positron emission tomography (PET) study by Castelli et al. (2000) in which six male volunteers were scanned during the presentation of 12 animations (four involving theory of mind animations, four involving goal-directed movement, and four random actions). After scanning, participants were asked to describe verbally what they thought was happening in each animation and the descriptions were scored in terms of mental state appreciation (the use of mental states in the explanation), appropriateness (how well the underlying story was understood), certainty of the explanation (the degree of hesitation in the explanation) and length (the number of phrases in the explanation). Participants attributed more intentionality to—and provided longer explanations for—the theory of mind animations compared to the goal-directed and random ones, but there was no difference in the appropriateness or certainty scores. In terms of regional cerebral blood flow, when the theory of mind animations were contrasted with the random ones, bilateral activity was found in the dorsomedial prefrontal cortex (Brodmann Area (BA) 9), as well as the temporoparietal junction (BA 22/39), the fusiform gyrus (BA 37), the temporal poles (BA 38) and the occipital gyrus (BA 19/18). Contrasting the theory of mind animations with the goal-directed ones resulted in activation of the same brain regions but to a lesser degree. The goal-directed versus random contrast was not reported. This was one of the first studies to suggest that the medial prefrontal cortex plays a role in understanding both simple and complex inner states portrayed through the animation of shapes. In a functional magnetic resonance imaging (fMRI) study, Gobbini et al. (2007) compared regional patterns of brain activation associated with the Animations Task and the Theory of Mind Stories (see Section 10.6). When the results of the theory of mind animations versus random actions baseline and the false belief stories versus physical stories baseline contrasts were compared, there was activity in the dorsal anterior cingulate (BA 9) but with only minimal overlap, as well as activating the supplementary motor area (BA 8), the temporal pole (BA 38), the middle and inferior temporal gyri (BA 37), the posterior cingulate cortex/precuneus (BA 7), and the inferior parietal lobule (BA 40). In addition, the Animations Task contrast revealed activation in the frontal operculum (BA 45), the superior temporal sulcus (BA 22) and the fusiform gyrus (BA 37), whereas the Theory of Mind Stories activated the superior (BA 9), middle (BA 44) and inferior frontal gyri (BA 47), and the temporoparietal junction (BA 39). The authors concluded that whereas some medial prefrontal activation was associated with the Animations Task, distinct patterns of activity were associated with these different mentalizing tasks.

Several neuroimaging studies have administered the Animations Task to individuals with high-functioning autism/Asperger syndrome. In a PET study with 10 individuals with autism/Asperger syndrome and 10 healthy controls matched in terms of verbal (the Quick test, Ammons and Ammons 1962) and non-verbal (Ravens Standard Progressive Matrices; Ravens 1958) abilities, Castelli et al. (2002) reported common activation in the dorsomedial prefrontal cortex (BA 9), the left inferior temporal gyrus (BA 37), left anterior fusiform gyrus (BA 20), right temporal pole (BA 38), and bilaterally in the superior temporal sulcus (BAs 21/22 and 22) and inferior occipital gyrus (BA 18) in both groups when the theory of mind animations were contrasted with the random actions). However, accompanying their significantly fewer and less appropriate mental state descriptions, the autistic group showed reduced activation compared to controls in all these regions (including the medial prefrontal cortex) except the left inferior temporal gyrus and bilateral inferior occipital gyrus.

The autism/Asperger syndrome group did not significantly differ from controls in their goal-directed or random action descriptions. In an fMRI study involving forced choice judgments (i.e., correct mental state response, incorrect mental state response, incorrect goal-directed response, and incorrect random action response) during scanning rather than the passive animation viewing adopted by Castelli et al. (2002), Kana et al. (2009) also reported reduced activation in the medial prefrontal cortex, as well as the anterior paracingulate cortex, anterior cingulate gyrus, and inferior orbital frontal gyrus in autistic individuals compared to healthy controls. Again, the autism and healthy control groups were matched in terms of their verbal and non-verbal abilities. Castelli et al. (2002) and Kana et al. (2009) propose that reduced functional connectivity between the medial prefrontal cortex and more posterior brain regions underlies the difficulties in attributing mental states found in autistic individuals.

To address whether the brain activation associated with the theory of mind and goal-directed animations does indeed reflect social interaction understanding rather than general problem-solving, Martin and Weisberg (2003) devised animations involving social interactions (e.g., dancing, playing, sharing) and mechanical interactions (e.g., bowling, a conveyor belt, pinball). During fMRI, 12 healthy participants were presented with the social and mechanical interactions. After each presentation, participants had to select the action depicted by the animation from four possible options. The results revealed that the right ventromedial prefrontal cortex (although more dorsally than Castelli et al. 2000, 2002), bilateral anterior and superior temporal sulcus, bilateral fusiform gyrus, and right amygdala were activated during the social but not mechanical interactions, providing further support that the medial prefrontal cortex activation is important for understanding social interactions depicted through animations.

10.1.4 Aging studies

To our knowledge, there is only one published study that has examined the influence of healthy adult aging on performance on the Animations Task (Moran et al. 2012) (Table 10.3). Thirty-one younger adults with a mean age of 23.0 years and 17 older adults with a mean age of 71.8 years performed three mentalizing tasks in the fMRI scanner: the Animations Task (Martin and Weisberg 2003), the Moral

Table 10.3 Animations Task: Aging studies

Study	n	Participant age groups (years)	Study type	Age effect
Moran et al. (2012)	31; 17	Younger, mean = 23.0 Older, mean = 71.8	Cross-sectional (neuroimaging)	Not reported

✓ = age effect found; X = age effect not found

Judgment task (Young et al., 2007), and the False Belief task (Zaitchik 1990; Saxe and Kanwisher 2003). When examining the age-related neural correlates of the Animations Task, the theory of mind > mechanical animations contrast revealed that younger adults activated the same brain regions as the original Martin and Weisberg (2003) study (i.e., the medial prefrontal cortex, bilateral inferior frontal gyrus, anterior superior temporal sulcus, bilateral temporoparietal junction, and precuneus). However, in older adults, only the right inferior frontal gyrus and temporal pole, bilateral temporoparietal junction, and precuneus were activated. Further, a direct contrast between younger and older adults performing the task showed significant age-related lower activation in the medial prefrontal cortex, bilateral inferior frontal gyrus, and right anterior superior temporal suclus. Moran et al. (2012) conclude that aging may result in declines in medial prefrontal functioning; indeed, age-related declines on other theory of mind tasks have been reported (for a review see Henry et al. 2013). One caveat of the study is that it did not record the responses of the younger and older adults performing the Animations Task. Bird et al. (2004) declare that they have conducted pilot work showing that older adults tend to provide more physical descriptions to explain the theory of mind animations than younger adults, but these data have not been published. Further work is needed to determine whether there are age-related effects on the behavioral performance on the task, and whether these are related to the putative age-related differences in BOLD activity.

10.1.5 Summary

Much of the work examining the localization of the processes associated with performing the Animations Task has involved neuroimaging studies of healthy individuals or individuals with autism. This work consistently associates the medial prefrontal cortex with task performance. The only lesion study to involve the Animations Task suggests that damage to the medial prefrontal cortex does not impair task performance. However, the patient in this study has a lesion which spares some of the more left subcortical structures (i.e., the left caudate nucleus, anterior limb of the internal capsule and putamen) which might explain her lack of impairment; thus, further lesion work is needed. In terms of aging, there is evidence to suggest that older adults have reduced medial prefrontal activation when performing the task, but work has not been published to determine whether this reduction in activation is associated with an age-related decline in performance.

10.2 Faux Pas Task

10.2.1 Task description

The Faux Pas Task (Stone et al. 1998) is widely used as a test of theory of mind, as it requires an understanding of the mental states of two (and sometimes three) individuals in a story. Participants should accurately detect and understand that someone has unintentionally said something that would hurt another person's feelings (i.e., they have made a "faux pas" or social slip). Therefore, the Faux Pas Task is thought to assess the affective component of theory of mind rather than the cognitive component of theory of mind.[1] Participants are presented with 10 stories in which a faux pas has occurred and 10 control stories in which there is no faux pas (see Box 10.2). To reduce the demands placed on working memory, the stories remain in front of the participants while performing the task. Participants are then asked questions tapping the detection of the faux pas and story comprehension.

10.2.2 Patient and lesion studies

Studies with brain-damaged participants indicate that Faux Pas Task performance is impaired following lesions that involve the ventromedial prefrontal cortex (Table 10.4). In their initial study, Stone et al. (1998) compared the Faux Pas performance of patients with orbitofrontal (BAs 10 and 11; one patient had a brain lesion extending into BA 9) and dorsolateral prefrontal (BAs 8, 9, 44, 45, and 46) damage to that of healthy controls. The researchers found that the patients with orbitofrontal lesions were impaired in integrating theory of mind inferences and the emotional understanding of the character who received the Faux Pas. More specifically, the orbitofrontal patients would answer that nothing awkward had been said, or, when they acknowledged that something awkward had been said, they performed poorly on the subsequent clarification questions. Yet, the orbitofrontal patients were able to answer the empathic questions. The poor performance of orbitofrontal patients was not due to comprehension deficits, as they answered the control questions correctly. Moreover, the orbitofrontal group could understand another person's mental state, as they performed well on simpler theory of mind tasks (e.g., first- and second-order false belief).[2] The results suggest that the orbitofrontal group had difficulty

---

[1] Brothers and Ring (1992) proposed a distinction between "cold" (cognitive) and "hot" (affective) components of theory of mind. Cognitive theory of mind is the ability to attribute thoughts and beliefs to another person without emotional understanding of their feelings. By contrast, affective theory of mind refers to the ability to understand another person's emotional state (Hynes et al. 2006; Shamay-Tsoory et al. 2007).

[2] The False Belief task assesses whether participants understand that someone else may hold a belief that is different from their own belief. Children aged three to four years may pass the simpler First Order False Belief task, which requires understanding that another person may hold a mistaken belief. After the age of six years, children may pass the more advanced Second Order False Belief task, which requires participants to understand one

Box 10.2 Example of a story used in the Faux Pas Task

Helen's husband was throwing a surprise party for her birthday. He invited Sarah, a friend of Helen's, and said, "Don't tell anyone, especially Helen." The day before the party, Helen was over at Sarah's and Sarah spilled some coffee on a new dress that was hanging over her chair. "Oh!" said Sarah, "I was going to wear this to your party!" "What party?" asked Helen. "Come on," said Sarah, "Let's go see if we can get the stain out."

Six types of questions are asked:

1: Faux pas detection: "Did someone say something s/he should not have said?"

2: Understanding the faux pas: "Who said something s/he should not have said?"

3: Understanding the recipient's mental state: "Why should s/he not have said it?"

4: Understanding the mental state of the character committing the faux pas: "Why did s/he say it?"

5: Control question: Both the faux pas and non-faux pas stories include one question relating to factual information about the stories, which do not require the inference of an individual's mental state.

6: Empathy question: Finally, an empathy question is asked to indicate how the character receiving the faux pas might feel. This question requires participants to articulate that the person who committed the faux pas is unaware that s/he said something they should not have said and that the subject of the faux pas might feel hurt or insulted.

Data from Valerie E. Stone, Simon Baron-Cohen, and Robert T. Knight, Frontal lobe contributions to theory of mind, *Journal of Cognitive Neuroscience*, 10(5), pp. 640–656, 1998.

relating their inference regarding another person's mental state to their understanding of the emotional implications. Stone et al. (1998) concluded that the ventromedial prefrontal cortex might be part of a broader circuit involving theory of mind understanding and that the ventromedial prefrontal cortex was involved in the affective aspects of the task. Roca et al. (2011) compared the performance of patients with frontal lesions and healthy controls on the Faux Pas Task. The frontal patients were grouped as those with and without damage

person's beliefs about what another person thinks (Wimmer and Perner 1983; Perner and Wimmer 1985).

Table 10.4 Faux Pas Task: Patient and lesion studies

Study	n	Patient/Control Groups	Study type	Brodmann Areas	FP	DL	OF	ACC
Stone et al. (1998)	5; 5; 1; 5	OF; DL; TC, HA	Lesion	8, 9, 10, 11, 45, 46, 47	✓		✓	
Lough et al. (2001)	1	fvFTD	Patient (single case)	–			✓	
Gregory et al. (2002)	19; 12; 16	fvFTD; AD; HA	Patient	–			✓	
Lough et al. (2002)	1	fvFTD	Patient (single case)	–		✓	✓	
Shamay-Tsoory et al. (2003)	12; 6; 17; 19	VM; DL; PC; HA	Lesion	6, 8, 9, 10, 11, 12, 24, 44, 45, 46	✓		✓	✓
Bird et al. (2004)	1	ACA	Lesion (single case)	–			X	X
Shamay-Tsoory et al. (2005a)	11; 7; 7; 16; 17	VM; DL; Mix; PC; HA	Lesion	6, 8, 9, 10, 11, 12, 24, 44, 45, 46	✓		✓	✓
Shamay-Tsoory et al. (2005b)	12; 7; 7; 13; 13	VM; DL; Mix; PC; HA	Lesion	6, 8, 9, 10, 11, 12, 24, 44, 45, 46	✓		✓	✓
Torralva et al. (2007)	20; 10	fvFTD; HA	Patient	–			✓	
Herold et al. (2009)	18; 21	schiz, HA	Structural (VBM)	10, 11	✓	✓		
Geraci et al. (2010)	11; 7; 20	VM; DL; HA	Lesion	8, 9, 10, 11, 12, 14, 24, 32, 43, 44, 45	✓		✓	✓
Lee et al. (2010)	9; 12; 5; 30	MPFC, LPFC, non-PFC, HC	Lesion	–			✓	
Roca et al. (2011)	3; 2; 5; 8; 3; 25	Inferior medial; superior medial; left lateral; right lateral; mix; HA	Lesion	10	✓			
Leopold et al. (2012)	30; 76; 55	VM; PC; HA	Lesion	–		✓	✓	✓

FP = frontal pole; DL = dorsolateral prefrontal cortex; OF = orbitofrontal cortex; ACC = anterior cingulate cortex; TC = temporal cortex; HA = healthy adults; fvFTD = frontal variant frontotemporal dementia; AD = Alzheimer's disease; VM = ventromedial prefrontal cortex; PC = posterior cortex; ACA = anterior cerebral artery infarct; mix = ventromedial and dorsolateral prefrontal cortex; schiz = patients with schizophrenia; MPFC = medial prefrontal cortex; LPFC = lateral prefrontal cortex; non-PFC = non-prefrontal cortex; ✓ = frontal region damaged and impairment found; X = frontal region damaged but no impairment.

involving the anterior prefrontal cortex (BA 10). Only patients with damage to BA 10 performed significantly more poorly on the Faux Pas Task compared to healthy controls, although neither frontal group significantly differed in their Faux Pas performance from one another.

Decline in Faux Pas understanding has also been reported in both single case and group studies of frontal variant frontotemporal dementia (fvFTD; Lough et al. 2001; Gregory et al. 2002; Lough and Hodges 2002; Torralva et al. 2007). Although FTD may involve extended frontal subregions, it is thought that in the early stages of the disease the atrophy involves mainly the superior medial prefrontal cortex and the orbitofrontal cortex (Kril and Halliday 2004). In line with this, Torralva et al. (2007) found impaired performance on all types of Faux Pas question (i.e., detection and understanding) in patients with early/ mild stages of fvFTD. In a different study, Gregory et al. (2002) investigated performance on the Faux Pas Task in a group of fvFTD patients whose atrophy predominantly involved the ventromedial prefrontal cortex. These patients were severely impaired on all theory of mind measures including the Faux Pas Task, and a close correspondence emerged between the degree of atrophy in the ventromedial prefrontal cortex and the theory of mind impairment. Furthermore, when a faux pas was detected, the patients often made errors on the subsequent clarifying questions, indicating that they did not recognize that the faux pas had been committed unintentionally. The control questions were answered correctly, indicating that their poorer performance on the Faux Pas stories was not due to poor comprehension.

A series of lesion studies by Shamay-Tsoory et al. (2003, 2005a, 2005b) also supports the role of the ventromedial prefrontal cortex, not the dorsolateral prefrontal cortex, in understanding others' mental states. The researchers investigated the Faux Pas performance of patients with prefrontal lesions divided into ventromedial prefrontal, dorsolateral prefrontal and mixed frontal damage, non-prefrontal patients, and healthy controls. The prefrontal group was significantly impaired compared to the non-prefrontal group and healthy controls. Further analysis showed that this was due to poorer performance of the ventromedial prefrontal patients compared to control groups. By contrast, the performance of the dorsolateral prefrontal group did not significantly differ from that of non-prefrontal patients and healthy controls.

A decline in performance on the Faux Pas Task has been recently been associated with damage to the left ventromedial prefrontal cortex (Leopold et al. 2012). This study assessed the performance of a group of Vietnam War veterans with focal penetrating traumatic brain injuries and healthy controls on affective and cognitive theory of mind tasks (Faux Pas Task, Section 10.2; Theory of Mind Stories, Section 10.6). The veterans were grouped as those with ventromedial prefrontal lesions (including left, right, or bilateral lesions) and those with posterior damage. The ventromedial prefrontal group performed more poorly than the individuals with posterior lesions and the healthy control group on the Faux Pas Task but not the Theory of Mind Stories. This suggests the role of the ventromedial prefrontal cortex in performing affective theory of mind tasks, including the Faux Pas Task. Poor performance on the Faux Pas Task was associated with left and bilateral but not right ventromedial prefrontal damage. The ventromedial prefrontal involvement in Faux Pas Task performance has also been reported in patients with schizophrenia (Feldman et al. 2009). The impaired task performance correlated with reduced gray matter of the left orbitofrontal superior gyrus, the right medial frontal gyrus, as well as the inferior temporal gyrus and the temporal poles. Another study investigated the performance on the Faux Pas Task of patients with prefrontal lesions following traumatic brain injury and healthy controls (Geraci et al. 2010). The prefrontal group included patients with focal damage predominantly involving the ventromedial prefrontal (i.e., mesial BAs 8, 9, 10, 24, and 32 as well as the orbital areas BAs 10, 11, 12, and 14) or the dorsolateral prefrontal cortex (BAs 8, 9, 43, 44, and 45). Only those with ventromedial prefrontal brain damage performed significantly more poorly on the task compared to healthy controls.

Further research has suggested that there is dissociation between the affective and cognitive theory of mind task demands of the Faux Pas Task (Blair and Cipolotti 2000; Hynes et al. 2006; Shamay-Tsoory and Aharon-Peretz 2007). Lee et al. (2010) investigated the affective (i.e., mental state understanding) and cognitive (i.e., faux pas detection) components of the Faux Pas Task by comparing the performance of patients with medial prefrontal lesions, patients with lateral prefrontal lesions, patients with non-prefrontal lesions, and healthy controls. Overall, all three lesion groups performed more poorly than healthy controls, with the medial prefrontal patients performing more poorly than the other two groups in terms of their Faux Pas total score (i.e., Faux Pas detection and question understanding), whereas no difference across groups emerged for the control questions. A further analysis of performance on the individual questions revealed that the medial prefrontal group performed more poorly than all other groups on the fourth question (i.e., Why did s/he say it?), whereas the three lesion groups did not differ significantly on the first three Faux Pas questions.

Despite the majority of lesion and patient evidence suggesting that the ventromedial prefrontal cortex is necessary to perform the Faux Pas Task, there is also the well-known case of patient GT who was able to perform the Faux Pas Task despite having a lesion in the orbital and medial frontal areas (Bird et al. 2004). As GT's lesion did not involve the entire ventromedial prefrontal cortex, this might explain her intact Faux Pas performance. Some of the ventromedial prefrontal patient groups assessed on the Faux Pas Task include individuals with lesions extending to the dorsal area of the prefrontal cortex. For example, in Stone et al's (1998) study, the orbitofrontal patient who was the most impaired on the Faux Pas Task had a lesion extending into the dorsolateral and ventrolateral prefrontal areas (BAs 9 and 47). Similarly, the ventromedial prefrontal group in Shamay-Tsoory et al's studies (2003, 2005a, 2005b) had dorsomedial prefrontal involvement (BA 9).

In summary, the evidence suggests that the ventromedial prefrontal cortex plays an important role in the ability to understand faux pas. Nevertheless, other brain areas (e.g., the dorsolateral prefrontal cortex) cannot be excluded in terms of playing a role in understanding others' mental states.

10.2.3 Neuroimaging studies

To our knowledge, no studies have examined the neural correlates of the Faux Pas Task using fMRI or PET. There has been research investigating the effect of repetitive transcranial magnetic stimulation (rTMS) on Faux Pas performance (Costa et al. 2008) (Table 10.5). Eleven healthy participants were administered inhibitory rTMS on the left and right dorsolateral prefrontal cortex and on the left and right temporal parietal junction prior to performing the Faux Pas Task. Participants' ability to attribute mental states to others was disrupted after rTMS over the left and right dorsolateral prefrontal cortex and right temporal parietal junction compared to sham. rTMS over the left temporal parietal junction did not disrupt mental state attribution. This suggests that the dorsolateral prefrontal cortex as well as the right temporal parietal junction are also important for Faux Pas Task performance.

10.2.4 Aging studies

Few studies have investigated the effect of healthy adult aging on Faux Pas Task performance, and the results are contradictory (Table 10.6). For example, MacPherson et al. (2002) compared the performance on the Faux Pas Task of healthy young (age range = 20–38 years), middle-aged (age range = 40–59 years), and older (age range = 61–80 years) adults, finding no

Table 10.5 Faux Pas Task: Neuroimaging studies

Study	n	Patient/ Control Groups	Study type	Brodmann Areas	FP	DL	OF	ACC
Costa et al. (2008)	11	HA	rTMS	–		✓		

FP = frontal pole; DL = dorsolateral prefrontal cortex; OF = orbitofrontal cortex; ACC = anterior cingulate cortex; HA = healthy adults; rTMS = repetitive transcranial magnetic stimulation; ✓ = frontal region involved.

Table 10.6 Faux Pas Task: Aging studies

Study	n	Participant age groups (years)	Study type	Age effect
MacPherson et al. (2002)	30; 30; 30	20–38; 40–59; 61–80	Cross-sectional (behavioral)	X
Wang and Su (2006)	30; 30	19–25; 62–77	Cross-sectional (behavioral)	✓
Halberstadt et al. (2011)	60; 61	18–35; 60–85	Cross-sectional (behavioral)	✓
Li et al. (2012)	28; 24; 28	19–22; 70–79; 70–86	Cross-sectional (behavioral)	✓
Wang and Su (2013)	32; 42; 32	20–35; 65,74; 75–85	Cross-sectional (behavioral)	X

✓ = age effect found; X = age effect not found

significant age difference. Wang and Su (2013) compared performance on Theory of Mind Stories that assessed cognitive theory of mind (e.g., bluff, double bluffs) and affective theory of mind (e.g., faux pas, white lies) in 32 young (age range = 20–35 years), 42 young-old (age range = 65–74 years) and 32 old-old (age range = 75–85 years) participants. Whereas both the young-old and the old-old groups performed significantly more poorly on the cognitive theory of mind stories than younger adults, no age effect was found for the affective Theory of Mind Stories which included faux pas. In an earlier study, Wang and Su (2006) compared the performance of younger (age range 19–25 years) and older (age range = 62–77 years) participants on the Faux Pas Task (i.e., affective theory of mind) and Theory of Mind Stories (i.e., Happé 1994): older adults were impaired on the Faux Pas Task, whereas the performance on the Theory of Mind Stories was not affected by aging. A meta-analysis by Henry et al. (2013) including five independent datasets, reported that performance on the Faux Pas Task declined significantly with age.

There has been some research on Faux Pas Task performance using visual rather than verbal stimuli. Halberstadt et al. (2011) developed a visual version of the Faux Pas Task consisting of 16 video clips featuring people at work. In half of the video clips, a character committed a faux pas, whereas in the remaining stimuli the behavior was socially appropriate. Participants were instructed to indicate the appropriateness of the behavior in each video clip on an 11-point scale, ranging from 0 (not socially appropriate at all) to 10 (entirely socially appropriate). Younger adults performed better on the faux pas and non-faux pas video clips than older adults.

The contradictory results in terms of the effects of age on theory of mind understanding have recently been explained in terms of individual differences (e.g., level of education) and cognitive decline. Li et al. (2012) compared the performance of a group of highly educated younger adults (mean age = 20.46 years; mean education = 15.11 years), a group of highly educated older participants (mean age = 76.29 years; mean education = 15.79 years), and a group of less-educated older individuals (mean age = 73.52 years; mean education = 9.71 years) on a series of theory of mind tasks which included two verbal tests, the Faux Pas Task and the False Belief Detection Task as well as a visual task, the Reading the Mind in the Eyes Task (Baron-Cohen et al. 2001). The study also included background measures of executive function (e.g., inhibition, shifting, and updating), speed of processing and memory to determine whether cognitive decline would mediate age differences on the theory of mind tasks. Older adults with a low level of education performed significantly more poorly compared to both younger and older participants with a higher level of education on the Faux Pas Task and the False Belief Task but not on the control questions and the Reading the Mind in the Eyes Task. By contrast, the performance of younger and older adults with a higher level of education did not significantly differ on any task. The findings suggest that a high level of education may compensate for an age effect on theory of mind understanding, at least in terms of verbal tasks. The results also indicate that the cognitive decline of older individuals mediates the age effect on Faux Pas performance. The younger group performed better than both the older groups on the background measures, indicating that even those older adults with a higher level of education demonstrated cognitive decline. An additional regression analysis showed that inhibition, updating, memory and speed processing mediated the age differences between young and older adults on the Faux Pas Task. These findings suggest that the Faux Pas Task is complex, relying on the ability to inhibit one's own perspective, to adopt the perspective of another person (e.g., a character in the story) and to update each scenario.

Overall, the results of the aging studies are contradictory and indicate that several factors may affect the Faux Pas performance in older individuals (e.g., cognitive abilities and level of education).

10.2.5 Summary

Although the evidence discussed supports the central role of the ventromedial prefrontal cortex in performing the Faux Pas Task, the involvement of other areas within the prefrontal cortex cannot be ruled out entirely. A review of the aging literature reveals contradictory results in terms of the effects of age on Faux Pas Task performance, and this may be due to individual differences (e.g., level of education) and test design (e.g., number and story type).

10.3 **Judgment of Preference Task**

10.3.1 **Task description**

The Judgment of Preference Task was originally developed and further modified to investigate theory of mind abilities in children with autistic spectrum disorder and patients with frontal variant frontotemporal dementia (fvFTD; Baron-Cohen et al. 1995; Snowden et al. 2003). The task assesses the ability to detect or decode mental states such as preferences on the basis of eye gaze direction (Sabbagh and Taylor 2000; Sabbagh 2004; Sabbagh et al., 2004; see Figure 10.2). By contrast with other theory of mind tasks, such as the Faux Pas Task (see Section 10.2) and Theory of Mind Stories (see Section 10.6), the Judgment of Preference Task involves forced-choice responses rather than open-ended questions. A typical task consists of a cartoon outline of a face

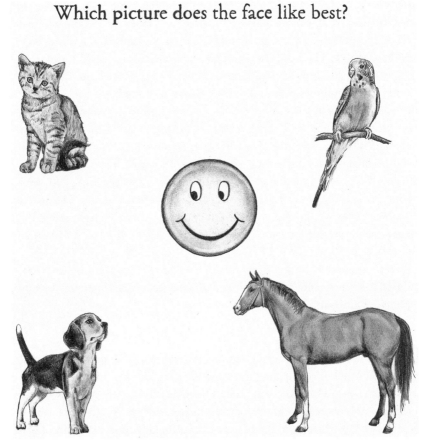

Which picture does the face like best?

Fig. 10.2 Example of the stimuli used in the Judgment of Preference Task.

presented in the middle of a computer screen and four colored pictures of objects belonging to the same semantic category in each corner of the screen. The eye gaze of the central face is directed towards one of the four objects. In the experimental condition, the task requires participants to indicate what object the central face "likes best." Three control conditions have also been developed (Snowden et al. 2003): (1) a physical (non-theory of mind) condition that requires participants to indicate what object the central face "is looking at"; (2) a distracting arrow condition in which an arrow pointing to one of the three objects that the face is not looking at is also presented; and (3) a condition whereby participants are simply asked to indicate their favorite object without the presence of the face.

It has been proposed that theory of mind can be subdivided into cognitive and affective aspects (e.g., Eslinger et al. 1996; Eslinger 1998; Blair and Cipolotti 2000). The former refers to the ability to understand others' thoughts and beliefs, whereas the latter refers to the ability to understand emotional responses. On this basis, a more recent version of the Judgment of Preference Task has been developed to investigate both cognitive and affective theory of mind (Yoni Task; Shamay-Tsoory and Aharon-Peretz 2007). The materials are the same as those used in the original version of the Judgment of Preference Task, but, to control for cognitive task demands, this version includes first- and second-order theory of mind trials. In the first-order theory of mind task, participants are instructed to indicate which object a central character, "Yoni," is referring to based on eye gaze and verbal cues. Three conditions are included: affective, cognitive, and physical. In the affective condition, both the face and the verbal cues provide emotional information (e.g., Yoni loves…), whereas in the cognitive condition, both the face expression and the words are emotionally neutral (e.g., Yoni is thinking of…). The physical condition requires the detection of a physical feature of the characters (e.g., Yoni is close to…). The same affective, cognitive, and physical conditions are used in the second-order theory of mind task except that an additional face is presented next to each of the four objects, and participants are required to understand the interaction between the four faces and the central character's mental state (see Figure 10.3).

10.3.2 **Patient and lesion studies**

Few studies have investigated the effects of focal prefrontal lesions on performance on the Judgment of Preference Task. However, the findings available suggest involvement of both the ventromedial prefrontal cortex and the dorsolateral prefrontal cortex when performing the task (Table 10.7). Snowden et al. (2003) assessed the performance of patients with FTD whose atrophy

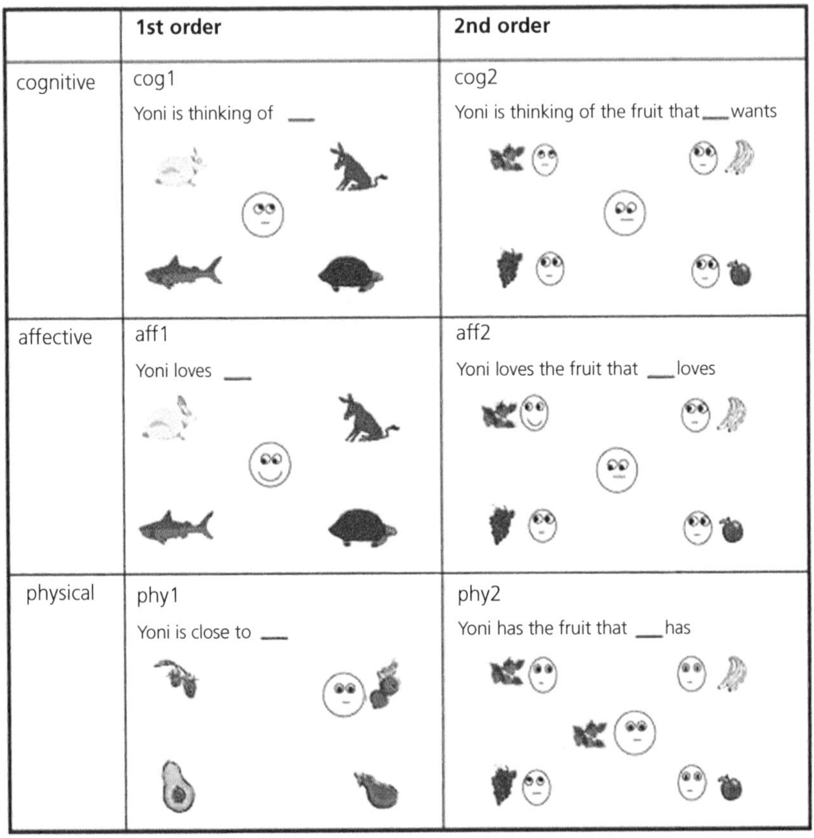

	1st order	2nd order
cognitive	cog1 Yoni is thinking of ___	cog2 Yoni is thinking of the fruit that ___wants
affective	aff1 Yoni loves ___	aff2 Yoni loves the fruit that ___loves
physical	phy1 Yoni is close to ___	phy2 Yoni has the fruit that ___has

Fig. 10.3 Stimuli used in the modified Judgment of Preference Task. Reprinted from *Neuropsychologia*, 45 (13), Elke Kalbe, Marius Schlegel, Alexander T. Sack, Dennis A. Nowak, Manuel Dafotakis, Christopher Bangard, Matthias Brand, Simone Shamay-Tsoory, Oezguer A. Onur, and Josef Kessler, Dissociating cognitive from affective theory of mind: A TMS study, pp. 769–80, Copyright (2010), with permission from Elsevier.

was largely characterized by changes in the orbitofrontal cortex, patients with Huntington's disease, and healthy controls. The FTD patients performed significantly more poorly on the task compared to both the Huntington's disease patients and healthy controls, selecting their favorite objects rather than the item the face "likes best." No deficits emerged in their ability to detect the eye gaze direction as measured in the "look at" conditions, indicating that their impaired performance was due to difficulty in using the eye gaze direction as a cue to infer the mental state of another individual. Despite these results, dorsolateral prefrontal involvement when performing the Judgment

Table 10.7 Judgment of Preference Task: Patient and lesion studies

Study	n	Patient/ Control Groups	Study type	Task	Brodmann Areas	FP	DL	OF	ACC
Snowden et al. (2003)	13; 13; 18	fvFTD; HD; HA	Patient	Baron-Cohen et al. (1995): Affective				✓	
Shamay-Tsoory and Aharon-Peretez (2007)	10; 9; 14; 17; 44	VM; DL; Mix; PC; HA	Lesion	Yoni: Affective	8, 9, 10, 11, 12, 14, 24, 32, 44, 45, 46	✓		✓	✓
Shamay-Tsoory et al. (2007)	24	VM; DL; Mix; NF; HA	Lesion		6, 8, 9, 10, 11, 12, 14, 24, 32, 44, 45, 46	✓		✓	✓

FP = frontal pole; DL = dorsolateral prefrontal cortex; OF = orbitofrontal cortex; ACC = anterior cingulate cortex; fvFTD = frontal variant frontotemporal dementia; HD = Huntington disease; HA = healthy adults; VM = ventromedial prefrontal cortex; Mix = dorsolateral and ventromedial prefrontal cortex; PC = posterior cortex; NF = non-frontal; ✓ = frontal region damaged and impairment found; X = frontal region damaged but no impairment.

of Preference Task cannot be ruled out, as a small number of the patients had more widespread frontal lobe involvement, extending into the dorsolateral prefrontal cortex.

More specific support for the role of the ventromedial prefrontal cortex on the Judgment of Preference Task has emerged from studies investigating patients with ventromedial prefrontal lesions, dorsolateral prefrontal lesions, mixed (i.e., both ventromedial and dorsolateral prefrontal lesions) or non-frontal lesions, and healthy controls on their ability to perform affective and cognitive theory of mind tasks (Shamay-Tsoory and Aharon-Peretez 2007; Shamay-Tsoory et al. 2007). All patient groups performed well on the first-order version of the Judgment of Preference Task. In the second-order version, the ventromedial prefrontal cortex and mixed groups performed significantly more poorly than the controls in the affective condition whereas the dorsolateral prefrontal and non-frontal groups performed similarly to healthy controls. However, even from these data, it is difficult to exclude the involvement of the dorsolateral prefrontal cortex, as the ventromedial prefrontal cortex patient group included patients with damage to mesial BA 9.

10.3.3 **Neuroimaging studies**

To our knowledge, no study has investigated the brain areas associated with performance on the Judgment of Preference Task. However, some insight into the brain areas involved might come from studies that have investigated the ability to follow eye gaze direction (Table 10.8). In an fMRI investigation, Hooker et al. (2003) instructed healthy adults to perform two tasks: in the eye gaze task, participants viewed faces whose eyes switched to different locations and then looked back to the viewer. In the arrow task, a dot was presented in the center of the screen and was then replaced by an arrow pointing in different directions. The task was to indicate whether the eyes/arrow were directed towards a given target location. The eye gaze condition activated several brain areas including the ventromedial prefrontal cortex (BA 10) and the dorsolateral prefrontal cortex (BA 46) compared to the arrow condition, which activated the dorsolateral prefrontal cortex only (BA 9).

Other studies have shown that the brain areas traditionally associated with theory of mind abilities are also activated when participants follow another person's eye gaze direction (e.g., the medial prefrontal cortex; Fletcher et al. 1995; Happé et al. 1996; Gallagher et al. 2000). Tasks that require the detection of eye gaze direction allow individuals to share the focus of attention (e.g., joint attention) and to draw inferences about another person's mental state (Baron-Cohen, 1995). In an fMRI investigation, Williams et al. (2005) showed that joint attention involves activation of the medial prefrontal cortex, suggesting that eye direction provides a cue to infer others' intentions.

More recent studies have investigated the effect of the temporary disruption of the prefrontal regions on the ability to understand affective and cognitive theory of mind (Kalbe et al. 2010; Krause et al. 2012; Lev-Ran et al. 2012). For example,

Table 10.8 Judgment of Preference Task: Neuroimaging studies

Study	n	Patient/ Control Groups	Study type	Task	Brodmann Areas	FP	DL	OF	ACC
Kalbe et al. (2010)	28	HA	rTMS	Yoni: Affective Yoni: Cognitive	8, 9				
Krause et al. (2012)	16	HA	rTMS	Yoni: Affective Yoni: Cognitive	–				
Lev-Ran et al. (2012)	13	HA	rTMS	Yoni: Affective	11, 12			✓	

FP = frontal pole; DL = dorsolateral prefrontal cortex; OF = orbitofrontal cortex; ACC = anterior cingulate cortex; HA = healthy adults; rTMS = repetitive transcranial magnetic stimulation; ✓ = frontal region involved.

in Kalbe et al.'s (2010) study, participants first received repetitive transcranial magnetic stimulation (rTMS) applied to the dorsolateral prefrontal cortex, and after the stimulation they performed the Judgment of Preference Task developed by Shamay-Tsoory and Aharon-Peretz (2007). rTMS affected performance on the cognitive but not the affective theory of mind or the physical control conditions. Although rTMS did not affect accuracy, the temporary disruption of the dorsolateral prefrontal cortex determined faster response times during performance of the cognitive theory of mind. The authors claimed that the dorsolateral prefrontal cortex may modulate the activity of the ventromedial prefrontal cortex and that its disruption would lead to more emotion-based responses and, thus, faster response times during the cognitive condition. Krause et al. (2012) also applied rTMS to the medial prefrontal cortex (mainly the dorsal region) of healthy participants. Overall, the temporary disruption of the medial prefrontal cortex did not affect cognitive or affective theory of mind performance on the Judgment of Preference Task. However, when the researchers included self-ratings of empathy, it appeared that rTMS affected the accuracy of affective theory of mind on the basis of the participant's empathic abilities. Accuracy decreased in those who reported high levels of empathy, whereas it increased in those with low empathic scores. These results suggest that the medial prefrontal cortex plays a role in processing affective theory of mind and that the effect of its disruption depends on the participant's baseline level of empathy.

10.3.4 Aging studies

At present, only two studies have investigated the impact of age on the Judgment of Preference Task (Table 10.9). Castelli et al. (2010) employed the version of the task devised by Snowden et al. (2003) and reported no significant age differences in performance, suggesting that the ability to attribute mental states on the basis of visual cues does not decrease with age. Duval et al. (2011) employed a modified version of Snowden et al.'s task, assessing the ability to identify others' preferences in a given context. In this version, the central face expressed

Table 10.9 Judgment of Preference Task: Aging studies

Study	n	Participant age groups (years)	Study type	Task	Age effect
Castelli et al. (2010)	12; 12	21–30; 60–78	Cross-sectional (behavioral)	Baron-Cohen et al. (1995): Affective	X
Duval et al. (2011)	25; 20; 25	21–34; 45–59; 61–83	Cross-sectional (behavioral)	Tom's Taste	✓

✓ = age effect found; X = age effect not found

its preference by either smiling or pouting (i.e., affective theory of mind) and its eyes were looking at a balloon, which contained the character's thoughts (i.e., cognitive theory of mind). The experimenter described a scenario and then asked a question related to the character's preferred object. For example, "Imagine you have kindly invited Tom to tea or coffee at home. What will you serve with it? Chocolates, oysters, crackers or madeleines?" (Duval et al. 2011, p. 632). The correct response required participants to consider simultaneously both the affective and cognitive theory of mind information. There was no significant difference between younger and middle-aged participants (mean age = 55.6 years) but both age groups performed significantly better than the older group (mean age = 70.4 years). The age effect disappeared when cognitive processes associated with the task (e.g., attention, shifting and updating) were controlled for. It seems that the Judgment of Preference Task is complex, susceptible to aging, and has a number of features reliant on executive abilities (e.g., the simultaneous manipulation of multiple sources of information).

10.3.5 Summary

The few studies that have investigated performance on the Judgment of Preference Task suggest that the ventromedial prefrontal cortex is preferentially involved in processing the affective components of the task. However, some evidence suggests that it is the dorsolateral prefrontal cortex that modulates this ventromedial prefrontal cortex activation in healthy adults, and further work is needed to clarify the role of the dorsolateral prefrontal cortex when performing the Judgment of Preference Task. Aging research suggests that the ability to understand others' mental states does not decrease until 70 years of age and that it is the cognitive demands rather than a decline in theory of mind abilities which underlies poor performance on the Judgment of Preference Task in older adults.

10.4 Reading the Mind in the Eyes Task

10.4.1 Task description

The Reading the Mind in the Eyes Task was originally developed by Baron-Cohen et al. (1997, 2001) to investigate the ability to attribute mental states to others in individuals with autism or Asperger syndrome. This ability to attribute beliefs, desires, and intentions to others, and to understand that someone else's mental states might differ from one's own is known as 'theory of mind'. The Reading the Mind in the Eyes Task is considered an advanced theory of mind test in that it requires understanding of complex mental states and how they are reflected in facial information around the eyes. The material consists of photographs depicting the eye region of the face (see Figure 10.4).

A.

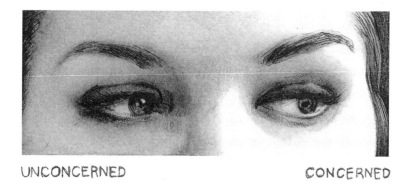

UNCONCERNED   CONCERNED

B.

JOKING   INSISTING

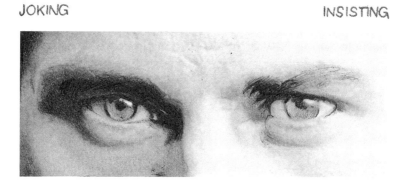

AMUSED   RELAXING

Fig. 10.4 Examples of stimuli used in Reading the Mind in the Eyes Task with (A) two mental state words (Baron-Cohen et al. 1999) and (B) four mental state words (Muller et al. 2010). (A) Reproduced from Simon Baron-Cohen, Howard A. Ring, Sally Wheelwright, Edward T. Bullmore, Mick J. Brammer, Andrew Simmons, and Steve C. R. Williams, Social intelligence in the normal and autistic brain: an fMRI study, *European Journal of Neuroscience*, 11(6), pp. 1891–1898, Figure 1 (top). © 1999, John Wiley & Sons, with permission. (B) Reprinted from *Cortex*, 46 (9), François Muller, Audrey Simion, Elsa Reviriego, Cédric Galera, Jean-Michel Mazaux, Michel Barat, and Pierre-Alain Joseph, Exploring theory of mind after severe traumatic brain injury, pp. 1088–1099, Copyright (2010), with permission from Elsevier.

Participants are typically instructed to indicate which of the two (Baron-Cohen et al. 1999) or four (Baron-Cohen et al. 2001) adjectives supplied best describes what the person in the photo is feeling or thinking.

10.4.2 Lesion and patient studies

Lesion studies investigating the localization of the processes associated with the Reading the Mind in the Eyes Task within the frontal lobes suggest that performance relies on the intactness of both the dorsolateral and ventrome-dial prefrontal cortex (Shaw et al. 2005; Geraci et al. 2010) (Table 10.10). For example, Shaw et al. (2005) investigated the performance of patients with focal brain damage in the dorsolateral prefrontal cortex or ventromedial prefrontal cortex on the Reading the Mind in the Eyes Task. Both dorsolateral and ventromedial prefrontal lesions were associated with poorer performance compared to healthy controls, suggesting that both these frontal subregions are involved in mental state processing. Similarly, Geraci et al. (2010) compared the performance of patients with focal prefrontal lesions following traumatic brain injury with healthy controls on the Reading the Mind in the Eyes Task.

Table 10.10 Reading the Mind in the Eyes Task: Patient and lesion studies

Study	n	Patient/ Control Groups	Study type	Brodmann Areas	FP	DL	OF	ACC
Lough et al. (2001)	1	fvFTD	Patient (single case)	–			X	
Gregory et al. (2002)	19; 12; 16	fvFTD; AD; HA	Patient	–				✓
Lough and Hodges (2002)	1; 16	fvFTD; HA	Patient	–			✓	✓
Shaw et al. (2005)	14; 9; 54; 91	VM; DL; TL; HA	Lesion	9, 10, 11, 12, 25, 46	✓	✓	✓	✓
Torralva et al. (2007)	20; 10	fvFTD; HA	Patient	–				✓
Hirao et al. (2008)	20; 20	schiz; HA	Patient (VBM)	9/32, 10, 11/25, 24/32, 47		✓		
Geraci et al. (2010)	11; 7; 20	VM; DL; HA		8, 9, 10, 11, 12, 14, 24, 32, 43, 44, 45	✓		✓	✓

FP = frontal pole; DL = dorsolateral prefrontal cortex; OF = orbitofrontal cortex; ACC = anterior cingulate cortex; fvFTD = frontal variant frontotemporal dementia; AD = Alzheimer's disease; HA = healthy adults; VM = ventromedial prefrontal cortex; TL = temporal lobes; schiz = schizophrenic patients; VBM = voxel-based morphometry; ✓ = frontal region damaged and impairment found; X = frontal region damaged but no impairment.

The frontal lesion group included patients whose lesion involved predominantly the dorsolateral prefrontal cortex or the ventromedial prefrontal cortex, whereas patients with more diffuse brain lesion were excluded on the basis of neuroradiological results. Geraci et al. (2010) found that both patient groups were impaired compared to healthy controls on the Reading the Mind in the Eyes Task.

Patient studies that have investigated performance on the Reading the Mind in the Eyes Task in patients with frontal variant frontotemporal dementia (fvFTD) provide further support for the view that both dorsal and ventral areas of the prefrontal cortex are involved in mental state attribution (Lough et al. 2001; Gregory et al. 2002; Lough and Hodges 2002; Torralva et al. 2007). Although FTD may affect distinct areas of the prefrontal cortex, it is thought that in the early stages of the disease, atrophy is mainly found in the superior medial and the orbitofrontal cortex (Kril and Halliday 2004). Gregory et al. (2002) assessed the performance of a group of fvFTD patients with predominately ventromedial prefrontal atrophy on a series of theory of mind tasks, including the two-word version of the Reading the Mind in the Eyes Task. fvFTD patients performed poorly compared to healthy controls, and there was a strong association between theory of mind performance and ventromedial prefrontal atrophy. However, although the brain damage was greater in the ventromedial prefrontal cortex, the dorsolateral prefrontal cortex was also affected. Similarly, Lough and Hodges (2002) reported the case of an fvFTD patient who was impaired on the Reading the Mind in the Eyes Task. Again, although his frontal involvement was mainly in the orbitofrontal cortex, the dorsolateral prefrontal cortex was also involved. These findings contrast with another fvFTD patient who performed normally on the Reading the Mind in the Eyes Task despite his frontal atrophy involving mainly the orbitofrontal cortex (Lough et al. 2001). This might suggest that damage to the orbitofrontal cortex alone is not sufficient to affect theory of mind processing. These studies suggest that the ability to attribute mental states accurately decreases when the brain damage involves both dorsolateral and ventromedial prefrontal cortex (Gregory et al. 2002; Lough and Hodges 2002).

Further evidence for the involvement of the lateral areas of the prefrontal cortex in performing the Reading the Mind in the Eyes Task has been provided by a voxel-based morphometry study with schizophrenic patients and healthy controls (Hirao et al. 2008). The authors found that the patient group performed significantly more poorly on the four-word version of the Reading the Mind in the Eyes Task compared to the control group. In addition, the patients' performance was accompanied by a reduction in gray matter concentration in the anterior and posterior dorsomedial prefrontal cortex (BAs 9/32 and 10), the ventromedial prefrontal cortex (BA 11/25), the ventrolateral prefrontal cortex (BA 47), the anterior cingulate cortex (BA 24/32), as well as the insula and the superior temporal gyrus. Further analysis revealed a significant association between task performance and the gray matter concentration in the dorsolateral (BA 8) and ventrolateral prefrontal cortex (BA 47).

The role of the lateral prefrontal brain areas in Reading the Mind in the Eye performance has been associated with the executive demands of the task. For example, Bull et al. (2008) investigated the relationship between executive functions and theory of mind using a dual task paradigm. Their participants performed the Reading the Mind in the Eyes Task under single and dual task conditions. For the dual conditions, three different secondary tasks were chosen that were thought to tap executive components: inhibition, updating, and switching. Performance was only disrupted by the secondary task thought to tap inhibition. The authors concluded that mental state attribution may require the inhibition of an initial strong response based on a first impression, and that this may explain the involvement of the lateral prefrontal cortex in Reading the Mind in the Eyes Task performance.

Altogether, the findings from lesion and patient studies suggest that both the dorsolateral and the ventromedial prefrontal cortex play a role in performing the Reading the Mind in the Eyes Task.

10.4.3 Neuroimaging studies

Only a handful of neuroimaging studies have investigated the brain regions associated with performance on the Reading the Mind in the Eyes Task (Table 10.11). Overall, the results of these studies have shown that the prefrontal cortex plays a central role in mental state attribution with both dorsolateral prefrontal and ventromedial prefrontal involvement (Baron-Cohen et al. 1999, 2006; Russell et al. 2000; Platek et al. 2004; Hill et al. 2007; Adams et al. 2010; Moor et al. 2012). In an early study, Baron-Cohen et al. (1999) investigated fMRI activity associated with performance on the Reading the Mind in the Eyes Task and a gender recognition task in autistic individuals and healthy controls. A network of temporal and prefrontal activation during mental state attribution was revealed, which included the left dorsolateral prefrontal cortex (BAs 44, 45, and 46) and the left medial prefrontal cortex (BA 9) in both groups. In addition, the inferior frontal gyrus (BA 44/45) was the only area of the prefrontal cortex significantly less activated in the autistic group compared to healthy controls. The dorsolateral prefrontal activation was interpreted in terms of the executive demands of the task, as it requires participants to match mental state words while looking at images of the eye region. Further analysis showed that the fMRI results were accompanied by poorer performance of the autistic individuals compared to the healthy controls on both the Reading the

Table 10.11 Reading the Mind in the Eyes Task: Neuroimaging studies

Study	n	Patient/ Control Groups	Study type	Brodmann Areas	FP	DL	OF	ACC
Baron-Cohen et al. (1999)	6; 12	Autistic; HA	fMRI	9, 44, 45, 46	✓			
Russell et al. (2000)	5; 7	schiz; HA	fMRI	9/44/45	✓			
Platek et al. (2004)	5	HA	fMRI	8, 9, 46	✓			
Sabbagh et al. (2004)	18	HA	ERPs	–			✓	
Baron-Cohen et al. (2006)	12; 12	pAS; HA	fMRI	44, 45				
Hill et al. (2007)	16; 8	ADF; HA	fMRI	10, 46	✓	✓		
Adams et al. (2010)	28	HA	fMRI	6, 6/8, 9, 32, 45, 47	✓			✓
Krause et al. (2012)	16	HA	rTMS	–	X			

FP = frontal pole; DL = dorsolateral prefrontal cortex; OF = orbitofrontal cortex; ACC = anterior cingulate cortex; HA = healthy adults; fMRI = functional magnetic resonance imaging; schiz = schizophrenic patients; ERPs = event-related potentials; PAS = parents of autistic individuals; ADF= alcohol dependent families; MDD = major depressive disorder; rTMS = repetitive transcranial magnetic stimulation; ✓ = frontal region involved.

Mind in the Eyes Task and the gender recognition task. The researchers noted, however, that the autistic group consisted of only six participants and that the performance on the gender control task has been shown to be preserved in a larger sample size (e.g., $n = 16$; Baron-Cohen et al. 1997).

It should also be noted that the neural activity associated with mental state attribution may have been due to the linguistic processing demands of the task (Baron-Cohen et al. 1999). To rule out the effect of linguistic processing on the ability to decode the mental state, an ERP study employed a modified version of the Reading the Mind in the Eyes Task in which the words and the eye region were not presented simultaneously (Sabbagh et al. 2004). Participants were first presented with a word related to a mental/emotional state or gender (male/female). A picture of the eye region then replaced the initial word and participants were instructed to indicate whether the word previously presented described the face. Two main components differentiated mental state attribution from gender discrimination: an anterior frontal component and a more posterior component. Low-resolution electromagnetic tomography showed that the orbitofrontal cortex and the temporal lobes were the most probable contributors to mental state attribution.

The findings from other fMRI investigations do not clearly identify any frontal region as being preferentially involved in Reading the Mind in the Eyes Task performance (Platek et al. 2004; Hill et al. 2007; Adams et al. 2010). For example, Adams et al. (2010) investigated Reading the Mind in the Eyes Task performance using fMRI in Japanese and American students. Both groups showed similar brain activation involving the anterior rostral medial prefrontal cortex (BAs 6 and 9), the inferior frontal gyrus (BAs 45 and 47), and the anterior cingulate cortex (BA 32). Using another version of the Reading the Mind in the Eyes Task in which the words were removed and participants were instructed to think of the mental state of the person in photo, Platek et al. (2004) reported activation of the middle and superior frontal gyri (BAs 8, 9, and 46). It has also been reported that repetitive transcranial magnetic stimulation (rTMS) of the medial prefrontal cortex does not disrupt Reading the Mind in the Eyes Task performance when compared to a sham condition, suggesting that this frontal region is not solely responsible for performance on the task (Krause et al. 2012).

In summary, the neuroimaging studies discussed do not implicate a single region of the frontal lobes in Reading the Mind in the Eyes Task performance—the dorsolateral prefrontal cortex, the ventromedial prefrontal cortex, and the anterior cingulate cortex have all been associated with task performance.

10.4.4 Aging studies

Most aging studies investigating Reading the Mind in the Eyes Task performance have reported a decline in the ability to attribute mental states to others as people age (Table 10.12). Indeed, a meta-analysis of Reading the Mind in the Eyes Task performance including seven datasets revealed that older adults perform significantly more poorly than younger adults (Henry et al. 2013). An earlier study compared younger and older adults' ability to recognize basic emotions taken from the Ekman and Friesen (1976) series and perform the Reading the Mind in the Eyes Task (Phillips et al. 2002a). The authors found an effect of age on both the basic emotion task and the Reading the Mind in the Eyes Task, with older adults performing more poorly than younger participants. The age effect remained significant after controlling for differences in years of education as well as fluid and crystallized intelligence. More recently, Pardini and Nichelli (2009) investigated age effects on the Reading the Mind in the Eyes Task in four age groups (20–25, 45–55, 55–65, and 70–75 years) with 30 participants in each age group. The poorer performance of older adults compared to younger participants on the ability to attribute accurately mental states to others appears to occur after the age of 55 years. However,

Table 10.12 Reading the Mind in the Eyes Task: Aging studies

Study	n	Participant age groups (years)	Study type	Age effect
Phillips et al. (2002a)	30; 30	20–40; 60–80	Cross-sectional (behavioral)	✓
Slessor et al. (2007)	40; 40	16–40; 60–74	Cross-sectional (behavioral)	✓
Bailey and Henry (2008)	36; 33	18–26; 62–82	Cross-sectional (behavioral)	✓
Bailey et al. (2008)	80; 49	19–25; 65–87	Cross-sectional (behavioral)	✓
Pardini and Nichelli (2009)	30; 30; 30; 30	20–25; 45–55; 55–65; 70–75	Cross-sectional (behavioral)	✓
Castelli et al. (2010)	12; 12	21–30; 60–78	Cross-sectional (neuroimaging)	X
Duval et al. (2011)	25; 20; 25	21–34; 45–59; 61–83	Cross-sectional (behavioral)	✓
Li et al. (2012)	28; 24; 28	19–22; 70–79; 70–86	Cross-sectional (behavioral)	X

✓ = age effect found; X = age effect not found

Slessor et al. (2007) demonstrated that not only were older adults significantly impaired compared to younger participants on the Reading the Mind in the Eyes Task, even when differences on vocabulary measures were controlled for, but also that older participants performed worse than younger adults on the control tasks (e.g., age and gender discrimination). This suggests that the decline with age is not specific to mentalizing. The authors suggested that the observed results were due to a more general deficit in other cognitive abilities such as switching, inhibition of impulsive responses, and working memory. Furthermore, Bailey and Henry (2008) and Bailey et al. (2008) found that older adults performed significantly more poorly than younger adults on the Reading the Mind in the Eyes Task, and that controlling for inhibitory capacity did not eliminate this age effect (Bailey and Henry 2008). However, the researchers found that the effect of age on the Reading the Mind in the Eyes Task was significantly reduced, concluding that inhibitory processes partially mediate this age effect. Duval et al. (2011) investigated age effects on a version of the Reading the Mind in the Eyes Task in which the eyes portrayed both basic and complex emotions. There was an age effect on the complex emotion version of the Reading the Mind in the Eyes Task but not the basic emotion version. The authors propose that complex emotions typically appear within a specific social context whereas basic ones do not, as they are universally recognized. As no context was supplied, it was suggested that understanding of complex emotions required greater cognitive effort.

Although most aging studies have reported a decline in the ability to attribute mental states to others as people age, some researchers have found no effect of age on Reading the Mind in the Eyes Task performance. For example, Castelli et al. (2010) reported no age differences between a group of 12 younger adults aged 21–30 years and 12 older adults aged 60–78 years. However, fMRI showed that the older group activated the frontal lobes to a greater extent than the younger groups, perhaps as compensation for decreased function in other brain areas. Similarly, Li et al. (2012) found no age effect on the Reading the Mind in the Eyes Task, yet less-educated older participants were impaired on other types of theory of mind tasks such as the Theory of Mind Stories and the Faux Pas Task compared to more highly educated older and younger adults. These contradictory results have been explained in terms of the different task demands. For example, Li et al. (2012) suggested that stories require participants to predict a behavior following a chain of actions, whereas the Reading the Mind in the Eyes Task requires participants only to attribute mental states. Overall, the majority of aging studies suggest that older participants perform more poorly than younger adults when performing the Reading the Mind in the Eyes Task. Such a decline with age may be attributed to deficits in executive abilities (e.g., matching words with images, inhibition of first impressions).

10.4.5 Summary

Performance on the Reading the Mind in the Eyes Task appears to rely on an extensive brain network including both the ventromedial and dorsolateral prefrontal cortex. Whereas the ventromedial prefrontal cortex is thought to play a role in the ability to understand other people's mental states through their eye gaze, the dorsolateral prefrontal cortex has been associated with the executive demands of the Reading the Mind in the Eyes Task (e.g., inhibition). The majority of studies examining the effects of healthy adult aging on the Reading the Mind in the Eyes Task have reported poorer performance in older compared to younger adults, although it is less clear whether this age effect is due to the executive or theory of mind demands of the task.

10.5 Cartoons Task

10.5.1 Task description

The Cartoons Task (Corcoran et al. 1997; Happé et al. 1999; Snowden et al. 2003) was developed as a first-order theory of mind task to assess the ability to understand a protagonist's beliefs or intentions (Bishop 1993; Mazza et al. 2001). The task consists of cartoon drawings taken from popular magazines (e.g., The New Yorker) illustrating either theory of mind jokes or physical jokes. The theory of mind jokes involve humor in which participants must understand a protagonist's false belief in order to appreciate the joke (e.g., a man mistakenly believes his son is joking about a monster that is actually on the staircase). The physical jokes can be understood in terms of the physical properties of the cartoon (e.g., a small boy in the scene is actually an adult scientist who has discovered the secret of eternal youth). Either the cartoons are presented one at a time with participants having to provide a verbal description of why the joke is funny (single cartoons), or pairs of cartoons are presented side by side, one cartoon containing a joke and the other cartoon having had the humor element replaced (cartoon pairs). Participants must choose which cartoon in the pair is funny and then describe why. The verbal description for the theory of mind cartoons should indicate that the participant correctly understood the mental states inferred in the cartoon (e.g., "did not know", "believed that"); for the physical cartoons, a physical account of the cartoon is adequate, as long as the participant does not simply name or identify the parts or actions in the cartoon. Verbal responses are transcribed and scored on a scale from 0 to 3: 0 for an incorrect or unrelated response; 1 point if the participant mentions the important parts of the cartoon without additional clarification; 2 points for an incomplete/implied explanation; and 3 points for a full and clear explanation. The cartoons remain in front of the participant until an explanation has been provided. Examples of the answers to the cartoons and their scoring are supplied in Happé et al. (1999).

This section focuses on the Cartoon Task and similar tasks that require non-verbal theory of mind understanding. Although the Cartoon Task also involves an element of humor appreciation, clinically it tends to be used to assess theory of mind abilities. We appreciate that there are several lesion and neuroimaging studies that have investigated humor appreciation (e.g., Shammi and Stuss 1999; Moran et al. 2004; Goel and Dolan 2007); however, these humor paradigms tend to be more experimental in nature and differ in the stimuli adopted from study to study (for a review see Clark and Warren 2014). To our knowledge, stimuli thought to assess humor appreciation with frontal localization evidence from both patient and neuroimaging studies have not yet been identified.

10.5.2 **Patient and lesion studies**

Whereas the established view is that the prefrontal cortex, notably the medial region, plays a key role in verbal theory of mind abilities (Gallagher and Frith 2003; Amodio and Frith 2006; Frith and Frith 2006), few lesion studies have assessed non-verbal theory of mind abilities (Table 10.13). Bibby and McDonald (2005) administered the single cartoons version of the Cartoons Task to 15

Table 10.13 Cartoons Task: Patient and lesion studies

Study	n	Patient/ Control Groups	Study type	Task	Brodmann Areas	FP	DL	OF	ACC
Happé et al. (2001)	1	OF	Lesion	Single cartoons: Cartoon pairs:	–			✓ ✓	
Bird et al. (2004)	1	ACA	Lesion (single case)	Single cartoons	–			X	X

FP = frontal pole; DL = dorsolateral prefrontal cortex; OF = orbitofrontal cortex; ACC = anterior cingulate cortex; ACA = anterior cerebral artery infarct; ✓ = frontal region damaged and impairment found; X = frontal region damaged but no impairment

individuals who had suffered traumatic brain injury, mainly involving the frontal and temporal lobes, and compared their performance with 15 healthy controls. The individuals with traumatic brain injury scored significantly more poorly than the controls on both the theory of mind and physical cartoons suggesting a general impairment in inference-making. When the famous case of patient GT, who had extensive medial prefrontal damage, was presented with the first two cartoons from the Cartoon Task during a neuropsychological assessment, she was able to explain the jokes successfully (Bird et al. 2004). Of course, the authors recognized that GT's damage did not involve the entire medial prefrontal cortex as she had sparing of the left caudate nucleus, anterior limb of the internal capsule, and putamen. Moreover, GT was not assessed formally on the Cartoons Task. Therefore, based on these findings, one cannot conclude that medial prefrontal damage does not impair performance on the task. In another single case study involving the Cartoons Task, Happé et al. (2001) assessed patient PB, a 76-year-old man, who had undergone a stereotactic anterior capsulotomy for the treatment of bipolar disorder. This surgical procedure involves lesioning the frontothalamic fibers connecting the midline thalamic nuclei and the orbitofrontal cortex. PB was assessed on both the single cartoons and cartoon pairs, performing significantly more poorly than healthy controls on the theory of mind versions of these tasks but not the physical ones. Compared to patient GT who had posterior medial orbitofrontal damage and seemed to understand theory of mind cartoons, patient PB's surgical procedure is more likely to have damaged the posterior lateral orbitofrontal cortex and resulted in deficits on the task. However, whereas the Happé et al. (2001) lesion study suggests that the orbitofrontal prefrontal region and its interactions with the thalamus may be important for performing the Cartoons Task, the extant data are insufficient to make strong claims about the frontal specificity of this task.

10.5.3 **Neuroimaging studies**

The Cartoons Task and similar cartoon theory of mind tasks have also been administered to healthy individuals in the PET and fMRI scanner (Table 10.14). In Gallagher et al. (2000), six participants were presented with theory of mind cartoons, physical cartoons, and jumbled pictures (images of randomly placed animals, people, and objects). During PET scanning, the participants had simply to look at each cartoon and consider its meaning. After scanning, participants had to describe verbally the meaning of each cartoon. In the theory of mind versus physical cartoons contrasts, and in the theory of mind cartoons versus random picture contrasts, Gallagher et al. (2000) found activation in the medial prefrontal gyrus (BA 8), right middle frontal gyrus (BA 6), the right temporo-parietal junction (BA 40), the precuneus (BA 7/31), and the fusiform (BA 20/36). Neuroimaging studies have also examined the neural correlates of a similar cartoon-related theory of

Table 10.14 Cartoons Task: Neuroimaging studies

Study	n	Patient/ Control Groups	Study type	Task	Brodmann Areas	FP	DL	OF	ACC
Brunet et al. (2000)	8	HA	PET	Comic strip	6, 8, 9, 10, 24, 32, 47	✓	✓		✓
Gallagher et al. (2000)	6	HA	PET	Single cartoons	6, 8				
Walter et al. (2004)	13	HA	fMRI	Social intentions: Private intentions:	8, 9, 10/32, 47; 24/32, 44/46		✓		✓ ✓
Völlm et al. (2006)	15	HA	fMRI	Comic strip	47			✓	
Ciaramidaro et al. (2007)	12	HA	fMRI	Comic strip Social intentions: Physical intentions:	–				✓ ✓
Samson et al. (2008)	17	HA	fMRI	Single cartoons	10/46, 32, 44			✓	✓
Sebastian et al. (2011)	16; 16	Adolescents; HA	fMRI	Comic strip Affective: Cognitive:	9, 10	✓			

FP = frontal pole; DL = dorsolateral prefrontal cortex; OF = orbitofrontal cortex; ACC = anterior cingulate cortex; HA = healthy adults; PET = positron emission tomography; fMRI = functional magnetic resonance imaging; ✓ = frontal region involved.

mind task called the Comic Strip Task (Sarfati et al. 1997; Brunet et al. 2000). Rather than requiring participants to understand theory of mind jokes from single cartoon frames, participants are presented with three pictures in a comic strip which represent a short story, and they should choose the logical ending to that story from three options by inferring the protagonist's intentions. When the theory of mind condition is contrasted with the physical condition, activity has been reported in the medial (BAs 8/9 and 9) and inferior (BA 47) regions of the prefrontal cortex, including the anterior cingulate cortex (BA 24), anterior temporal regions bilaterally (BAs 21 and 22), and the left cerebellum (Brunet et al 2000), as well as the orbitofrontal cortex (BA 47), the temporal parietal junction (BA 19/22/39) and temporal cortex (BAs 21 and 22; Völlm et al. 2006). In another fMRI study using the Comic Strip Task, Sebastian et al. (2011) examined the activation associated with cognitive theory of mind cartoons (i.e., an inference is made based on the intentions or belief of one individual and his/her acquaintance) and affective theory of mind cartoons (i.e., an inference is made based on how one individual will react to another individual's feelings). Both theory of mind conditions were contrasted with a physical condition but medial prefrontal activation (BAs 9 and 10) was specific only to the affective condition, not the cognitive condition. It has also been shown by Samson et al. (2008) that the activation patterns associated with non-verbal cartoon understanding are specific to mental state attribution rather than to humor processing. Some other neuroimaging studies suggest further specialization associated with the Comic Strip Task when different types of intentions are considered such as private intentions (e.g., changing a light bulb to read a book) versus social and communicative intentions (e.g., preparing dinner for another character yet to arrive). Private intentions activate the "typical" theory of mind regions (i.e., the medial prefrontal cortex, the temporo-parietal junction and the precuneus), but social intentions additionally activate the dorsal anterior cingulate (Walter et al. 2004; Ciaramidaro et al. 2007). To conclude, the neuroimaging evidence suggests that the dorsomedial prefrontal cortex plays an important role in understanding mentalizing from non-verbal cartoons.

10.5.4 **Aging studies**

The only study to examine the effects of age on the Cartoons Task involved 30 younger adults (mean age = 25.7 years) and 30 older adults (mean age = 72.5 years; Keightley et al. 2006) (Table 10.15). Participants were presented with single theory of mind and physical cartoons and were asked to

Table 10.15 Cartoons Task: Aging studies

Study	n	Participant age groups (years)	Study type	Task	Age effect
Keightley et al. (2006)	30; 30	Younger, mean = 25.7 Older, mean = 72.5	Cross-sectional (behavioral)	Single cartoons	✓
Duval et al. (2011)	25; 25; 25	21–34; 45–59; 61–83	Cross-sectional (behavioral)	Comic strip	✓

✓ = age effect found; X = age effect not found

provide a brief written description of their meaning. Unlike Happé et al.'s (1999) study, the description was not scored using a three-point scale; instead only one point was awarded for each correct answer. Keightley et al. (2006) found that the older adults performed significantly more poorly than the younger adults on both the theory of mind and physical cartoons. They associated this impairment with a decline in memory rather than in social processing, since the younger adults' delayed recall memory scores on the Hopkins Verbal Learning test predicted performance on the theory of mind cartoons and the cartoon stimuli were removed before participants provided their explanations. Using the Comic Strip Task, Duval et al. (2011) assessed 25 younger (mean age = 23.80 years), 25 middle-aged (mean age = 52.55 years), and 25 older participants (mean age = 70.14 years). Again, the older participants performed significantly more poorly than the younger participants (and the middle-aged) on both the theory of mind and physical comic strips, but age only had an indirect effect on performance. The authors also showed that performance on the Comic Strip Task was predicted by executive abilities including shifting (Part B of the Trail-Making Test), updating (Running Span Task) and inhibition (Stroop Test).

10.5.5 Summary

The majority of studies have investigated theory of mind abilities using verbal measures such as the Faux Pas Task (Section 10.2) and the Theory of Mind Stories (Section 10.6). The few studies examining the localization of non-verbal theory of mind abilities assessed through cartoons suggest a role for the medial and orbital prefrontal cortex. In healthy aging, studies have shown that older adults are poorer at understanding theory of mind cartoons, but this age-related decline may be the result of a decline in other cognitive processes such as memory or executive abilities rather than a specific social processing impairment.

10.6 **Theory of Mind Stories**

10.6.1 **Task description**

The Theory of Mind Stories were developed to investigate the ability to mentalize (i.e., understand other people's beliefs) in individuals with autism (Happé 1994; Fletcher et al. 1995). Participants are presented with two types of stories that they should read silently to themselves before each story is removed and a question asked about the story. Theory of mind stories require participants to infer the mental state of a character in the story; and physical or non-mental (control) stories assess whether participants have an overall understanding of the story (see Box 10.3 for examples). These physical stories also require participants to make inferences beyond the information provided in the story. However, they differ from the theory of mind stories in that their understanding does not require the attribution of a mental state. More recently, it has been

---

Box 10.3 **Examples of theory of mind and physical stories**

Example: Theory of Mind Story

"A burglar who has just robbed a shop is making his getaway. As he is running home, a policeman on his beat sees him drop his glove. He doesn't know the man is a burglar, he just wants to tell him he dropped his glove. But when the policeman shouts out to the burglar, "Hey, you! Stop!," the burglar turns round, sees the policeman and gives himself up. He puts his hands up and admits that he did the break-in at the local shop".
Question: Why did the burglar do that?

Example: Non-Mental Story

"A burglar is about to break into a jewelers shop. He skillfully picks the lock on the shop door. Carefully he crawls under the electronic detector beam. If he breaks this beam it will set off the alarm. Quietly he opens the door of the store-room and sees the gems glittering. As he reaches out, however, he steps on something soft. He hears a screech and something small and furry runs out past him, towards the shop door. Immediately the alarm sounds."
Question: Why did the alarm go off?

Data from Francesca Happé, Hiram Brownell, and Ellen Winner, Acquired "theory of mind" impairments following stroke, *Cognition*, 70(3), pp. 211–240, doi: 10.1016/S0010-0277(99)00005-0, 1999.

proposed that theory of mind abilities consist of cognitive and affective components (e.g., Blair and Cipolotti 2000; Hynes et al. 2006).

Cognitive theory of mind refers to the ability to understand cognitive mental states (i.e., false beliefs), whereas affective theory of mind refers to the ability to understand others' emotions (Blair and Cipolotti 2000). Based on this view, the Theory of Mind Stories developed by Happé (1994) are thought to tap cognitive aspects of theory of mind processing, whereas other stories commonly used, such as the Faux Pas Task (Stone et al. 1998) are thought to tap affective theory of mind (Kalbe et al. 2007).

One consideration when administering the Theory of Mind Stories to assess theory of mind abilities is that this test relies on verbal output to demonstrate understanding of the stories. Participants who are less willing or able to provide a long description to explain the story (e.g., patients with amyotrophic lateral sclerosis) might be scored as having poor theory of mind abilities even if such a deficit does not exist. Therefore, clinicians may prefer not to use Theory of Mind Stories to assess theory of mind abilities in patients with poor spontaneous speech.

10.6.2 Patient and lesion studies

Few studies have examined the effect of focal frontal lobe damage on performance on the Theory of Mind Stories (Table 10.16). Snowden et al. (2003) administered Happé et al.'s stories (1999) to nine individuals with frontal variant frontotemporal dementia (fvFTD) whose lesions predominantly involved the orbitofrontal cortex, four fvFTD with more widespread frontal involvement

Table 10.16 Theory of Mind Stories: Patient and lesion studies

Study	n	Patient/Control Groups	Study type	Brodmann Areas	FP	DL	OF	ACC
Blair and Cipolotti (2000)	1	TBI	Lesion (single case)	–			X	
Snowden et al. (2003)	13; 13; 18	fvFTD; HD; HA	Patient	–			✓	
Bird et al. (2004)	1	ACA	Lesion (single case)	–			X	X
Leopold et al. (2012)	30; 76; 55	VM; PC; HA	Lesion	–	X		X	X

FP = frontal pole; DL = dorsolateral prefrontal cortex; OF = orbitofrontal cortex; ACC = anterior cingulate cortex; TBI = traumatic brain injury; fvFTD = frontal variant frontotemporal dementia; HD = Huntington's disease; HA = healthy adults; ACA = anterior cerebral artery infarct; posterior cortex; VM = ventromedial prefrontal cortex; PC = posterior cortex; ✓ = frontal region damaged and impairment found; X = frontal region damaged but no impairment.

and 18 healthy controls. The fvFTD patients were impaired on the Theory of Mind Stories compared to the healthy control group. However, Blair and Cipolotti (2000) administered the Theory of Mind Stories to patient JS who suffered trauma to the right frontal region resulting in bilateral orbitofrontal damage. Patient JS was not impaired on the Theory of Mind Stories. Moreover, Bird et al. (2004) reported ceiling performance on the original Theory of Mind Stories in a patient who suffered an anterior cerebral artery infarction and whose damage extended from the orbitofrontal cortex to the genu of the corpus callosum and included the anterior cingulate gyrus as well as the medial superior frontal sulcus. Bird et al. (2004) acknowledged that patient GT's lesion spared some of the ventromedial prefrontal cortex and this might explain her intact theory of mind abilities. More recently, Leopold et al. (2012) compared the performance of a group of patients with ventromedial prefrontal lesions (n = 30) and patients with more posterior brain damage (n = 76) and healthy controls (n = 55) on the Theory of Mind Stories (see Section 10.6) and the Faux Pas Task (see Section 10.2). The ventromedial prefrontal patient group performed significantly more poorly than the posterior patients and the healthy control group on the Faux Pas Task but not on the Theory of Mind Stories. Therefore, the evidence from patient and lesion studies is not sufficient to conclude that the ventromedial prefrontal cortex is necessary for successful performance on the Theory of Mind Stories.

10.6.3 Neuroimaging studies

Several neuroimaging studies have examinedthe role of the the prefrontal cortex when performing the Theory of Mind Stories task compared to the non-Theory of Mind physical stories (e.g., Fletcher et al. 1995; Gallagher et al. 2000; Table 10.17). In an early PET study, Happé et al. (1996) compared the brain activation of patients with Asperger syndrome and healthy adults on the Theory of Mind Stories and physical control stories. Individuals with Asperger syndrome were impaired on the Theory of Mind Stories but not on the control stories compared to healthy controls. These findings were accompanied by differences in brain activation. Both Asperger syndrome individuals and healthy controls activated the temporal pole, which has been associated with theory of mind abilities (e.g., Frith and Frith 2003, 2006; Gallagher and Frith 2003). However, a difference emerged in the activation of the medial prefrontal cortex, with BA 8/9 activated only in healthy adults (Happé et al. 1996). By contrast, Asperger syndrome patients showed activation of a more ventral area of the medial prefrontal cortex, BA 9/10. This same area was also activated in healthy controls, although to a lesser degree than BA 8/9. The greater activation of BA 9/10 in Asperger syndrome patients was interpreted by Happé et al.

Table 10.17 Theory of Mind Stories: Neuroimaging studies

Study	n	Patient/ Control Groups	Study type	Task	Brodmann Areas	FP	DL	OF	ACC
Fletcher et al. (1995)	6	HA	PET		8, 9				✓
Happé et al. (1996)	5; 6	AS; HA	PET		9/10				
Gallagher et al. (2000)	6	HA	fMRI		8/9				
Vogeley et al. (2001)	8	HA	fMRI		–				✓
Hynes et al. (2006)	20	HA	fMRI	Cognitive: Affective:	9/10, 10, 11; 9/10, 10, 11, 25, 47, 47/10	✓	✓ ✓	✓
Gobbini et al. (2007)	12	HA	fMRI		9, 10, 47				

FP = frontal pole; DL = dorsolateral prefrontal cortex; OF = orbitofrontal cortex; ACC = anterior cingulate cortex; HA = healthy adults; PET = positron emission tomography; AS = Asperger's syndrome; fMRI = functional magnetic resonance imaging; ✓ = frontal region involved.

(1996) as indicating that Asperger syndrome patients relied more on reasoning processes to infer mental states.

PET and fMRI studies involving healthy participants have also reported activation of the left medial frontal gyrus (BA 8) extending into BA 9, the anterior cingulate cortex, and to a lesser extent the inferior frontal area (BA 9/10) associated with Theory of Mind Stories performance (Fletcher et al. 1995; Happé et al. 1996; Gallagher et al. 2000; Vogeley et al. 2001). Additional activation in the ventral (BAs 10 and 47) areas of the prefrontal cortex has also been reported in an fMRI study comparing brain activation associated with two widely used tests of theory of mind: Theory of Mind Stories and the Animations Task (see Section 10.1; Gobbini et al. 2007).[3] Whereas researchers did indeed demonstrate activation of the typical theory of mind-related BA 8, 9, and 9/10 regions when contrasting the theory of mind stories with the physical stories, their findings suggested that more ventral prefrontal regions might also be involved in this task.

[3] Gobbini et al. (2007) investigated brain activation associated with a task which required the understanding of mental states (i.e., goals and intentions) expressed by the movement of geometrical shapes.

The activation of different areas within the prefrontal cortex while performing Theory of Mind Stories has also been investigated in relation to the cognitive and affective components of theory of mind (Blair and Cipolotti 2000; Hynes et al. 2006). Hynes et al. (2006) investigated cognitive theory of mind (i.e., false beliefs) using the Theory of Mind Stories developed by Happé (1994) and modified by Fletcher et al. (1995), but also developed 14 affective Theory of Mind Stories which assessed emotional state attribution and required participants to understand someone else's feelings (see Box 10.4). In line with previous neuroimaging results (e.g., Happé et al. 1996; Gobbini et al. 2007), Hynes et al. (2006) reported activation in the medial prefrontal cortex including the left medial superior frontal gyrus (BA 9/10) and the right superior rostral gyrus (BA 10) when performing both cognitive and affective types of theory of mind stories. However, the results showed greater medial (BAs 11 and 25) and orbital (BA 47) activation associated with the affective compared to the cognitive theory of mind stories. Cognitive theory of mind was instead associated with activation of the right anterior inferior frontal gyrus and right frontal pole (BAs 47/10 and 10). These findings suggest that performance on Theory of Mind Stories—particularly affective stories—mainly activate more medial regions of the prefrontal cortex.

Studies investigating performance on Theory of Mind Stories have employed slightly different methodologies. Some studies have instructed participants to read the story silently to themselves for a limited time (e.g., 25 s), the story is then removed and participants are asked to answer a question about the story (Fletcher et al. 1995; Gallagher et al. 2000; Vogeley et al. 2001). By contrast, more recent studies have reduced the cognitive demands of the Theory of Mind Stories by allowing participants to take as long as they need to read each passage (Hynes et al. 2006) and present them with multiple-choice responses (Hynes

---

Box 10.4 Example of an Affective Theory of Mind Story

"Ruth is driving away from Debbie's place when Debbie's cat runs suddenly into the road. She hits the brakes, but feels her car go over something. She stops and checks to see whether she has killed the cat. She finds that she ran over a bump in the road, and that the cat is safely on the other side of the road".

Question: How does Ruth feel?

Data from Catherine A. Hynes, Abigail A. Baird, and Scott T. Grafton, Differential role of the orbital frontal lobe in emotional versus cognitive perspective-taking, *Neuropsychologia*, 44(3), pp. 374–383, doi: 10.1016/j. neuropsychologia.2005.06.011, 2006.

et al. 2006; Gobbini et al. 2007). This might explain why these more recent studies report additional activation in BAs 10 and 47 whereas earlier studies do not.

10.6.4 **Aging studies**

Studies investigating the effect of age on the ability to perform the Theory of Mind Stories have reported contrasting results (Table 10.18). Happé et al. (1998) was the first study that explicitly examined age differences in performance on Theory of Mind Stories. They found that older adults performed better than younger participants on the theory of mind stories, whereas no age difference emerged on the control stories. The authors attributed these results

Table 10.18 Theory of Mind Stories: Aging studies

Study	*n*	Participant age groups (years)	Study type	Age effect
Happé et al. (1998)	52; 15; 19	16–30; 21–30; 61–80	Cross-sectional (behavioral)	✓
Saltzman et al. (2000)	8; 9	18.58–25.91; 49.50–79.67	Cross-sectional (behavioral)	X
Maylor et al. (2002)	25; 25; 25	16–29; 60–74; 75–89	Cross-sectional (behavioral)	✓
Sullivan and Ruffman (2004a)	25; 25; 25	16–29; 60–74; 75–89	Cross-sectional (behavioral)	✓
German et al. (2006)	27; 20	18–26; 62–90	Cross-sectional (behavioral)	✓
Keightley et al. (2006)	30; 30	Younger, mean = 25.7 Older, mean = 72.5	Cross-sectional (behavioral)	✓
Wang and Su (2006)	30; 30	19–25; 62–77	Cross-sectional (behavioral)	X
McKinnon and Moscovitch (2007)	12; 12	Younger, mean = 20.16 Older, mean = 78.18	Cross-sectional (behavioral)	✓
Slessor et al. (2007)	40; 40	16–40; 60–74	Cross-sectional (behavioral)	X
Charlton et al. (2009)	106	50–90	Correlational (neuroimaging)	✓
Castelli et al. (2010)	12; 12	21–30; 60–78	Cross-sectional (behavioral)	✓
Rakoczy et al. (2012)	27; 20	19–28; 60–91	Cross-sectional (behavioral)	✓

✓ = age effect found; X = age effect not found

to greater social sensitivity in older adults. However, studies since then have reported similar rather than age-related improvement on the Theory of Mind Stories in younger and older adults (Saltzman et al. 2000; Wang and Su 2006; Slessor et al. 2007) and there are also studies that have reported poorer performance in older compared to younger adults (Maylor et al. 2002; Sullivan and Ruffman 2004a; German and Hehman 2006; Keightley et al. 2006; Charlton et al. 2009; Castelli et al. 2010; Henry et al. 2013). Maylor et al. (2002) investigated performance on the Theory of Mind Stories in young (16–29 years), young-old (60–74 years), and old-old (75–89 years) healthy adults who performed the task under two conditions. In the memory load condition, participants were instructed to read the story and then the story was removed before the question was asked; and a no-memory load condition in which the story and the question were presented together and participants were instructed that they could refer back to the story when answering the question. The results showed that younger adults performed significantly better than both the two older groups in the memory-load condition. By contrast, only the old-old group was impaired when the memory demands were reduced, whereas the younger and young-older participants performed similarly. In line with this result, other studies have shown that older adults perform well when they are allowed to keep the story in front them to answer the questions (Saltzman et al. 2000; Slessor et al. 2007). For example, Slessor et al. (2007) found no age difference on theory of mind task performance when participants were presented with the stories, questions, and response options at once, and when they remained in front of the participant until a response was made. These findings suggest that performance on the Theory of Mind Stories may be affected by the memory demands of the task and that this memory demand may underlie age differences found on the task.

Further work has suggested that performance on the Theory of Mind Stories is mediated by executive abilities, intelligence, and information processing speed (Sullivan and Ruffman 2004a; McKinnon and Moscovitch 2007; Slessor et al. 2007; Charlton et al. 2009; Rakoczy et al. 2012). For example, Rakoczy et al. (2012) administered the Theory of Mind Stories as well as tests of executive function (e.g., the Trail-Making Test, the Stroop Test), processing speed, and crystallized intellectual abilities to 27 younger adults aged between 19 and 28 years and to 20 older adults aged between 60 and 91 years. Whereas a significant effect of age was found on Theory of Mind Stories, this effect was mediated by executive abilities but not processing speed or crystallized intelligence. In another study, Sullivan and Ruffman (2004a) examined the relationship between performance on the Theory of Mind Stories, and fluid and crystallized intelligence in younger and older participants. The authors found an age-related difference on theory of mind performance with older adults performing more poorly than younger adults on the Theory of Mind Stories but not the control stories. However, once fluid intelligence was accounted for, this age difference disappeared, suggesting that theory of mind abilities may be partially mediated by fluid intelligence. By contrast, the results did not change when crystallized intelligence was controlled for. On the basis of these results, the better performance of older compared to younger adults in Happé et al. (1998) may be due to the inclusion of high-functioning older adults. Nevertheless, Happé et al. (1998) question this as a possible explanation for their improved theory of mind performance with age, since their older adults did not perform better on the control stories. Moreover, when Slessor et al. (2007) controlled for vocabulary using the Mill Hill Vocabulary Scale (Raven et al. 1998), a crystallized intelligence test, a significant decline in the older group's theory of mind performance emerged. These findings suggest that the older participants perform well on the Theory of Mind Stories due to their high cognitive abilities. Therefore, the literature would support the view that older adults perform poorly on the Theory of Mind Stories due to general intellectual functions, memory, executive abilities and attentional demands.

10.6.5 Summary

Few patient or lesion studies have sought to determine the regions within the frontal lobes that are important for performing Theory of Mind Stories. Those patient studies that have made the attempt do not provide conclusive evidence of ventromedial prefrontal lesions producing impairments on Theory of Mind Stories. By contrast, there appears to be some agreement among fMRI and PET studies that the left medial frontal gyrus (BA 8), the inferior frontal area (BA 9/10) and the anterior cingulate cortex are activated when performing this theory of mind task. When responses to the Theory of Mind Stories require multiple choice responses rather than answering the questions internally, additional activation in the ventral (BAs 10 and 47) areas of the prefrontal cortex has been demonstrated. Studies of cognitive aging and Theory of Mind Stories have produced mixed results, with some studies reporting age-related improvement, some reporting age-related decline, and some reporting similar performance between younger and older adults. However, further work has suggested that intellectual and executive abilities as well as memory demands may underlie age effects on Theory of Mind Stories.

Appendix

Summary Table

Table A1 Degree of involvement of frontal subregions when performing the frontal tasks

	Frontal pole	Dorsolateral	Orbitofrontal	Anterior cingulate
Abstraction				
Brixton Spatial Anticipation Test		+		
Proverb Interpretation Task	+	+		
Initiation and inhibition				
AX-Continuous Performance Task		++	+	++
Go/No-Go Tasks	+	+++	+	+++
Hayling Sentence Completion Task		+		++
Stimulus–response compatibility tasks		++		+++
Verbal fluency tasks		+++		++
Mental flexibility				
Goal Neglect Task				
Reversal Learning Task		+	+++	++
Trail Making Test		+++		+
Wisconsin Card Sorting Test		+++	+	++
Multi-tasking				
Six Elements Task and Multiple Errands Task	+	+	+	
Problem-solving and judgment				
Cognitive Estimation Task			+	
Recency and temporal order discrimination	+	+++		+
Tower tests	++	+++		+++

(continued)

Table A1 Continued

	Frontal pole	Dorsolateral	Orbitofrontal	Anterior cingulate
Working memory				
Digit Span Backwards		+++		+
Target/response delay tasks	+	+++	+	+
N-Back Task	+	+++	+	+
Self-Ordered Pointing Task		+++		+
Emotional processing				
Emotion identification		+	++	+
Social decision-making				
Implicit Association Task	+	++	+	++
Iowa Gambling Task	+	++	++	++
Moral Decision-Making	+		++	++[a]
Ultimatum Game	++	++	++	++
Theory of mind				
Animations Task			+	+
Faux Pas Task	+		+++	+
Judgment of Preference Task	+		+	+
Reading the Mind in the Eyes Task		++	++	+
Cartoons Task		+	+	+
Theory of Mind Stories			+	+

+ = a little evidence; ++ = some evidence; = +++ considerable evidence.

[a]Specifically ventral portions of the medial prefrontal cortex that include ventral anterior cingulate.

References

Abell F, Happé F and Frith U (2000). Do triangles play tricks? Attribution of mental states to animated shapes in normal and abnormal development. *Cognitive Development*, **15**, 1–20.

Abrahams S, Goldstein LH, Kew JJM, Brooks DJ, Lloyd CM, Frith CD and Leigh PN (1996). Frontal lobe dysfunction in amyotrophic lateral sclerosis. A PET study. *Brain*, **119**(6), 2105–2120.

Abrahams S, Goldstein LH, Simmons A, Brammer MJ and Williams SCR, Giampietro VP, Andrew CM and Leigh PN (2003). Functional magnetic resonance imaging of verbal fluency and confrontation naming using compressed image acquisition to permit overt responses. *Human Brain Mapping*, **20**(1), 29–40.

Abrahams S, Goldstein LH, Simmons A, Brammer M, Williams SCR, Giampietro V and Leigh PN (2004). Word retrieval in amyotrophic lateral sclerosis: a functional magnetic resonance imaging study. *Brain*, **127**(7), 1507–1517.

Adams RB, Rule NO, Franklin RG, Wang E, Stevenson MT, Yoshikawa S, Nomura M, Sato W, Kveraga K and Ambady N (2010). Cross-cultural reading the mind in the eyes: an fMRI investigation. *Journal of Cognitive Neuroscience*, **22**(1), 97–108.

Adrover-Roig D and Barceló F (2010). Individual differences in aging and cognitive control modulate the neural indexes of context updating and maintenance during task switching. *Cortex*, **46**(4), 434–450.

Agostini C (1914). Tumori dei lobi frontali e criminalità. *Archivio di Antropologia Criminale, Psichiatrie e Medecina Legale*, **35**, 544–558.

Albert MS, Wolfe J and Lafleche G (1990). Differences in abstraction ability with age. *Psychology and Aging*, **5**(1), 94–100.

Alderman N, Burgess PW, Knight C and Henman C (2003). Ecological validity of a simplified version of the multiple errands shopping test. *Journal of the International Neuropsychological Society*, **9**(1), 31–44.

Alegre M, Gurtubay IG, Labarga A, Iriarte J, Valencia M and Artieda J (2004). Frontal and central oscillatory changes related to different aspects of the motor process: a study in go/no-go paradigms. *Experimental Brain Research*, **159**(1), 14–22.

Aleman A and van't Wout M (2008). Repetitive transcranial magnetic stimulation over the right dorsolateral prefrontal cortex disrupts digit span task performance. *Neuropsychobiology*, **57**(1–2), 44–48.

Alexander MP, Stuss DT, Shallice T, Picton TW and Gillingham S (2005). Impaired concentration due to frontal lobe damage from two distinct lesion sites. *Neurology*, **65**(4), 572–579.

Alexander MP, Gillingham S, Schweizer T and Stuss DT (2012). Cognitive impairments due to focal cerebellar injuries in adults. *Cortex*, **48**(8), 980–990.

Allamanno N, Della Sala S, Laiacona M, Pasetti C and Spinnler H (1987). Problem-solving ability in aging: normative data on a nonverbal test. *Italian Journal of Neurological Sciences*, **8**, 111–119.

Allen G, McColl R, Barnard H, Ringe WK, Fleckenstein J and Cullum CM (2005). Magnetic resonance imaging of cerebellar-prefrontal and cerebellar-parietal functional connectivity. *NeuroImage*, **28**(**1**), 39–48.

Allen MD, Owens TE, Fong AK and Richards DR (2011). A functional neuroimaging analysis of the Trail Making Test B: implications for clinical Application. *Behavioural Neurology*, **24**, 159–171.

Allen R and Brosgole L (1993). Facial and auditory affect recognition in senile geriatrics, the normal elderly and young adults. *International Journal of Neuroscience*, **68**, 33–42.

Allman JM, Watson KK, Tetreault NA and Hakeem AY (2005). Intuition and autism: a possible role for Von Economo neurons. *Trends in Cognitive Sciences*, **9**(**8**), 367–373.

Amiez C and Petrides M (2007). Selective involvement of the mid-dorsolateral pre-frontal cortex in the coding of the serial order of visual stimuli in working memory. *Proceedings of the National Academy of Sciences of the USA*, **104**(**34**), 13786–13791.

Ammons RB and Ammons CH (1962). *The Quick Test*. Psychological Test Specialists, Missoula, MT.

Amodio DM and Frith CD (2006). Meeting of minds: the medial frontal cortex and social cognition. *Nature Review Neuroscience*, **7**, 268–277.

Amunts K, Weiss PH, Mohlberg H, Pieperhoff P, Eickhoff S, Gurd JM, Marshall JC, Shah NJ, Fink GR and Zilles K (2004). Analysis of neural mechanisms underlying verbal flu-ency in cytoarchitectonically defined stereotaxic space—the role of Brodmann areas 44 and 45. *NeuroImage*, **22**(**1**), 42–56.

Anderson CV, Bigler ED and Blatter DD (1995). Frontal lobe lesions, diffuse damage and neuropsychological functioning in traumatic brain-injured patients. *Journal of Clinical and Experimental Neuropsychology*, **17**(**6**), 900–908.

Anderson SW, Damasio H, Jones RD and Tranel D (1991). Wisconsin Card Sorting Test performance as a measure of frontal lobe damage. *Journal of Clinical and Experimental Neuropsychology*, **13**, 909–922.

Anderson SW, Barrash J, Bechara A and Tranel D (2006). Impairments of emotion and real-world complex behavior following childhood- or adult-onset damage to ventro-medial prefrontal cortex. *Journal of the International Neuropsychological Society*, **12**(**2**), 224–235.

Andrés P and Van der Linden M (2000). Age-related differences in supervisory attentional system functions. *Journal of Gerontology*, **55B**(**6**), 373–380.

Andrés P and Van der Linden M (2001). Supervisory attentional system in patients with focal frontal lesions. *Journal of Clinical and Experimental Neuropsychology*, **23**(**2**), 225–239.

Andrews JA, Hampson SE, Greenwald AG, Gordon J and Widdop C (2010). Using the Implicit Association Test to assess children's implicit attitudes toward smoking. *Journal of Applied Social Psychology*, **40**(**9**), 2387–2406.

Andrews SC, Hoy KE, Enticott PG, Daskalakis ZJ and Fitzgerald PB (2011). Improving working memory: the effect of combining cognitive activity and anodal transcranial direct current stimulation to the left dorsolateral prefrontal cortex. *Brain Stimulation*, **4**(**2**), 84–89.

Anonymous (1851). Remarkable case of injury. *American Phrenology Journal*, **13**, 89.

Ardila A, Ostrosky-Solis F, Rosselli M and Gómez C (2000). Age-related cognitive decline during normal aging: the complex effect of education. *Archives of Clinical Neuropsychology*, **15**(**6**), 495–513.

Ardila A, Rosselli M and Rosas P (1989). Neuropsychological assessment of illiterates. Visuospatial and memory abilities. *Brain and Cognition*, **11**, 147–166.

Arnsten AFT and Contant TA (1992). Alpha-2 adrenergic agonists decrease distractibility in aged monkeys performing the delayed response task. *Psychopharmacology*, **108**(1–2), 159–169.

Arnsten AFT and Goldman-Rakic PS (1985). Alpha 2-adrenergic mechanisms in prefrontal cortex associated with cognitive decline in aged nonhuman primates. *Science*, **230**(4731), 1273–1276.

Aron AR, Fletcher PC, Bullmore ET, Sahakian BJ and Robbins TW (2003). Stop-signal inhibition disrupted by damage to right inferior frontal gyrus in humans. *Nature Neuroscience*, **6**(2), 115–116.

Asahi S, Okamoto Y, Okada G, Yamawaki S and Yokota N (2004). Negative correlation between right prefrontal activity during response inhibition and impulsiveness: a fMRI study. *European Archives of Psychiatry and Clinical Neuroscience*, **254**(4), 245–251.

Ashendorf L and McCaffrey RJ (2007). Exploring age-related decline on the Wisconsin Card Sorting Test. *The Clinical Neuropsychologist*, **22**(2), 262–272.

Ashendorf L, Jefferson AL, O'Connor MK, Chaisson C, Green RC and Stern RA (2008). Trail Making Test errors in normal aging, mild cognitive impairment, and dementia. *Archives of Clinical Neuropsychology*, **23**(2), 129–137.

Audenaert K, Brans B, Van Laere K, Lahorte P, Versijpt J, van Heeringen K and Dierckx R (2000). Verbal fluency as a prefrontal activation probe: a validation study using 99mTc-ECD brain SPET. *European Journal of Nuclear Medicine*, **27**(12), 1800–1808.

Auriacombe S, Fabrigoule C, Lafont S, Jacqmin-Gadda H and Dartigues JF (2001). Letter and category fluency in normal elderly participants: a population-based study. *Aging, Neuropsychology, and Cognition*, **8**(2), 98–108.

Axelrod BN and Millis SR (1994). Preliminary standardization of the Cognitive Estimation Test. *Assessment*, **1**, 269–274.

Baddeley A (1992). Working memory. *Science*, **255**, 556–559.

Baddeley A (1996). Exploring the central executive. *Quarterly Journal of Experimental Psychology*, **49A**(1), 5–28.

Baddeley A (2012). Working memory: theories, models, and controversies. *Annual Review of Psychology*, **63**, 1–29.

Baena E, Allen PA, Kaut KP and Hall RJ (2010). On age differences in prefrontal function: the importance of emotional/cognitive integration. *Neuropsychologia*, **48**(1), 319–333.

Bailey PE and Henry JD (2008). Growing less empathic with age: disinhibition of the self-perspective. *Journals of Gerontology. Series B, Psychological Sciences and Social Sciences*, **63**(4), P219–P226.

Bailey PE, Henry JD and Von Hippel W (2008). Empathy and social functioning in late adulthood. *Aging & Mental Health*, **12**(4), 499–503.

Bailey PE, Ruffman T and Rendell PG (2013). Age-related differences in social economic decision making: The ultimatum game. *Journals of Gerontology, Series B, Psychological Sciences and Social Sciences*, **68**(3), 356–363.

Baird A, Dewar B-K, Critchley H, Gilbert SJ, Dolan RJ and Cipolotti L (2006). Cognitive functioning after medial frontal lobe damage including the anterior cingulate cortex: a preliminary investigation. *Brain and Cognition*, **60**(2), 166–175.

Baker SC, Rogers RD, Owen AM, Frith CD, Dolan RJ, Frackowiak RSJ and Robbins TW (1996). Neural systems engaged by planning: a PET study of the Tower of London task. *Neuropsychologia*, **34**, 515–526.

Baldo J and Shimamura A (2000). Spatial and color working memory in patients with lateral prefrontal cortex lesions. *Psychobiology*, **28**(2), 156–167.

Baldo JV, Schwartz S, Wilkins D and Dronkers NF (2006). Role of frontal versus temporal cortex in verbal fluency as revealed by voxel-based lesion symptom mapping. *Journal of the International Neuropsychological Society*, **12**(6), 896–900.

Baldo JV, Schwartz S, Wilkins DP and Dronkers NF (2010). Double dissociation of letter and category fluency following left frontal and temporal lobe lesions. *Aphasiology*, **24**(12), 1593–1604.

Barbas H (1995). Pattern in the cortical distribution of prefrontally directed neurons with divergent axons in the rhesus monkey. *Cerebral Cortex*, **5**(2), 158–165.

Barbas H (2000). Connections underlying the synthesis of cognition, memory, and emotion in primate prefrontal cortices. *Brain Research Bulletin*, **52**(5), 319–330.

Barceló F and Knight RT (2002). Both random and perseverative errors underlie WCST deficits in prefrontal patients. *Neuropsychologia*, **40**(3), 349–356.

Barch DM, Braver TS, Nystrom LE, Forman SD, Noll DC and Cohen JD (1997). Dissociating working memory from task difficulty in human prefrontal cortex. *Neuropsychologia*, **35**(10), 1373–1380.

Barch DM, Braver TS, Sabb FW and Noll DC (2000). Anterior cingulate and the monitoring of response conflict: evidence from an fMRI study of overt verb generation. *Journal of Cognitive Neuroscience*, **12**(2), 298–309.

Barch DM, Braver TS, Akbudak E, Conturo T, Ollinger J and Snyder A (2001a). Anterior cingulate cortex and response conflict: effects of response modality and processing domain. *Cerebral Cortex*, **11**, 837–848.

Barch DM, Carter CS, Braver TS, Sabb FW, MacDonald A, Noll DC and Cohen JD (2001b). Selective deficits in prefrontal cortex function in medication-naive patients with schizophrenia. *Archives of General Psychiatry*, **58**(3), 280–288.

Barker II FG (1995). Phineas among the phrenologists: the American crowbar case and nineteenth-century theories of cerebral localization. *Journal of Neurosurgery*, **82**, 672–682.

Barnes DE, Targer IB, Satariano WA and Yaffe K (2004). The relationship between literacy and cognition in well-educated elders. *Journals of Gerontology, Series A, Medical Sciences and Biological Sciences*, **59A**, 390–395.

Baron-Cohen S (1995). *Mindblindness: An Essay on Autism and Theory of Mind*. Bradford Books, MIT Press, Cambridge, MA.

Baron-Cohen S, Campbell R, Karmiloff-Smith A, Grant J and Walker J (1995). Are children with autism blind to the mentalistic significance of the eyes? *British Journal of Developmental Psychology*, **13**, 379–398.

Baron-Cohen S, Jolliffe T, Mortimore C and Robertson M (1997). Another advanced test of theory of mind: evidence from very high functioning adults with autism or Asperger syndrome. *Journal of Child Psychology and Psychiatry, and Allied Disciplines*, **38**(7), 813–822.

Baron-Cohen S, Ring H, Wheelwright S, Bullmore ET, Brammer MJ, Simmons A and Williams SC (1999). Social intelligence in the normal and autistic brain: an fMRI study. *European Journal of Neuroscience*, **11**(6), 1891–1898.

Baron-Cohen S, Wheelwright S, Hill J, Raste Y and Plumb I (2001). The "Reading the Mind in the Eyes" Test, revised version: a study with normal adults, and adults with Asperger syndrome or high-functioning autism. *Journal of Child Psychology and Psychiatry, and Allied Disciplines*, **42**(2), 241–251.

Baron-Cohen S, Ring H, Chitnis X, Wheelwright S, Gregory L, Williams S, Brammer M and Bullmore E (2006). fMRI of parents of children with Asperger Syndrome: a pilot study. *Brain and Cognition*, **61**(1), 122–130.

Barrash J, Tranel D and Anderson SW (2000). Acquired personality disturbances associated with bilateral damage to the ventromedial prefrontal region. *Developmental Neuropsychology*, **18**(3), 355–381.

Barrett NA, Large MM, Smith GL, Michie PT, Karayanidis F, Kavanagh DJ, Fawdry R, Henderson D and O'Sullivan BT (2001). Human cortical processing of colour and pattern. *Human Brain Mapping*, **13**(4), 213–225.

Barry D, Bates ME and Labouvie E (2008). FAS and CFL forms of verbal fluency differ in difficulty: a meta-analytic study. *Applied Neuropsychology*, **15**(2), 97–106.

Barry D and Petry N (2008). Predictors of decision-making on the Iowa Gambling Task: independent effects of lifetime history of substance use disorders and performance on the Trail Making Test. *Brain and Cognition*, **66**(3), 243–252.

Bartus RT, Fleming D and Johnson HR (1978). Aging in the rhesus monkey: debilitating effects on short-term memory. *Journal of Gerontology*, **33**(6), 858–871.

Bartus RT, Dean III RL and Fleming DL (1979). Aging in the rhesus monkey: effects on visual discrimination learning and reversal learning. *Journal of Gerontology*, **34**, 209–219.

Bartzokis G, Beckson M, Lu PH, Nuechterlein KH, Edwards N and Mintz J (2001). Age-related changes in frontal and temporal lobe volumes in men: a magnetic resonance imaging study. *Archives of General Psychiatry*, **58**(5), 461–465.

Basho S, Palmer ED, Rubio MA, Wulfeck B and Müller RA (2007). Effects of generation mode in fMRI adaptations of semantic fluency: paced production and overt speech. *Neuropsychologia*, **45**(8), 1697–1706.

Bastin C and Van der Linden M (2005). Memory for temporal context: effects of ageing, encoding instructions, and retrieval strategies. *Memory*, **13**(1), 95–109.

Bauer RH and Fuster JM (1976). Delayed-matching and delayed-response deficit from cooling dorsolateral prefrontal cortex in monkeys. *Journal of Comparative and Physiological Psychology*, **90**(3), 293–302.

Baxter MG, Parker A, Lindner CC, Izquierdo AD and Murray EA (2000). Control of response selection by reinforce value requires interaction of amygdala and orbital prefrontal cortex. *Journal of Neuroscience*, **20**, 4311–4319.

Beadle JN, Paradiso S, Kovach C, Polgreen L, Denburg NL and Tranel D (2012). Effects of age-related differences in empathy on social economic decision-making. *International Psychogeriatrics*, **24**(5), 822–833.

Beauchamp MH, Dagher A, Aston JA and Doyon J (2003). Dynamic functional changes associated with cognitive skill learning of an adapted version of the Tower of London task. *Neuroimage*, **20**(3), 1649–1660.

Bechara A, Damasio AR, Damasio H and Anderson SW (1994). Insensitivity to future consequences following damage to human prefrontal cortex. *Cognition*, **50**(1–3), 7–15.

Bechara A, Tranel D, Damasio H and Damasio AR (1996). Failure to respond autonomically to anticipated future outcomes following damage to prefrontal cortex. *Cerebral Cortex*, **6**(2), 215–225.

Bechara A, Damasio H, Tranel D and Damasio AR (1997). Deciding advantageously before knowing the advantageous strategy. *Science*, **275**(5304), 1293–1295.

Bechara A, Damasio H, Tranel D and Anderson SW (1998). Dissociation of working memory from decision making within the human prefrontal cortex. *Journal of Neuroscience*, **18**(1), 428–437.

Bechara A, Damasio H, Damasio AR and Lee GP (1999). Different contributions of the human amygdala and ventromedial prefrontal cortex to decision-making. *Journal of Neuroscience*, **19**(13), 5473–5481.

Bechara A, Damasio H and Damasio AR (2000). Emotion, decision making and the orbitofrontal cortex. *Cerebral Cortex*, **10**(3), 295–307.

Bechara A, Dolan S, Denburg N, Hindes A, Anderson SW and Nathan PE (2001). Decision-making deficits, linked to a dysfunctional ventromedial prefrontal cortex, revealed in alcohol and stimulant abusers. *Neuropsychologia*, **39**(4), 376–389.

Bechara A, Damasio H, Tranel D and Damasio AR (2005). The Iowa Gambling Task and the somatic marker hypothesis: some questions and answers. *Trends in Cognitive Sciences*, **9**(4), 159–164.

Beckmann M, Johansen-Berg H and Rushworth MF (2009). Connectivity-based parcellation of human cingulate cortex and its relation to functional specialization. *Journal of Neuroscience*, **29**(4), 1175–1190.

Beer JS, Heerey EA, Keltner D, Scabini D and Knight RT (2003). The regulatory function of self-conscious emotion: insights from patients with orbitofrontal damage. *Journal of Personality and Social Psychology*, **85**(4), 594–604.

Beer JS, Stallen M, Lombardo MV, Gonsalkorale K, Cunningham WA and Sherman JW (2008). The Quadruple Process model approach to examining the neural underpinnings of prejudice. *NeuroImage*, **43**(4), 775–783.

Beglinger LJ, Unverzagt FW, Beristain X and Kareken D (2008). An updated version of the Weigl discriminates adults with dementia from those with mild impairment and healthy controls. *Archives of Clinical Neuropsychology*, **23**(2), 149–156.

Beliak AAM, Mansueti L, Strauss E and Dixon RA (2006). Performance on the Hayling and Brixton tests in older adults: norms and correlates. *Archives of Clinical Neuropsychology*, **21**, 141–149.

Bellgrove MA1, Hester R and Garavan H (2004). The functional neuroanatomical correlates of response variability: evidence from a response inhibition task. *Neuropsychologia*, **42**(14), 1910–1916.

Benton AL (1968). Differential behavioral effects in frontal lobe disease. *Neuropsychologia*, **6**(1), 53–60.

Benton AL, Hamsher KD and Sivan AB (1994). *Multilingual Aphasia Examination*. AJA Associates, Iowa City, IA.

Berent-Spillson A, Persad CC, Love T, Tkaczyk A, Wang H, Reame NK, Frey KA, Zubieta JK and Smith YR (2010). Early menopausal hormone use influences brain regions used for visual working memory. *Menopause*, **17**(4), 692–699.

Berlin HA, Rolls ET and Kischka U (2004). Impulsivity, time perception, emotion and reinforcement sensitivity in patients with orbitofrontal cortex lesions. *Brain*, **127**(5), 1108–1126.

Berman KF, Ostrem JL, Randolph C, Gold J, Goldberg TE, Coppola R, Carson RE, Herscovitch P and Weinberger DR (1995). Physiological activation of a cortical network during performance of the Wisconsin Card Sorting Test: a positron emisson tomography study. *Neuropsychologia*, **33**, 1027–1046.

Berry DS and Springer K (1993). Structure, motion, and preschoolers' perceptions of social causality. *Ecological Psychology*, **5**, 273–283.

Berry DS, Misovich SJ, Kean KJ and Baron RM (1992). Effects of disruption of structure and motion on perceptions of social causality. *Personality and Social Psychology Bulletin*, **18**, 237–244.

Best M, Williams JM and Coccaro EF (2002). Evidence for a dysfunctional prefrontal circuit in patients with an impulsive aggressive disorder. *Proceedings of the National Academy of Sciences of the USA*, **99**(**12**), 8448–8453.

Bialystok E, Craik FI, Klein R and Viswanathan M (2004). Bilingualism, aging and cognitive control: evidence from the Simon task. *Psychology and Aging*, **19**(**2**), 290–303.

Bibby H and McDonald S (2005). Theory of mind after traumatic brain injury. *Neuropsychologia*, **43**(**1**), 99–114.

Bielak AA, Mansueti L, Strauss E and Dixon RA (2006). Performance on the Hayling and Brixton tests in older adults: norms and correlates. *Archives of Clinical Neuropsychology*, **21**(**2**), 141–149.

Billingsley RL, Simos PG, Castillo EM, Sarkari S, Breier JI, Pataraia E and Papanicolaou AC (2004). Spatio-temporal cortical dynamics of phonemic and semantic fluency. *Journal of Clinical and Experimental Neuropsychology*, **26**(**8**), 1031–1043.

Bird CM, Castelli F, Malik O, Frith U and Husain M (2004). The impact of extensive medial frontal lobe damage on "Theory of Mind" and cognition. *Brain*, **127**(**4**), 914–928.

Birn RM, Kenworthy L, Case L, Caravella R, Jones TB, Bandettini PA and Martin A (2010). Neural systems supporting lexical search guided by letter and semantic category cues: a self-paced overt response fMRI study of verbal fluency. *NeuroImage*, **49**(**1**), 1099–1107.

Birnbaum SG, Yuan PX, Wang M, Vijayraghavan S, Bloom AK, Davis DJ, Gobeske KT, Sweatt JD, Manji HK and Arnsten AF (2004). Protein kinase C overactivity impairs prefrontal cortical regulation of working memory. *Science*, **306**(**5697**), 882–884.

Bishop DVM (1993). Annotation: autism, executive functions and theory of mind: a neuropsychological perspective. *Journal of Child Psychology and Psychiatry*, **34**(**3**), 279–293.

Black DN, Stip E, Bédard M, Kabay M, Paquette I and Bigras MJ (2000). Leukotomy revisited: late cognitive and behavioral effects in chronic institutionalized schizophrenics. *Schizophrenia Research*, **43**(**1**), 57–64.

Black FW and Strub RL (1978). Digit repetition performance in patients with focal brain damage. *Cortex*, **14**(**1**), 12–21.

Blair RJ and Cipolotti L (2000). Impaired social response reversal. A case of "acquired sociopathy". *Brain*, **123**(**6**), 1122–1141.

Blair RJ, Morris JS, Frith CD, Perrett DI and Dolan RJ (1999). Dissociable neural responses to facial expressions of sadness and anger. *Brain*, **122**(**5**), 883–893.

Bloom PA and Fischler I (1980). Completion norms for 329 sentence contexts. *Memory and Cognition*, **38**, 631–642.

Bogdanova Y and Cronin-Golomb A (2011). Neurocognitive correlates of apathy and anxiety in Parkinson's disease. *Parkinson's Disease*, **1**, 1–9.

Boghi A, Rasetti R, Avidano F, Manzone C, Orsi L, D'Agata F, Caroppo P, Bergui M, Rocca P, Pulvirenti L, Bradac GB, Bogetto F, Mutani R and Mortara P (2006). The effect of gender on planning: an fMRI study using the Tower of London task. *Neuroimage*, **33**(3), 999–1010.

Bokura H, Yamaguchi S and Kobayashi S (2001). Electrophysiological correlates for response inhibition in a Go/NoGo task. *Clinical Neurophysiology*, **112**(12), 2224–2232.

Boll TJ and Reitan RM (1973). Effect of age on performance of the Trail Making Test. *Perceptual and Motor Skills*, **36**, 691–694.

Bolla KI, Gray S, Resnick SM, Galante R and Kawas C (1998). Category and letter fluency in highly educated older adults. *The Clinical Neuropsychologist*, **12**(3), 330–338.

Bolla KI, Lindgren KN, Bonaccorsy C and Bleecker ML (1990). Predictors of verbal fluency (FAS) in the healthy elderly. *Journal of Clinical Psychology*, **46**(5), 623–628.

Bolla KI, Eldreth DA, Matochik JA and Cadet JL (2004). Sex-related differences in a gambling task and its neurological correlates. *Cerebral Cortex*, **14**(11), 1226–1232.

Bolton GE and Zwick R (1995). Anonymity versus punishment in ultimatum bargaining. *Games and Economic Behavior*, **10**, 95–121.

Boone KB, Ghaffarian S, Lesser IM, Hill-Gutierrez E and Berman NG (1993). Wisconsin Card Sorting Test performance in healthy, older adults: relationship to age, sex, education, and IQ. *Journal of Clinical Psychology*, **49**(1), 54–60.

Booth JR, Burman DD, Meyer JR, Lei Z, Trommer BL, Davenport ND, Li W, Parrish TB, Gitelman DR and Mesulam MM (2003). Neural development of selective attention and response inhibition. *Neuroimage*, **20**(2), 737–751.

Bopp KL and Verhaeghen P (2005). Aging and verbal memory span: a meta-analysis. *The Journals of Gerontology, Series B, Psychological Sciences and Social Sciences*, **60**(5), P223–P233.

Borg JS, Hynes C, Van Horn J, Grafton S and Sinnott-Armstrong W (2006). Consequences, action and intention as factors in moral judgements: an fMRI investigation. *Journal of Cognitive Neuroscience*, **18**, 803–817.

Borkowski JG, Benton AL and Spreen O (1967). Word fluency and brain damage. *Neuropsychologia*, **5**(2), 135–140.

Borod JC, Yecker SA, Brickman AM, Moreno CR, Sliwinski M, Foldi NS, Alpert M and Welkowitz J (2004). Changes in posed facial expression of emotion across the adult life span. *Experimental Aging Research*, **30**, 305–331.

Botvinick MM (2007). Conflict monitoring and decision making: reconciling two perspectives on anterior cingulate function. *Cognitive, Affective & Behavioral Neuroscience*, **7**(4), 356–366.

Botvinick MM, Cohen JD and Carter CS (2004). Conflict monitoring and anterior cingulate cortex: an update. *Trends in Cognitive Sciences*, **8**(12), 539–546.

Bowman CH and Turnbull OH (2003). Real versus facsimile reinforcers on the Iowa Gambling Task. *Brain and Cognition*, **53**(2), 207–210.

Bowman CH, Evans CEY and Turnbull OH (2005). Artificial time constraints on the Iowa Gambling Task: the effects on behavioural performance and subjective experience. *Brain and Cognition*, **57**(1), 21–25.

Brammer MJ, Bullmore ET, Simmons A, Williams SCR, Grasby PM, Howard RJ, Woodruff PWR and Rabe-Hesketh S (1997). Generic brain activation mapping in functional magnetic resonance imaging: a nonparametric approach. *Magnetic Resonance Imaging*, **15**(7), 763–770.

Brand M, Kalbe E and Kessler J (2002). Test zum kognitiven Schätzen (TKS). Hogrefe, Göttingen.

Brand M, Fujiwara E, Borsutzky S, Kalbe E, Kessler J and Markowitsch HJ (2005a). Decision-making deficits of Korsakoff patients in a new gambling task with explicit rules: associations with executive functions. *Neuropsychology*, **19**(3), 267–277.

Brand M, Kalbe E, Labudda K, Fujiwara E, Kessler J and Markowitsch HJ (2005b). Decision-making impairments in patients with pathological gambling. *Psychiatry Research*, **133**(1), 91–99.

Brand M, Labudda K and Markowitsch HJ (2006). Neuropsychological correlates of decision-making in ambiguous and risky situations. *Neural Networks*, **19**(8), 1266–1276.

Braver TS and Bongiolatti SR (2002). The role of frontopolar cortex in subgoal processing during working memory. *NeuroImage*, **15**(3), 523–536.

Braver TS, Barch DM, Gray JR, Molfese DL and Snyder A (2001a). Anterior cingulate cortex and response conflict: effects of frequency, inhibition, and errors. *Cerebral Cortex*, **11**(9), 825–836.

Braver TS, Barch DM, Kelley WM, Buckner RL, Cohen NJ, Miezin FM, Snyder AZ, Ollinger JM, Akbudak E, Conturo TE and Petersen SE (2001b). Direct comparison of prefrontal cortex regions engaged by working and long-term memory tasks. *NeuroImage*, **14**(1), 48–59.

Braver TS, Barch DM, Keys BA, Carter CS, Cohen JD, Kaye JA, Janowsky JS, Taylor SF, Yesavage JA, Mumenthaler MS, Jagust WJ and Reed BR (2001c). Context processing in older adults: evidence for a theory relating cognitive control to neurobiology in healthy aging. *Journal of Experimental Psychology: General*, **130**(4), 746–763.

Brazzelli M, Colombo N, Della Sala S and Spinnler H (1994). Spared and impaired cognitive abilities after bilateral frontal damage. *Cortex*, **30**, 27–51.

Breiter HC and Rosen BR (1999). Functional magnetic resonance imaging of brain reward circuitry in the human. *Annals of the New York Academy of Sciences*, **877**(3), 523–547.

Breteler MM, van Amerongen NM, van Swieten JC, Claus JJ, Grobbee DE, van Gijn J, Hofman A and van Harskamp F (1994). Cognitive correlates of ventricular enlargement and cerebral white matter lesions on magnetic resonance imaging. The Rotterdam Study. *Stroke*, **25**(6), 1109–1115.

Brickman AM, Paul RH, Cohen RA, Williams LM, MacGregor KL, Jefferson AL, Tate DF, Gunstad J and Gordon E (2005). Category and letter verbal fluency across the adult lifespan: relationship to EEG theta power. *Archives of Clinical Neuropsychology*, **20**(5), 561–573.

Britton JC, Taylor SF, Sudheimer KD and Liberzonb I (2006). Facial expressions and complex IAPS pictures: common and differential networks. *NeuroImage*, **31**, 906–919.

Brodmann K (1909). *Vergleichende Lokalisationslehre der Großhirnrinde in ihren Prinzipien dargestellt auf Grund des Zellenbaues*. Barth, Leipzig. English translation available in LJ Garey (1994). *Brodmann's Localization in the Cerebral Cortex*. Smith Gordon, London.

Brosgole L and Weisman J (1995). Mood recognition across the ages. *International Journal of Neuroscience*, **82**, 169–189.

Brothers L and Ring B (1992). A neuroethological framework for the representation of minds. *Journal of Cognitive Neuroscience*, **4**(2), 107–118.

Brotis AG, Kapsalaki EZ, Paterakis K, Smith JR and Fountas KN (2009). Historic evolution of open cingulectomy and stereotactic cingulotomy in the management of medically intractable psychiatric disorders, pain and drug addiction. *Stereotactic and Functional Neurosurgery*, **87**(5), 271–291.

Brunet E, Sarfati Y, Hardy-Baylé MC and Decety J (2000). A PET investigation of the attribution of intentions with a nonverbal task. *NeuroImage*, **11**(2), 157–166.

Bryan J and Luszcz MA (2000). Measures of fluency as predictors of incidental memory among older adults. *Psychology and Aging*, **15**(3), 483–489.

Bryan, J and Luszcz MA (2001). Adult age differences in Self-Ordered Pointing task performance: contributions from working memory, executive function and speed of information processing. *Journal of Clinical and Experimental Neuropsychology*, **23**(5), 608–619.

Bryan J, Luszcz M and Crawford JR (1997). Verbal knowledge and speed of information processing as mediators of age differences in verbal fluency performance among older adults. *Psychology and Aging*, **12**(3), 473–478.

Buchsbaum BR, Greer S, Chang WL and Berman KF (2005). Meta-analysis of neuroimaging studies of the Wisconsin card-sorting task and component processes. *Human Brain Mapping*, **25**(1), 35–45.

Buelow MT and Suhr JA (2009). Construct validity of the Iowa Gambling Task. *Neuropsychology Review*, **19**(1), 102–114.

Bugg JM, Zook NA, DeLosh EL, Davalos DB and Davis HP (2006). Age differences in fluid intelligence: contributions of general slowing and frontal decline. *Brain and Cognition*, **62**(1), 9–16.

Bugg JM, DeLosh EL, Davalos DB and Davis HP (2007). Age differences in Stroop interference: contributions of general slowing and task-specific deficits. *Aging, Neuropsychology & Cognition*, **14**, 155–167.

Bull R, Phillips LH and Conway CA (2008). The role of control functions in mentalizing: dual-task studies of theory of mind and executive function. *Cognition*, **107**(2), 663–672.

Bullard SE, Fein D, Gleeson MK, Tischer N, Mapou RL and Kaplan (2004). The Biber Cognitive Estimation Test. *Archives of Clinical Neuropsychology*, **19**, 835–846.

Bunge SA, Kahn I, Wallis JD, Miller EK and Wagner AD (2003). Neural circuits subserving the retrieval and maintenance of abstract rules. *Journal of Neurophysiology*, **90**(5), 3419–3428.

Burgess PW (1997). Theory and methodology in executive function research. In P Rabbitt, ed., *Methodology of Frontal and Executive Functions*, pp. 81–116. Psychology Press, Hove.

Burgess PW (2011). Frontopolar cortex: constraints for theorizing. *Trends in Cognitive Sciences*, **15**(6), 242.

Burgess PW and Shallice T (1994). Fractionation of the frontal lobe syndrome. *Revue de Neuropsychologie*, **4**, 345–370.

Burgess PW and Shallice T (1996a). Bizarre responses, rule detection and frontal lobe lesions. *Cortex*, **32**(2), 241–259.

Burgess PW and Shallice T (1996b). Response suppression, initiation and strategy use following frontal lobe lesions. *Neuropsychologia*, **34**(4), 263–273.

Burgess PW, Veitch E, de Lacy Costello A and Shallice T (2000). The cognitive and neuroanatomical correlates of multitasking. *Neuropsychologia*, **38**(6), 848–63.

Burgess PW, Simons JW, Dumontheil I and Gilbert SJ (2005). The gateway hypothesis of rostral PFC function. In J Duncan, L Phillips and P McLeod, eds, *Measuring the Mind: Speed, Control and Age*, pp. 217–248. Oxford University Press, Oxford.

Burgess PW, Alderman N, Volle E, Benoit RG and Gilbert SJ (2009). Mesulam's frontal lobe mystery re-examined. *Restorative Neurology and Neuroscience*, **27**(5), 493–506.

Burzynska AZ, Nagel IE, Preuschhof C, Gluth S, Bäckman L, Li SC, Lindenberger U and Heekeren HR (2011). Cortical thickness is linked to executive functioning in adulthood and aging. *Human Brain Mapping*, **33**(7), 1607–1620.

Bush G, Luu P and Posner MI (2000). Cognitive and emotional influences in anterior cingulate cortex. *Trends in Cognitive Science*, **4**(6), 215–222.

Bushara KO, Weeks RA, Ishii K, Catalan MJ, Tian B, Rauschecker JP and Hallett M (1999). Modality-specific frontal and parietal areas for auditory and visual spatial localization in humans. *Nature Neuroscience*, **2**(8), 759–766.

Butler KM, Zacks RT and Henderson JM (1999). Suppression of reflexive saccades in younger and older adults: age comparisons on an antisaccade task. *Journal of Memory and Cognition*, **27**, 584–591.

Butters MA, Kaszniak AW, Glisky EL, Eslinger PJ and Schacter DL (1994). Recency discrimination deficits in frontal lobe patients. *Neuropsychology*, **8**, 343–353.

Byrnes MA and Spitz HH (1977). Performance of retarded adolescents and nonretarded children on the Tower of Hanoi problem. *American Journal on Mental Deficiency*, **81**, 561–569.

Cabeza R (2002). Hemispheric asymmetry reduction in older adults: the HAROLD model. *Psychology and Aging*, **17**, 85–100.

Cabeza R, Mangels J, Nyberg L, Habib R, Houle S, McIntosh AR and Tulving E (1997). Brain regions differentially involved in remembering what and when: a PET study. *Neuron*, **19**(4), 863–870.

Cabeza R, Anderson ND, Houle S, Mangels JA and Nyberg L (2000). Age-related differences in neural activity during item and temporal-order memory retrieval: a positron emission tomography study. *Journal of Cognitive Neuroscience*, **12**(1), 197–206.

Caetano MS, Horst NK, Harenberg L, Liu B, Arnsten AFT and Laubach M (2012). Lost in transition: aging-related changes in executive control by the medial prefrontal cortex. *The Journal of Neuroscience*, **32**(11), 3765–3777.

Calder AJ, Young AW, Keane J and Dean M (2000). Configural information in facial expression perception. *Journal of Experimental Psychology. Human Perception and Performance*, **26**(2), 527–551.

Calder AJ, Lawrence AD and Young AW (2001). Neuropsychology of fear and loathing. *Nature Reviews Neuroscience*, **2**(5), 352–363.

Calder AJ, Keane J, Manly T, Sprengelmeyer R, Scott S, Nimmo-Smith I and Young AW (2003). Facial expression recognition across the adult life span. *Neuropsychologia*, **41**(2), 195–202.

Caldú X, Vendrell, P Bartrés-Faz D, Clemente I, Bargalló N, Jurado MA, Serra-Grabulosa JM and Junqué C (2007). Impact of the COMT Val108/158 Met and DAT genotypes on prefrontal function in healthy subjects. *NeuroImage*, **37**(4), 1437–1444.

Callicott JH, Bertolino A, Mattay VS, Langheim FJ, Duyn J, Coppola R, Goldberg TE and Weinberger DR (2000). Physiological dysfunction of the dorsolateral prefrontal cortex in schizophrenia revisited. *Cerebral Cortex*, **10**(11), 1078–1092.

Campbell AW (1905). *Histological Studies on the Localisation of Cerebral Function.* Cambridge University Press, Cambridge.

Canavan AG, Passingham RE, Marsden CD, Quinn N, Wyke M and Polkey CE (1989). Sequence ability in parkinsonians, patients with frontal lobe lesions and patients who have undergone unilateral temporal lobectomies. *Neuropsychologia*, **27**(**6**), 787–798.

Cantor-Graae E, Warkentin S, Franzen G and Risberg J (1993). Frontal lobe challenge: a comparison of activation procedures during rCBF measurements in normal subjects. *Cognitive and Behavioral Neurology*, **6**(**2**), 83–92.

Capitani E (1997) Normative data and neuropsychological assessment. Common problems in clinical practice and research. *Neuropsychological Rehabilitation*, **7**(**4**), 295–310.

Capitani E, Della Sala S, Lucchelli F, Soave P and Spinnler H (1988). Gottschaldt's hidden figure test: sensitivity of perceptual attention to aging and dementia. *Journal of Gerontology*, **43**(**6**), 157–163.

Capitani E, Della Sala S, Logie RH and Spinnler H (1992). Recency, primacy and deficits of memory: reappraising and standardising the serial position curve. *Cortex*, **28**, 315–342.

Capitani E, Laiacona M and Basso A (1998). Phonetically cued word-fluency, gender differences and aging: a reappraisal. *Cortex*, **34**, 779–783.

Cardebat D, Demonet JF, Viallard G, Faure S, Puel M and Celsis P (1996). Brain functional profiles in formal and semantic fluency tasks: a SPECT study in normals. *Brain and Language*, **52**(**2**), 305–313.

Carlson S, Martinkauppi S, Rämä P, Salli E, Korvenoja A and Aronen HJ (1998). Distribution of cortical activation during visuospatial n-back tasks as revealed by functional magnetic resonance imaging. *Cerebral Cortex*, **8**(**8**), 743–752.

Carter CS and van Veen V (2007). Anterior cingulate cortex and conflict detection: An update of theory and data. *Cognitive, Affective and Behavioural Neuroscience*, **7**(**4**), 367–379.

Carter CS, Braver TS, Barch DM, Botvinick MM, Noll D and Cohen JD (1998). Anterior cingulate cortex, error detection, and the online monitoring of performance. *Science*, **280**, 747–749.

Carter CS, Macdonald AM, Botvinick M, Ross LL, Stenger VA, Noll DD and Cohen JD (2000). Parsing executive processes: strategic vs. evaluative functions of the anterior cingulate cortex. *Proceedings of the National Academy of Science of the USA*, **97**(**4**), 1944–1948.

Casey BJ, Trainor RJ, Orendi JL, Schubert AB, Nystrom LE, Giedd JN, Castellanos FX, Haxby JV, Noll DC, Cohen JD, Forman SD, Dahl RE and Rapoport JL (1997). A developmental functional MRI study of prefrontal activation during performance of a Go-No-Go Task. *Journal of Cognitive Neuroscience*, **9**(**6**), 835–847.

Castelli F, Happé F, Frith U and Frith C (2000). Movement and mind: a functional imaging study of perception and interpretation of complex intentional movement patterns. *Neuroimage*, **12**(**3**), 314–325.

Castelli F, Frith C, Happé F and Frith U (2002). Autism, Asperger syndrome and brain mechanisms for the attribution of mental states to animated shapes. *Brain*, **125**(**8**), 1839–1849.

Castelli I, Baglio F, Blasi V, Alberoni M, Falini A, Liverta-Sempio O, Nemni R and Marchetti A (2010). Effects of aging on mindreading ability through the eyes: an fMRI study. *Neuropsychologia*, **48**(**9**), 2586–2594.

Catani M (2007). From hodology to function. *Brain*, **130**(3), 602–605.

Catani M and ffytche DH (2005). The rises and falls of disconnection syndromes. *Brain*, **128**, 2224–2239.

Catani M and Stuss DT (2012a). Frontal lobes. *Cortex*, **48**(1), 1–132.

Catani M and Stuss DT (2012b). Frontal lobes. *Cortex*, **48**(2), 133–292.

Catani M and Thiebaut de Schotten M (2008). A diffusion tensor imaging tractography atlas for virtual in vivo dissections. *Cortex*, **44**(8), 1105–1132.

Catani M, Dell'Acqua F, Vergani F, Malik F, Hodge H, Roy P, Valabregue R and Thiebaut de Schotten M (2012). Short frontal lobe connections of the human brain. *Cortex*, **48**(2), 273–291.

Cattaneo Z, Mattavelli G, Platania E and Papagno C (2011). The role of the prefrontal cortex in controlling gender-stereotypical associations: a TMS investigation. *NeuroImage*, **56**(3), 1839–1846.

Cazalis F, Valabrègue R, Pélégrini-Issac M, Asloun S, Robbins TW and Granon S (2003). Individual differences in prefrontal cortical activation on the Tower of London planning task: implication for effortful processing. *European Journal of Neuroscience*, **17**(10), 2219–2225.

Cazalis F, Feydy A, Valabrègue R, Pélégrini-Issac M, Pierot L and Azouvi P (2006). fMRI study of problem-solving after severe traumatic brain injury. *Brain Injury*, **20**(10), 1019–1028.

Channon S and Crawford S (1999). Problem-solving in real-life-type situations: the effects of anterior and posterior lesions on performance. *Neuropsychologia*, **37**, 757–770.

Channon S and Crawford S (2000). The effects of anterior lesions on performance on a story comprehension test: left anterior impairment on a theory of mind-type task. *Neuropsychologia*, **38**, 1006–1017.

Chao LL and Knight RT (1997). Prefrontal deficits in attention and inhibitory control with aging. *Cerebral Cortex*, **7**, 63–69.

Charlton RA, Barrick TR, Markus HS and Morris RG (2009). Theory of mind associations with other cognitive functions and brain imaging in normal aging. *Psychology and Aging*, **24**(2), 338–348.

Charness N (1987). Component processes in bridge bidding and novel problem-solving tasks. *Canadian Journal of Psychology*, **41**, 223–243.

Chase HW, Clark L, Sahakian BJ, Bullmore ET and Robbins TW (2008). Dissociable roles of prefrontal subregions in self-ordered working memory performance. *Neuropsychologia*, **46**(11), 2650–2661.

Chaytor N and Schmitter-Edgecombe M (2004). Working memory and aging: a cross-sectional and longitudinal analysis using a self-ordered pointing task. *Journal of the International Neuropsychological Society*, **10**(4), 489–503.

Chee MW, Sriram N, Soon CS and Lee KM (2000). Dorsolateral prefrontal cortex and the implicit association of concepts and attributes. Neuroreport, **11**(1), 135–140.

Chen WJ, Hsiao CK, Hsiao LL and Hwu HG (1998). Performance of the Continuous Performance Test among community samples. *Schizophrenia Bulletin*, **24**(1), 163–174.

Chikazoe J (2010). Localizing performance of go/no-go tasks to prefrontal cortical subregions. *Current Opinions in Psychiatry*, **23**(3), 267–272.

Chikazoe J, Jimura K, Asari T, Yamashita K, Morimoto H, Hirose S, Miyashita Y and Konishi S (2009). Functional dissociation in right inferior frontal cortex during performance of go/no-go task. *Cerebral Cortex*, **19**(1), 146–152.

Chiu Y-C and Lin C-H (2007). Is deck C an advantageous deck in the Iowa Gambling Task? *Behavioral and Brain Functions*, **3**, 37–47.

Ciaramelli E, Muccioli M, Ladavas E and di Pellegrino G (2007). Selective deficit in personal moral judgement following damage to ventromedial prefrontal cortex. *Social Cognitive and Affective Neuroscience*, **2**, 84–92.

Ciaramidaro A, Adenzato M, Enrici I, Erk S, Pia L, Bara BG and Walter H (2007). The intentional network: how the brain reads varieties of intentions. *Neuropsychologia*, **45**(13), 3105–3113.

Cicerone KD and Tanenbaum LN (1997). Disturbance of social cognition after traumatic orbitofrontal brain injury. *Archives of Clinical Neuropsychology*, **12**(2), 173–188.

Cilia R, Siri C, Marotta G, De Gaspari D, Landi A, Mariani CB, Benti R, Isaias IU, Vergani F, Pezzoli G and Antonini A (2007). Brain networks underlining verbal fluency decline during STN-DBS in Parkinson's disease: an ECD-SPECT study. *Parkinsonism & Related Disorders*, **13**(5), 290–294.

Cima M, Tonnaer F and Hauser MD (2010). Psychopaths know right from wrong but don't care. *Social Cognitive and Affective Neuroscience*, **5**, 59–67.

Clark CN and Warren JD (2014). The neurology of humour. *Advances in Clinical Neuroscience and Rehabilitation*, **V13**(7), 9–11.

Clark CR, Veltmeyer MD, Hamilton RJ, Simms E, Paul R, Hermens D and Gordon E (2004). Spontaneous alpha peak frequency predicts working memory performance across the age span. *International Journal of Psychophysiology*, **53**(1), 1–9.

Clark L, Manes F, Antoun N, Sahakian BJ and Robbins TW (2003). The contributions of lesion laterality and lesion volume to decision-making impairment following frontal lobe damage. *Neuropsychologia*, **41**(11), 1474–1483.

Coccaro EF, McCloskey MS, Fitzgerald DA and Phan KL (2007). Amygdala and orbitofrontal reactivity to social threat in individuals with impulsive aggression. *Biological Psychiatry*, **62**(2), 168–178.

Cohen JD, Braver TS and O'Reilly RC (1996). A computational approach to prefrontal cortex, cognitive control and schizophrenia: recent developments and current challenges. *Philosophical Transactions of the Royal Society of London, Series B, Biological Sciences*, **351**(1346), 1515–1527.

Cohen JD, Perlstein W, Braver T, Nystrom LE, Noll DC, Jonides J and Smith EE (1997). Temporal dynamics of brain activation during a working memory task. *Nature*, **386**, 604–608.

Cohen MX, Ridderinkhof KR, Haupt S, Elger CE and Fell J (2008). Medial frontal cortex and response conflict: evidence from human intracranial EEG and medial frontal cortex lesion. *Brain Research*, 1238, 127–142.

Cohen RA, Kaplan RF, Moser DJ, Jenkins MA and Wilkinson H (1999). Impairments of attention after cingulotomy. *Neurology*, **53**(4), 819–824.

Cole MW, Yeung N, Freiwald WA and Botvinick M (2009). Cingulate cortex: diverging data from humans and monkeys. *Trends in Neurosciences*, **32**(11), 566–574.

Collette F, Van der Linden M, Delfiore G, Degueldre C, Luxen A and Salmon E (2001). The functional anatomy of inhibition processes investigated with the Hayling Task. *NeuroImage*, **14**, 258–267.

Collette F, Hogge M, Salmon E and Van der Linden M (2006). Exploration of the neural substrates of executive functioning by functional neuroimaging. *Neuroscience*, **139**, 209–221.

Comali PE Jr, Wapner S and Werner H (1962). Interference effects of Stroop Colour-Word Test in childhood, adulthood and aging. *Journal of Genetic Psychology*, **100**, 47–53.

Cook IA, Bookheimer SY, Mickes L, Leuchter AF and Kumar A (2007). Aging and brain activation with working memory tasks: an fMRI study of connectivity. *International Journal of Geriatric Psychiatry*, **22**(4), 332–342.

Cools R, Clark L, Owen AM and Robbins TW (2002a). Defining the neural mechanisms of probabilistic reversal learning using event-related functional magnetic resonance imaging. *Journal of Neuroscience*, **22**(11), 4563–4567.

Cools R, Stefanova E, Barker RA, Robbins TW and Owen AM (2002b). Dopaminergic modulation of high-level cognition in Parkinson's disease: the role of the prefrontal cortex revealed by PET. *Brain*, **125**, 584–594.

Corcoran R, Cahill C and Frith CD (1997). The appreciation of visual jokes in people with schizophrenia: a study of "mentalizing" ability. *Schizophrenia Research*, **24**(3), 319–327.

Costa A, Torriero S, Olivieri M and Caltagirone C (2008). Prefrontal and temporo-parietal involvement in taking others' perspective: TMS evidence. *Behavioural Neurology*, **19**, 71–74.

Coull JT, Cheng RK and Meck WH (2011). Neuroanatomical and neurochemical substrates of timing. *Neuropsychopharmacology*, **36**(1), 3–25.

Cox SR, Ferguson KJ, Royle NA, Shenkin SD, MacPherson SE, MacLullich AMJ, Deary IJ and Wardlaw JM (2014). A systematic review of brain frontal lobe parcellation techniques in magnetic resonance imaging. *Brain Structure and Function*, **219**(1), 1–22.

Craik FIM and Bialystok E (2006). Planning and task management in older adults: cooking breakfast. *Memory & Cognition*, **34**(6), 1236–1249.

Crawford JR, Bryan J, Luszcz M, Obonsawin MC and Stewart L (2000). The executive decline hypothesis of cognitive aging: do executive deficits qualify as differential deficits and do they mediate age-related memory decline? *Aging, Neuropsychology, and Cognition*, **7**(1), 9–31.

Crawford S and Channon S (2002). Dissociation between performance on abstract tests of executive function and problem solving in real-life-type situations in normal aging. *Aging & Mental Health*, **6**(1), 12–21.

Crescentini C, Seyed-Allaei S, De Pisapia N, Jovicich J, Amati D and Shallice T (2011). Mechanisms of rule acquisition and rule following in inductive reasoning. *Journal of Neuroscience*, **31**(21), 7763–7774.

Critchley HD, Mathias CJ, Josephs O, O'Doherty J, Zanini S, Dewar B-K, Cipolotti L, Shallice T and Dolan RJ (2003). Human cingulate cortex and autonomic control: converging neuroimaging and clinical evidence. *Brain*, **126**(10), 2139–2152.

Crossley M, D'Arcy C and Rawson NS (1997). Letter and category fluency in community-dwelling Canadian seniors: a comparison of normal participants to those with dementia of the Alzheimer or vascular type. *Journal of Clinical and Experimental Neuropsychology*, **19**(1), 52–62.

Crosson B, Sadek JR, Maron L, Gökçay D, Mohr CM, Auerbach EJ, Freeman AJ, Leonard CM and Briggs RW (2001). Relative shift in activity from medial to lateral frontal cortex during internally versus externally guided word generation. *Journal of Cognitive Neuroscience*, **13**(2), 272–283.

Cubelli R and Della Sala S (2011). The purposes of neuropsychological assessment and how to achieve them. *Advances in Clinical Neuroscience & Rehabilitation*, **11**(1), 36–37.

Cubelli R, Beschin N and Della Sala S (2011). Ipsilateral neglect for non-verbal stimuli following left brain damage. *Cortex*, **47**(7), 899–901.

Cubelli R, Pedrizzi S and Della Sala S (in press). The role of cognitive neuropsychology in clinical settings: the example of a single case of deep dyslexia. In J Macniven, ed., *Neuropsychological Formulation: A Clinical Casebook*. Springer Science+Business Media, Inc., New York/Berlin.

Cuenod CA, Bookheimer SY, Hertz-Pannier L, Zeffiro TA, Theodore WH and LeBihan D (1995). Functional MRI during word generation, using conventional equipment: a potential tool for language localization in the clinical environment. *Neurology*, **45**(10), 1821–1827.

Culbertson WC, Moberg PJ, Duda JE, Stern MB and Weintraub D (2004). Assessing the executive function deficits of patients with Parkinson's disease: utility of the Tower of London—Drexel. *Assessment*, **11**(1), 27–39.

Curtis CE, Zald DH and Pardo JV (2000). Organization of working memory within the human prefrontal cortex: a PET study of self-ordered object working memory. *Neuropsychologia*, **38**, 1503–1510.

Curtis CE, Rao VY and D'Esposito M (2004). Maintenance of spatial and motor codes during oculomotor delayed response tasks. *Journal of Neuroscience*, **24**(16), 3944–3952.

Czernochowski D, Fabiani M and Friedman D (2008). Use it or lose it? SES mitigates age-related decline in a recency/recognition task. *Neurobiology of Aging*, **29**, 945–958.

Dagher A, Owen AM, Boecker H and Brooks DJ (1999). Mapping the network for planning: a correlational PET activation study with the Tower of London task. *Brain*, **122**, 1973–1987.

Dagher A, Owen AM, Boecker H and Brooks DJ (2001). The role of the striatum and hippocampus in planning. A PET activation study in Parkinson's disease. *Brain*, **124**, 1020–1032.

Dalton JC (1859–1871). *A Treatise on Human Physiology*. HC Lea, Philadelphia.

Damasio AR, Tranel D and Damasio H (1991). Somatic markers and the guidance of behavior: theory and preliminary testing. In HS Levin, HM Eisenberg and AL Benton, eds, *Frontal Lobe Function and Dysfunction*, pp. 217–229. Oxford University Press, New York.

Dan H, Dan I, Sano T, Kyutoku Y, Oguro K, Yokota H, Tsuzuki D and Watanabe E (2013). Language-specific cortical activation patterns for verbal fluency tasks in Japanese as assessed by multichannel functional near-infrared spectroscopy. *Brain and Language*, **126**(2), 208–216.

Danielmeier C, Elchele T, Forstmann BU, Tittgemeyer M and Ullsperger M (2011). Poster medial frontal cortex activity predicts post-error adaptations in task-related visual and motor areas. *Journal of Neuroscience*, **31**(5), 1780–1789.

Daum I, Gräber S, Schugens MM and Mayes AR (1996). Memory dysfunction of the frontal type in normal ageing. *Neuroreport*, **7**(15–17), 2625–2628.

Davidson DJ, Zacks RT and Williams CC (2003). Stroop interference, practice, and aging. *Neuropsychology, Development & Cognition B*, **10**(2), 85–98.

Davidson PSR, Gao FQ, Mason WP, Winocur G and Anderson ND (2008). Verbal fluency, Trail Making, and Wisconsin Card Sorting Test performance following right frontal lobe tumor resection. *Journal of Clinical and Experimental Neuropsychology*, **30**(1), 18–32.

Deakin J, Aitken M, Robbins T and Sahakian BJ (2004). Risk taking during decision-making in normal volunteers changes with age. *Journal of the International Neuropsychological Society*, **10**(4), 590–598.

Décary A and Richer F (1995). Response selection deficits in frontal excisions. *Neuropsychologia*, **33**(10), 1243–1253.

de Chastelaine M, Wang TH, Minton B, Muftuler LT and Rugg MD (2011). The effects of age, memory performance, and callosal integrity on the neural correlates of successful associative encoding. *Cerebral Cortex*, **21**(9), 2166–2176.

Delis DC, Kaplan E and Kramer J (2001). *Delis-Kaplan Executive Function System: Examiner's Manual*. The Psychological Corporation, San Antonio, TX.

De Jong R (2001). Adult age differences in goal activation and goal maintenance. *European Journal of Cognitive Psychology*, **13**, 71–89.

Della Sala S (2009). Dr. Strangelove syndrome. *Cortex*, **45**(10), 1278–1279.

Della Sala S, Laiacona M, Spinnler H and Ubezio MC (1992). A cancellation test: its reliability in assessing attentional deficits in Alzheimer's disease. *Psychological Medicine*, **22**, 885–901.

Della Sala S, Laiacona M, Trivelli C and Spinnler H (1995). Poppelreuter-Ghent's Overlapping Figures test: its sensitivity to age, and its clinical use. *Archives of Clinical Neuropsychology*, **10**, 511–534.

Della Sala S, Gray C, Spinnler H and Trivelli C (1998a). Frontal lobe functioning in man: the riddle revisited. *Archives of Clinical Neuropsychology*, **13**, 663–682.

Della Sala S, Gray C and Trivelli C (1998b). Putative functions of the prefrontal cortex: historical perspectives and new horizons. In G Mazzoni and TO Nelson, eds, *Metacognition and Cognitive Neuropsychology*, pp. 53–95. LEA, Hove.

Della Sala S, MacPherson SE, Phillips LH, Sacco L and Spinnler H (2003). How many camels are there in Italy? Cognitive estimates standardised on the Italian population. *Neurological Sciences*, **24**, 10–15.

Della Sala S, MacPherson SE, Phillips LH, Sacco L and Spinnler H (2004). The role of semantic memory on the Cognitive Estimation Task: evidence from Alzheimer's Disease and healthy adult aging. *Journal of Neurology*, **251**, 156–164.

Demakis GJ (2003). A meta-analytic review of the sensitivity of the Wisconsin Card Sorting Test to frontal and lateralized frontal brain damage. *Neuropsychology*, **17**(2), 255–264.

Demakis GJ (2004) Frontal lobe damage and tests of executive processing: a meta-analysis of the Category Test, Stroop Test, and Trail-Making Test. *Journal of Clinical and Experimental Neuropsychology*, **26**(3), 441–450.

den Braber A, Ent Dv, Blokland GA, van Grootheest DS, Cath DC, Veltman DJ, de Ruiter MB and Boomsma DI (2008). An fMRI study in monozygotic twins discordant for obsessive-compulsive symptoms. *Biological Psychology*, **79**, 91–102.

Denburg NL, Tranel D and Bechara A (2005). The ability to decide advantageously declines prematurely in some normal older persons. *Neuropsychologia*, **43**(7), 1099–1106.

De Pellegrino G, Ciaramelli E and Ladavas E (2007). The regulation of cognitive control following rostral anterior cingulate cortex lesion in humans. *Journal of Cognitive Neuroscience*, **19**(2), 275–286.

De Renzi E, Faglioni P, Savoiardo M and Vignolo LA (1966). The influence of aphasia and the hemisphere side of cerebral lesion on abstract thinking. *Cortex*, **2**, 399–420.

de Ruiter MB, Veltman DJ, Goudriaan AE, Oosterlaan J, Sjoerds Z and van den Brink W (2009). Response perseveration and ventral prefrontal sensitivity to reward and punishment in male problem gamblers and smokers. *Neuropsychopharmacology*, **34**(4), 1027–1038.

D'Esposito M and Postle BR (1999). The dependence of span and delayed-response performance on prefrontal cortex. *Neuropsychologia*, **37**(11), 1303–1315.

D'Esposito M, Aguirre GK, Zarahn E, Ballard D, Shin RK and Lease J (1998). Functional MRI studies of spatial and nonspatial working memory. *Brain Research. Cognitive Brain Research*, **7**(1), 1–13.

Devinsky O, Morrell MJ and Vogt BA (1995). Contributions of anterior cingulate cortex to behaviour. *Brain*, **118**, 279–306.

Devlin JT and Poldrack RA (2007). In praise of tedious anatomy. *NeuroImage*, **37**(4),1033–1041.

De Zubicaray GI, Chalk JB, Rose SE, Semple J and Smith GA (1997). Deficits on self ordered tasks associated with hyperostosis frontalis interna. *Journal of Neurology, Neurosurgery, and Psychiatry*, **63**(3), 309–314.

De Zubicaray GI, Andrew C, Zelaya FO, Williams SC and Dumanoir C (2000). Motor response suppression and the prepotent tendency to respond: a parametric fMRI study. *Neuropsychologia*, **38**(9), 1280–1291.

Diamond A and Goldman-Rakic P (1989). Comparison of human infants and rhesus monkeys on Piaget's AB task: evidence for dependence on dorsolateral prefrontal cortex. *Experimental Brain Research*, **74**, 24–40.

Dias EC, Foxe JJ and Javitt DC (2003). Changing plans: a high density electrical mapping study of cortical control. *Cerebral Cortex*, **13**(7), 701–715.

Dias R, Robins TW and Roberts AC (1997). Dissociable forms of inhibitory control within prefrontal cortex with an analog of the Wisconsin Card Sort Test: restriction to novel situations and independence from "on-line" processing. *Journal of Neuroscience*, **17**, 9285–9297.

Dimitrov M, Phipps M, Zahn TP and Grafman J (1999). A thoroughly modern Gage. *Neurocase*, **5**(4), 345–354.

di Pellegrino G, Ciaramelli E and Làdavas E (2007). The regulation of cognitive control following rostral anterior cingulate cortex lesion in humans. *Journal of Cognitive Neuroscience*, **19**(2), 275–286.

Dixit NK, Gerton BK, Kohn P, Meyer-Lindenberg A and Berman KF (2000). Age-related changes in rCBF activation during an N-back working memory paradigm occur prior to age 50. *NeuroImage*, **11**(5), S94.

Dobbins IG, Rice HJ, Wagner AD and Schacter DL (2003). Memory orientation and success: separable neurocognitive components underlying episodic recognition. *Neuropsychologia*, **41**(3), 318–333.

Dobbs AR and Rule BG (1989). Adult age differences in working memory. *Psychology and Aging*, **4**(4), 500–503.

Donkers FC and van Boxtel GJ (2004). The N2 in go/no-go tasks reflects conflict monitoring not response inhibition. *Brain and Cognition*, **56**(2), 165–176.

Drewe EA (1974). The effect of type and area of brain lesion on Wisconsin Card Sorting Test Performance. *Neuropsychologia*, **12**, 159–170.

Driscoll I, Davatzikos C, An Y, Wu X, Shen D, Kraut M and Resnick SM (2009). Longitudinal pattern of regional brain volume change differentiates normal aging from MCI. *Neurology*, **72**, 1906–1913.

Dubois B, Slachevsky A, Litvan I and Pillon B (2000). The FAB: a Frontal Assessment Battery at bedside. *Neurology*, **55**, 1621–1626.

Dudukovic NM and Wagner AD (2007). Goal-dependent modulation of declarative memory: neural correlates of temporal recency decisions and novelty detection. *Neuropsychologia*, **45**(**11**), 2608–2620.

Dufouil C, Alpérovitch A and Tzourio C (2003). Influence of education on the relationship between white matter lesions and cognition. *Neurology*, **60**(**5**), 831–836.

Dumontheil I, Thompson R and Duncan J (2011). Assembly and use of new task rules in fronto-parietal cortex. *Journal of Cognitive Neuroscience*, **23**, 168–182.

Duncan J (2006). Brain mechanisms of attention. *Quarterly Journal of Experimental Psychology*, **59**, 2–27.

Duncan J (2010). The multiple-demand (MD) system of the primate brain: mental programs for intelligent behaviour. *Trends in Cognitive Sciences*, **14**(**4**), 172–179.

Duncan J (2013). The structure of cognition: attentional episodes in mind and brain. *Neuron*, **80**, 35–80.

Duncan J and Owen AM (2000). Common regions of the human frontal lobe recruited by diverse cognitive demands. *Trends in Neurosciences*, **23**(**10**), 475–483.

Duncan J and Miller EK (2002). Cognitive focus through adaptive neural coding in the primate prefrontal cortex. In DT Stuss and R Knight, eds, *Principles of Frontal Lobe Functions*, pp. 278–292. Oxford University Press, New York.

Duncan J, Emslie H, Williams P, Johnson R and Freer C (1996). Intelligence and the frontal lobe: the organization of goal-directed behaviour. *Cognitive Psychology*, **30**, 257–303.

Duncan J, Johnson R, Swales M and Freer C (1997). Frontal lobe deficits after head injury: unity and diversity of function. *Cognitive Neuropsychology*, **14**, 713–741.

Duncan J, Seitz RJ, Kolodny J, Bor D, Herzog H, Ahmed A, Newell FN and Emslie H (2000). A neural basis for general intelligence. *Science*, **289**, 457–460.

Duncan J, Parr A, Woolgar A, Thompson R, Bright P, Cox S, Bishop S and Nimmo-Smith I (2008). Goal neglect and Spearman's g: competing parts of a complex task. *Journal of Experimental Psychology: General*, **137**, 131–148.

Dunn BD, Dalgleish T and Lawrence AD (2006). The somatic marker hypothesis: a critical evaluation. *Neuroscience and Biobehavioral Reviews*, **30**(**2**), 239–271.

Durston S, Thomas KM, Worden MS, Yang Y and Casey BJ (2002). The effect of preceding context on inhibition: an event-related fMRI study. *NeuroImage*, **16**(**2**), 449–453.

Dursun SM, Robertson HA, Bird D, Kutcher D and Kutcher SP (2002). Effects of ageing on prefrontal temporal cortical network function in healthy volunteers as assessed by COWA: an exploratory survey. *Progress in Neuro-Psychopharmacology & Biological Psychiatry*, **26**, 1007–1010.

Dutilh G, Vandekerckhove J, Forstmann BU, Keuleers E, Brysbaert M and Wagenamkers E-J (2012). Testing theories of post-error slowing. *Attention, Perception & Psychophysics*, **74**, 454–465.

Duval C, Piolino P, Bejanin A, Eustache F and Desgranges B (2011). Age effects on different components of theory of mind. *Consciousness and Cognition*, **20**(**3**), 627–642.

Ebner NC and Johnson MK (2009). Young and older emotional faces: are there age group differences in expression identification and memory? *Emotion*, **9**(3), 329–339.

Ecker A (1869). *Die Hirnwindungen des Menschen*. Vieweg, Braunschweig.

Ecker A (1873). *On the Convolutions of the Human Brain*. Smith Elder, London.

Egner T (2008). Multiple conflict-driven control mechanisms in the human brain. *Trends in Cognitive Sciences*, **12**(10), 374–80.

Ekman P and Friesen WV (1976). *Pictures of Facial Affect*. Consulting Psychologists, Palo Alto, CA.

Ekstrom RB, French JW, Harman HH and Derman D (1976). *Manual for Kit of Factor Referenced Cognitive Tests*. Educational Testing Service, Princeton, NJ.

Elfgren CI and Risberg J (1998). Lateralized frontal blood flow increases during fluency tasks: influence of cognitive strategy. *Neuropsychologia*, **36**(6), 505–512.

Elgamal S, Roy E and Sharratt MT (2011). Age and verbal fluency: the mediating effect of speed of processing. *Canadian Geriatrics Journal*, **14**(3), 66–72.

Elliott R and Dolan RJ (1999). Differential neural responses during performance of matching and nonmatching to sample tasks at two delay intervals. *Journal of Neuroscience*, **19**(12), 5066–5073.

Elliott R, Frith CD and Dolan RJ (1997). Differential neural response to positive and negative feedback in planning and guessing tasks. *Neuropsychologia*, **35**(10), 1395–1404.

Elliott R, Dolan RJ and Frith CD (2000). Dissociable functions in the medial and lateral orbitofrontal cortex: evidence from human neuroimaging studies. *Cerebral Cortex*, **10**(3), 308–317.

Eriksen BA and Eriksen CW (1974). Effects of noise letters upon the identification of a target letter in a nonsearch task. *Perception & Psychophysics*, **16**(1), 143–149.

Eslinger PJ (1998). Neurological and neuropsychological bases of empathy. *European Neurology*, **39**, 193–199.

Eslinger PJ and Damasio AR (1985). Severe disturbance of higher cognition after bilateral frontal lobe ablation: patient EVR. *Neurology*, **35**(12), 1731–1741.

Eslinger PJ and Grattan LM (1993). Frontal lobe and frontal-striatal substrates for different forms of cognitive flexibility. *Neuropsychologia*, **31**, 17–28.

Eslinger PJ, Satish U and Grattan LM (1996). Alterations in cognitive and affectively based empathy after cerebral damage. *Journal of the International Neuropsychological Society*, **2**, 15.

Esposito G, Kirkby BS, Van Horn JD, Ellmore TM and Berman KF (1999). Context-dependent, neural system-specific neurophysiological concomitants of ageing: mapping PET correlates during cognitive activation. *Brain*, **122**(5), 963–979.

Ethofer T, Anders S, Erb M, Herbert C, Wiethoff S, Kissler J, Grodd W and Wildgruber D (2006). Cerebral pathways in processing of affective prosody: a dynamic causal modeling study. *NeuroImage*, **30**(2), 580–587.

Etkin A, Egner, T, Peraza DM, Kandel ER and Hirsch J (2006). Resolving emotional conflict: a role for the rostral anterior cingulate cortex in modulating activity in the amygdala. *Neuron*, **51**, 1–12.

Exner C, Weniger G and Irle E (2004). Cerebellar lesions in the PICA but not SCA territory impair cognition. *Neurology*, **63**(11), 2132–2135.

Fabiani M and Friedman D (1997). Dissociations between memory for temporal order and recognition memory in aging. *Neuropsychologia*, **35**(2), 129–141.

Falkenstein M, Hoormann J and Hohnsbein J (1999). ERP components in Go/Nogo tasks and their relation to inhibition. *Acta Psychologica*, **101**(2–3), 267–291.

Falkenstein M, Hoormann J and Hohnsbein J (2001). Changes of error-related ERPs with age. *Experimental Brain Research*, **138**(2), 258–262.

Falkenstein M, Hoormann J and Hohnsbein J (2002). Inhibition-related ERP components: variation with modality, age, and time-on-task. *Journal of Psychophysiology*, **16**, 167–175.

Fallgatter AJ and Strik WK (1998). Frontal brain activation during the Wisconsin Card Sorting Test assessed with two-channel near-infrared spectroscopy. *European Archives of Psychiatry and Clinical Neuroscience*, **248**(5), 245–249.

Farrimond S, Knight RG and Titov N (2006). The effects of aging on remembering intentions: performance on a simulated shopping task. *Applied Cognitive Psychology*, **20**(4), 533–555.

Feldmann D, Schuepbach D, von Rickenbach B, Theodoridou A and Hell D (2006). Association between two distinct executive tasks in schizophrenia: a functional transcranial Doppler sonography study. *BMC Psychiatry*, **6**, 25.

Fellows LK and Farah MJ (2003). Ventromedial frontal cortex mediates affective shifting in humans: evidence from a reversal learning paradigm. *Brain*, **126**(8), 1830–1837.

Fellows LK and Farah MJ (2005a). Is anterior cingulate cortex necessary for cognitive control? *Brain*, **128**(4), 788–796.

Fellows LK and Farah MJ (2005b). Different underlying impairments in decision-making following ventromedial and dorsolateral frontal lobe damage in humans. *Cerebral Cortex*, **15**, 58–63.

Fernandez-Duque D and Black SE (2005). Impaired recognition of negative facial emotions in patients with frontotemporal dementia. *Neuropsychologia*, **43**(11), 1673–1687.

Feuchtwanger E (1923). *Monographien aus dem Gesamtgebiete der Neurologie und Psychiatrie, Vol. 38*. Julius Springer, Berlin.

ffytche DH and Catani M (2005). Beyond localisation: from hodology to function. *Philosophical Transactions of the Royal Society of London, Series B: Biological Sciences*, **360**, 767–779.

Fichman HC, Fernandes CS, Nitrini R, Lourenço RA, de Paiva EM and Cathery-Goulart MT (2009). Age and educational level effects on the performance of normal elderly on category verbal fluency tasks. *Dementia & Neuropsychologia*, **3**(1), 49–54.

Finan J (1942). Delayed response with pre-delay reenforcement in monkeys after the removal of the frontal lobes. *American Journal of Psychology*, **55**(2), 202–214.

Fincham JM, Carter CS, van Veen V, Stenger VA and Anderson JR (2002). Neural mechanisms of planning: a computational analysis using event-related fMRI. *Proceedings of the National Academy of Sciences of the USA*, **99**(5), 3346–3351.

Fine C and Blair RJR (2000). Mini review: the cognitive and emotional effects of amygdala damage. *Neurocase*, **6**, 435–450.

Fitzgerald PB, Benitez J, de Castella A, Daskalakis ZJ, Brown TL and Kulkarni J (2006). A randomized, controlled trial of sequential bilateral repetitive transcranial magnetic stimulation for treatment-resistant depression. *American Journal of Psychiatry*, **163**(1), 88–94.

Fitzgerald PB, Srithiran A, Benitez J, Daskalakis ZZ, Oxley TJ, Kulkarni J and Egan GF (2008). An fMRI study of prefrontal brain activation during multiple tasks in patients with major depressive disorder. *Human Brain Mapping*, **29**(4), 490–501.

Fjell AM, Westlye LT, Amlien I, Espeseth T, Reinvang I, Raz N, Agartz I, Salat DH, Greve DN, Fischl B, Dale AM and Walhovd KB (2009). High consistency of regional cortical thinning in aging across multiple samples. *Cerebral Cortex*, **19**(9), 2001–2012.

Fletcher PC, Happé F, Frith U, Baker SC, Dolan RJ, Frackowiak RS and Frith CD (1995). Other minds in the brain: a functional imaging study of "theory of mind" in story comprehension. *Cognition*, **57**, 109–128.

Floden D, Vallesi A and Stuss DT (2011). Task context and frontal lobe activation in the Stroop task. *Journal of Cognitive Neuroscience*, **23**(4), 867–879.

Forbes CE, Cameron KA, Grafman J, Barbey A, Solomon J, Ritter W and Ruchkin DS (2012). Identifying temporal and causal contributions of neural processes underlying the Implicit Association Test (IAT). *Frontiers in Human Neuroscience*, **6**, 320.

Fork M, Bartels C, Ebert AD, Grubich C, Synowitz H and Wallesch CW (2005). Neuropsychological sequelae of diffuse traumatic brain injury. *Brain Injury*, **19**(2), 101–108.

Foville AL (1844). *Traité Complet de L'anatomie, de la Physiologie et de la Pathologie du Système Nerveux Cérébro-Spinal*. Fortin, Masson & Cie, Paris.

Frackowiak RSJ, Friston KJ, Frith CD, Dolan RJ and Mazziotta JC (1997). *Human Brain Function*. Academic Press, San Diego.

Fozard JL and Weinert JR (1972). Absolute judgments of recency for pictures and nouns after various numbers of intervening items. *Journal of Experimental Psychology*, **95**(2), 472–474.

Fozard JL, Vercryssen M, Reynolds SL, Hancock PA and Quilter RE (1994). Age differences and changes in reaction time: the Baltimore Longitudinal Study of Aging. *Journal of Gerontology*, **49**(4), P179–P189.

Freedman DJ and Assad JA (2011). A proposed common neural mechanism for categorization and perceptual decisions. *Nature Neuroscience*, **14**(2), 143–146.

Freedman M and Oscar-Berman M (1986). Bilateral frontal lobe disease and selective delayed response deficits in humans. *Behavioral Neuroscience*, **100**(3), 337–342.

Freeman W and Watts JW (1942). *Psychosurgery. Intelligence, Emotion and Social Behavior Following Prefrontal Lobotomy for Mental Disorders*. Charles C. Thomas, Springfield, IL.

Friedman L, Kenny JT, Wise L, Wu D, Stuve T, Miller D, Jesberger J and Lewin JS (1998). Brain activation during silent word generation evaluated with functional MRI. *Brain and Language*, **64**(2), 231–256.

Fristoe NM, Salthouse TA and Woodard JL (1997). Examination of age-related deficits on the Wisconsin Card Sorting Test. *Neuropsychology*, **11**, 428–436.

Frith CD (2000). The role of dorsolateral prefrontal cortex in the selection of action as revealed by functional imaging. In S Monsell and J Driver, eds, *Control of Cognitive Processes: Attention and Performance XVIII*, pp. 549–565. MIT Press, Cambridge, MA.

Frith CD and Frith U (2006). The neural basis of mentalizing. *Neuron*, **50**(4), 531–534.

Frith CD, Friston KJ, Liddle PF and Frackowiak RSJ (1991). A PET study of word finding. *Neuropsychologia*, **29**(12), 1137–1148.

Frith U and Frith CD (2003). Development and neurophysiology of mentalizing. *Philosophical Transactions of the Royal Society, London, Series B, Biological Sciences*, **358**(1431), 459–473.

Fu CHY, Kevin M, Steve CRW, Chris A, Vythelingum GN and McGuire PKM (2002). A functional magnetic resonance imaging study of overt letter verbal fluency using a clustered acquisition sequence: greater anterior cingulate activation with increased task demand. *NeuroImage*, **17**(2), 871–879.

Fukui H, Murai T, Fukuyama H, Hayashi T and Hanakawa T (2005). Functional activity related to risk anticipation during performance of the Iowa Gambling Task. *NeuroImage*, **24**(1), 253–259.

Funahashi S, Bruce CJ and Goldman-Rakic PS (1993). Dorsolateral prefrontal lesions and oculomotor delayed-response performance: evidence for mnemonic "scotomas". *Journal of Neuroscience*, **13**(4), 1479–1497.

Fuster JM (1999). Synopsis of function and dysfunction of the frontal lobe. *Acta Psychiatrica Scandinavica, Supplementum*, **395**, 51–57.

Fuster JM (2000). Executive frontal functions. *Experimental Brain Research*, **133**(1), 66–70.

Fuster JM (2013). Cognitive functions of the prefrontal cortex. In DT Stuss and RT Knight, eds, *Principles of Frontal Lobe Function*, pp. 11–22. Oxford University Press, New York.

Gaillard WD, Hertz–Pannier L, Mott SH, Barnett AS, LeBihan D and Theodore WH (2000). Functional anatomy of cognitive development: fMRI of verbal fluency in children and adults. *Neurology*, **54**(1), 180–185.

Gaillard WD, Sachs BC, Whitnah JR, Ahmad Z, Balsamo LM, Petrella JR, Braniecki SH, McKinney CM, Hunter K, Xu B and Grandin CB (2003). Developmental aspects of language processing: fMRI of verbal fluency in children and adults. *Human Brain Mapping*, **18**(3), 176–185.

Gallagher HL and Frith CD (2003). Functional imaging of "theory of mind". *Trends in Cognitive Sciences*, **7**(2), 77–83.

Gallagher HL, Happé F, Brunswick N, Fletcher PC, Frith PC and Frith CD (2000). Reading the mind in cartoons and stories: an fMRI study of "theory of mind" in verbal and nonverbal tasks. *Neuropsychologia*, **38**, 11–21.

Gamboz N, Borella E and Brandimonte MA (2009) The role of switching, inhibition and working memory in older adults' performance in the Wisconsin Card Sorting Test. *Aging, Neuropsychology, and Cognition*, **16**(3), 260–284.

Garavan H, Ross TJ and Stein EA (1999). Right hemispheric dominance of inhibitory control: an event-related functional MRI study. *Proceedings of the National Academy of Sciences, of the USA*, **96**(14), 8301–8306.

Garavan H, Ross TJ, Murphy K, Roche RA and Stein EA (2002). Dissociable executive functions in the dynamic control of behavior: inhibition, error detection, and correction. *Neuroimage*, **17**(4), 1820–1829.

Garavan, H, Ross, TJ, Kaufman J and Stein EA (2003). A midline dissociation between error-processing and response-conflict monitoring. *NeuroImage*, **20**(2), 1132–1139.

Garden SE, Phillips LH and MacPherson SE (2001). Midlife aging, open-ended planning, and laboratory measures of executive function. *Neuropsychology*, **15**(4), 472–482.

Gaudino EA, Geisler MW and Squires NK (1995). Construct validity in the Trail Making Test: what makes Part B harder? *Journal of Clinical and Experimental Neuropsychology*, **17**, 529–535.

Gazzaniga MS (2000). *The New Cognitive Neurosciences*, 2nd edn. MIT Press, Cambridge, MA.

Geerlings MI, Appelman AP, Vincken KL, Mali WP and van der Graaf Y; SMART Study Group (2009). Association of white matter lesions and lacunar infarcts with executive functioning: the SMART-MR study. *American Journal of Epidemiology*, **170**(9), 1147–1155.

George MS, Ketter TA, Gill DS, Haxby JV, Ungerleider LG, Herscovitch P and Post RM (1993). Brain regions involved in recognizing facial emotion or identity: an oxygen-15 PET study. *Journal of Neuropsychiatry and Clinical Neurosciences*, **5**(**4**), 384–394.

Geraci A, Surian L, Ferraro M and Cantagallo A (2010). Theory of Mind in patients with ventromedial or dorsolateral prefrontal lesions following traumatic brain injury. *Brain Injury*, **24**(7–8), 978–987.

German TP and Hehman JA (2006). Representational and executive selection resources in "theory of mind": evidence from compromised belief-desire reasoning in old age. *Cognition*, **101**(**1**), 129–152.

Gerton BK, Brown TT, Meyer-Lindenberg A, Kohn P, Holt JL, Olsen RK and Berman KF (2004). Shared and distinct neurophysiological components of the digits forward and backward tasks as revealed by functional neuroimaging. *Neuropsychologia*, **42**(**13**), 1781–1787.

Ghahremani DG, Moterosso J, Jentsch JD, Bilder RM and Poldrack RA (2010). Neural components underlying behavioural flexibility in human reversal learning. *Cerebral Cortex*, **20**(**8**), 1843–1852.

Gibbs RW Jr and Beitel D (1995). What proverb understanding reveals about how people think. *Psychological Bulletin*, **118**(**1**), 133–154.

Gilbert SJ, Spengler S, Simons JS, Steele JD, Lawrie SM, Frith CD and Burgess PW (2006). Functional specialization within rostral prefrontal cortex (area 10): a meta-analysis. *Journal of Cognitive Neuroscience*, **18**(**6**), 932–948.

Gilhooly K, Phillips L, Wynn V, Logie R and Della Sala S (1999). Planning processes and age in the 5-disc Tower of London task. *Thinking and Reasoning*, **5**, 339–361.

Gilhooly KJ, Wynn VE, Phillips LH, Logie RH and Della Sala S (2002). Visuo-spatial and verbal working memory in the five-disc Tower of London task: an individual-differences approach. *Thinking and Reasoning*, **8**(**3**), 165–178.

Gillespie DC, Evans RI, Gardener EA and Bowen A (2002). Performance of older adults on tests of cognitive estimation. *Journal of Clinical and Experimental Neuropsychology*, **24**, 286–293.

Gläscher J, Hampton AN and O'Doherty JP (2009). Determining a role for ventromedial prefrontal cortex in encoding action-based value signals during reward-related decision making. *Cerebral Cortex*, **19**, 483–495.

Gläscher J, Adolphs R, Damasio H, Bechara A, Rudrauf D, Calamia M, Paul LK and Tranel D (2012). Lesion mapping of cognitive control and value-based decision making in the prefrontal cortex. *Proceedings of the National Academy of Sciences of the USA*, **109**(**36**), 14681–14686.

Glenn AL, Raine A and Schug RA (2009). The neural correlates of moral decision-making in psychopathy. *Molecular Psychiatry*, **14**, 5–9.

Glickstein M, Arora H and Sperry R (1963). Delayed-response performance following optic tract section, unilateral frontal lesion, and commissurotomy. *Journal of Comparative and Physiological Psychology*, **56**(**1**), 11–18.

Gobbini MI, Koralek AC, Bryan RE, Montgomery KJ and Haxby JV (2007). Two takes on the social brain: a comparison of theory of mind tasks. *Journal of Cognitive Neuroscience*, **19**(**11**), 1803–1814.

Godefroy O, Lhullier C and Rousseaux M (1996). Non-spatial attention disorders in patients with frontal or posterior brain damage. *Brain*, **119**(**1**), 191–202.

Goel V and Dolan RJ (2007). Social regulation of affective experience of humor. *Journal of Cognitive Neuroscience*, **19(9)**, 1574–1580.

Gold J, Berman K, Randolph C, Goldberg TE and Weinberger DR (1996). PET validation of a novel prefrontal task: delayed response alternation. *Neuropsychology*, **10(1)**, 3–10.

Goldberg TE, Berman KF, Randolph C, Gold JM and Weinberger DR (1996). Isolating the mnemonic component in spatial delayed response: a controlled PET 15O-labeled water regional cerebral blood flow study in normal humans. *NeuroImage*, **3(1)**, 69–78.

Goldman-Rakic PS, Funahashi S and Bruce CJ (1990). Neocortical memory circuits. *Cold Spring Harbor Symposia on Quantitative Biology*, **55**, 1025–1038.

Goldstein B, Obrzut JE, John C, Ledakis G and Armstrong CL (2004). The impact of frontal and non-frontal brain tumor lesions on Wisconsin Card Sorting Test performance. *Brain and Cognition*, **54**, 110–116.

Goldstein K and Scheerer M (1941). Abstract and concrete behavior: an experimental study with special tests. *Psychological Monographs*, **53(2)**, 2.

Goldstein LH, Bernard S, Fenwick PB, Burgess PW and McNeil J (1993). Unilateral frontal lobectomy can produce strategy application disorder. *Journal of Neurology, Neurosurgery & Psychiatry*, **56(3)**, 274–276.

Gomez-Beldarrain M, Harries C, Garcia-Monco JC, Ballus E and Grafman J (2004). Patients with right frontal lesions are unable to assess and use advice to make predictive judgments. *Journal of Cognitive Neuroscience*, **16(1)**, 74–89.

Gonsalkorale K, Sherman JW and Klauer KC (2009). Aging and prejudice: diminished regulation of automatic race bias among older adults. *Journal of Experimental Social Psychology*, **45**, 410–414.

Gorham D (1956). A proverbs test for clinical and experimental use. *Psychological Reports*, **2**, 1–12.

Gorno-Tempini ML, Pradelli S, Serafini M, Pagnoni G, Baraldi P, Porro C, Nicoletti R, Umità C and Nichelli P (2001). Explicit and incidental facial expression processing: an fMRI study. *NeuroImage*, **14(2)**, 465–473.

Gottwald B, Wilde B, Mihajlovic Z and Mehdorn HM (2004). Evidence for distinct cognitive deficits after focal cerebellar lesions. *Journal of Neurology, Neurosurgery & Psychiatry*, **75**, 1524–1531.

Gourovitch ML, Kirkby BS, Goldberg TE, Weinberger DR, Gold JM, Esposito G, Van Horn JD and Berman KF (2000). A comparison of rCBF patterns during letter and semantic fluency. *Neuropsychology*, **14(3)**, 353–360.

Gouveia PAR, Brucki SMD, Malheiros SMF and Bueno OFA (2007). Disorders in planning and strategy application in frontal lobe lesion patients. *Brain and Cognition*, **63(3)**, 240–246.

Gozzi M, Raymont V, Solomon J, Koenigs M and Grafman J (2009). Dissociable effects of prefrontal and anterior temporal cortical lesions on stereotypical gender attitudes. *Neuropsychologia*, **47(10)**, 2125–2132.

Grady CL, McIntosh AR, Bookstein F, Horwitz B, Rapoport SI and Haxby JV (1998). Age-related changes in regional cerebral blood flow during working memory for faces. *NeuroImage*, **8(4)**, 409–425.

Grant DA and Berg EA (1948). A behavioral analysis of degree of reinforcement and ease of shifting to new responses in a Weigl-type card-sorting problem. *Journal of Experimental Psychology*, **38**, 404–411.

Greene JD, Sommerville RB, Nystrom LE, Darley JM and Cohen JD (2001). An fMRI investigation of emotional engagement in moral judgement. *Science*, **293**, 2105–2108.

Greene JD, Nystrom LE, Engell AD, Darley JM and Cohen JD (2004). The neural bases of cognitive conflict and control in moral judgement. *Neuron*, **44**, 389–400.

Greene JD, Morelli SA, Lowenberg K, Nystrom LE and Cohen JD (2008). Cognitive load selectively interferes with utilitarian moral judgement. *Cognition*, **107**, 1144–1154.

Greenwald AG and Banaji MR (1995). Implicit social cognition: attitudes, self-esteem, and stereotypes. *Psychological Review*, **102**(1), 4–27.

Greenwald AG, McGhee DE and Schwartz JL (1998). Measuring individual differences in implicit cognition: the implicit association test. *Journal of Personality and Social Psychology*, **74**(6), 1464–1480.

Gregory C, Lough S, Stone V, Erzinclioglu S, Martin L, Baron-Cohen S and Hodges JR (2002). Theory of mind in patients with frontal variant frontotemporal dementia and Alzheimer's disease: theoretical and practical implications. *Brain*, **125**(4), 752–764.

Greve KW (2001). The WCST-64: a standardized short-form of the Wisconsin Card Sorting Test. *The Clinical Neuropsychologist*, **15**(2), 228–234.

Griesmayr B, Gruber WR, Klimesch W and Sauseng P (2010). Human frontal midline theta and its synchronization to gamma during a verbal delayed match to sample task. *Neurobiology of Learning and Memory*, **93**(2), 208–215.

Gross C and Weiskrantz L (1962). Evidence for dissociation of impairment on auditory discrimination and delayed response following lateral frontal lesions in monkeys. *Experimental Neurology*, **476**, 453–476.

Grossi D, Santangelo G, Barbarulo AM, Vitale C, Castaldo G, Proto MG, Siano P, Barone P and Trojano L (2013). Apathy and related executive syndromes in dementia associated with Parkinson's disease and in Alzheimer's disease. *Behavioural Neurology*, **27**(4), 515–522.

Grossman AB, Woolley-Levine S, Bradley WG and Miller RG (2007). Detecting neurobehavioral changes in amyotrophic lateral sclerosis. *Amyotrophic Lateral Sclerosis*, **8**(1), 56–61.

Grossman M, Eslinger PJ, Troiani V, Anderson C, Avants B, Gee JC, McMillan C, Massimo L, Khan A and Antani S (2010). The role of ventral medial prefrontal cortex in social decisions: converging evidence from fMRI and frontotemporal lobar degeneration. *Neuropsychologia*, **48**, 3505–3512.

Gunning-Dixon FM, Gur RC, Perkins AC, Schroeder L, Turner T, Turetsky BI, Chan RM, Loughead JW, Alsop DC, Maldjian J and Gur RE (2003). Age-related differences in brain activation during emotional face processing. *Neurobiology of Aging*, **24**(2), 285–295.

Gurd JM, Amunts K, Weiss PH, Zafiris O, Zilles K, Marshall JC and Fink GR (2002). Posterior parietal cortex is implicated in continuous switching between verbal fluency tasks: an fMRI study with clinical implications. *Brain*, **125**(5), 1024–1038.

Guth W, Schmittberger R and Schwarze B (1982). An experimental analysis of ultimatum bargaining. *Journal of Economic Behavior and Organization*, **3**(4), 367–388.

Haaland KY, Vranes LF, Goodwin JS and Garry PJ (1987) Wisconsin Card Sorting Test performance in a healthy elderly population. *Journal of Gerontology*, **42**, 345–346.

Hajcak G, McDonald N and Simons RF (2003). To err is autonomic: error-related brain potentials, ANS activity, and post-error compensatory behaviour. *Psychophysiology*, **40**(6), 895–903.

Halari R, Sharma T, Hines M, Andrew C, Simmons A and Kumari V (2006). Comparable fMRI activity with differential behavioural performance on mental rotation and overt verbal fluency tasks in healthy men and women. *Experimental Brain Research*, **169**(1), 1–14.

Halberstadt J, Ruffman T, Murray J, Taumoepeau M and Ryan M (2011). Emotion perception explains age-related differences in the perception of social gaffes. *Psychology and Aging*, **26**(1), 133–136.

Hale JB, Hoeppner JB and Fiorello CA (2002). Analyzing digit span components for assessment of attention processes. *Journal of Psychoeducational Assessment*, **20**, 128–143.

Hamdan AC and Hamdan ELR (2009). Effects of age and education level on the Trail Making Test in a healthy Brazilian sample. *Psychology & Neuroscience*, **2**(2), 199–203.

Hampshire A, Gruszka A, Fallon SJ and Owen AM (2008). Inefficiency in self-organized attentional switching in the normal aging population is associated with decreased activity in the ventrolateral prefrontal cortex. *Journal of Cognitive Neuroscience*, **20**, 1670–1686.

Hampshire A, Thompson R, Duncan J and Owen AM (2011). Lateral prefrontal cortex subregions make dissociable contributions during fluid reasoning. *Cerebral Cortex*, **21**, 1–10.

Hampton AN, Bossaerts P and O'Doherty JP (2006). The role of the ventromedial prefrontal cortex in abstract state-based inference during decision making in humans. *Journal of Neuroscience*, **26**(32), 8360–8367.

Happé FGE (1994). An advanced test of theory of mind: understanding of story characters' thoughts and feelings by able autistic, mentally handicapped, and normal children and adults. *Journal of Autism and Developmental Disorders*, **24**(2), 129–154.

Happé F, Ehlers S, Fletcher P, Frith U, Johansson M, Gillberg C, Dolan R, Frackowiak R and Frith C (1996). "Theory of mind" in the brain. Evidence from a PET scan study of Asperger syndrome. *Neuroreport*, **8**(1), 197–201.

Happé FG, Winner E and Brownell H (1998). The getting of wisdom: theory of mind in old age. *Developmental Psychology*, **34**(2), 358–362.

Happé F, Brownell H and Winner E (1999). Acquired "theory of mind" impairments following stroke. *Cognition*, **70**(3), 211–240.

Happé F, Malhi GS and Checkley S (2001). Acquired mind-blindness following frontal lobe surgery? A single case study of impaired "theory of mind" in a patient treated with stereotactic anterior capsulotomy. *Neuropsychologia*, **39**, 83–90.

Harenski CL and Hamann S (2006). Neural correlates of regulating negative emotions related to moral violations. *NeuroImage*, **30**, 313–324.

Harlé KM and Sanfey AG (2012). Social economic decision-making across the lifespan: an fMRI investigation. *Neuropsychologia*, **50**(7), 1416–1424.

Harlow JM (1848). Passage of an iron rod through the head. *The Boston Medical and Surgical Journal*, **39**, 389–383.

Harmer CJ, Thilo KV, Rothwell JC and Goodwin GM (2001). Transcranial magnetic stimulation of medial-frontal cortex impairs the processing of angry facial expressions. *Nature Neuroscience*, **4**(1), 17–18.

Harrison BJ, Pujol J, Lopez-Sola M, Hernández-Ribas R, Deus J, Ortiz H, Soriano-Mas C, Yucel M, Pantelis C and Cardoner N (2008). Consistency and functional specialization in the default mode brain network. *Proceedings of the National Academy of Sciences of the USA*, **105**, 9781–9786.

Hartman M, Bolton E and Fehnel SE (2001). Accounting for age differences on the Wisconsin Card Sorting Test: decreased working memory, not flexibility. *Psychology and Aging*, **16**(3), 385–399.

Hashimoto R, Meguro K, Lee E, Kasai M, Ishii H and Yamaguchi S (2006). Effect of age and education on the Trail Making Test and determination of normative data for Japanese elderly people: the Tajiri Project. *Psychiatry and Clinical Neurosciences*, **60**, 422–428.

Haug H and Eggers R (1991). Morphometry of the human cortex cerebri and corpus striatum during aging. *Neurobiology of Aging*, **12**(4), 336–338; discussion 352–355.

Heaton RK, Chelune GJ, Talley JL, Kay GG and Curtis G (1993). *Wisconsin Card Sorting Test Manual: Revised and Expanded*. Psychological Assessment Resources, Odessa, FL.

Hebb D (1949). *The Organization of Behavior*. Wiley & Sons, New York.

Heberlein AS, Padon AA, Gillihan SJ, Farah MJ and Fellows LK (2008). Ventromedial frontal lobe plays a critical role in facial emotion recognition. *Journal of Cognitive Neuroscience*, **20**(4), 721–733.

Hedden T, Park DC, Nisbett R, Ji LJ, Jing Q and Jiao S (2002). Cultural variation in verbal versus spatial neuropsychological function across the life span. *Neuropsychology*, **16**(1), 65–73.

Heider F and Simmel M (1944). An experimental study of apparent behavior. *American Journal of Psychology*, **57**, 243–259.

Heilbronner RL, Henry GK, Buck P, Adams RL and Fogle T (1991). Lateralized brain damage and performance on Trail Making A and B, Digit Span Forward and Backward, and TPT Memory and Location. *Archives of Clinical Neuropsychology*, **6**(4), 251–258.

Heim S, Eickhoff SB and Amunts K (2008). Specialisation in Broca's region for semantic, phonological, and syntactic fluency? *NeuroImage*, **40**(3), 1362–1368.

Heinzel S, Metzger FG, Ehlis AC, Korell R, Alboji A, Haeussinger FB, Hagen K, Maetzler W, Eschweiler GW, Berg D and Fallgatter AJ; TREND Study Consortium (2013). Aging-related cortical reorganization of verbal fluency processing: a functional near-infrared spectroscopy study. *Neurobiology of Aging*, **34**(2), 439–450.

Henry JD and Crawford JR (2004). A meta-analytic review of verbal fluency performance following focal cortical lesions. *Neuropsychology*, **18**(2), 284–295.

Henry JD and Phillips LH (2006). Covariates of production and perseveration on tests of phonemic, semantic and alternating fluency in normal aging. *Aging, Neuropsychology, and Cognition*, **13**(3–4), 529–551.

Henry JD, Phillips LH, Ruffman T and Bailey PE (2013). A meta-analytic review of age differences in theory of mind. *Psychology and Aging*, **28**(3), 826–839.

Herndon JG, Moss MB, Rosene DL and Killiany RJ (1997). Patterns of cognitive decline in aged rhesus monkeys. *Behaviour and Brain Research*, **87**, 25–34.

Herold R, Feldmann A, Simon M, Tényi T, Kövér F, Nagy F, Varga E and Fekete S (2009). Regional gray matter reduction and theory of mind deficit in the early phase of schizophrenia: a voxel-based morphometric study. *Acta Psychiatrica Scandanavica*, **119**(3), 199–208.

Hester RL, Kinsella GJ and Ong B (2004a). Effect of age on forward and backward span tasks. *Journal of the International Neuropsychological Society*, **10**(4), 475–481.

Hester RL, Murphy K, Foxe JJ, Foxe DM, Javitt DC and Garavan H (2004b). Predicting success: patterns of cortical activation and deactivation prior to response inhibition. *Journal of Cognitive Neuroscience*, **16**(5), 776–785.

Hester RL, Kinsella GJ, Ong B and McGregor J (2005). Demographic influences on baseline and derived scores from the Trail Making Test in healthy older Australian Adults. *The Clinical Neuropsychologist*, **19**(1), 45–54.

Hill SY, Kostelnik B, Holmes B, Goradia D, McDermott M, Diwadkar V and Keshavan M (2007). fMRI BOLD response to the eyes task in offspring from multiplex alcohol dependence families. *Alcoholism: Clinical and Experimental Research*, **31**(12), 2028–2035.

Hillert DG and Buračas GT (2009). The neural substrates of spoken idiom comprehension. *Language and Cognitive Processes*, **24**(9), 1370–1391.

Hirao K, Miyata J, Fujiwara H, Yamada M, Namiki C, Shimizu M, Sawamoto N, Fukuyama H, Hayashi T and Murai T (2008). Theory of mind and frontal lobe pathology in schizophrenia: a voxel-based morphometry study. *Schizophrenia Research*, **105**(1), 165–174.

Hirshorn EA and Thompson-Schill S (2006). Role of the left inferior frontal gyrus in covert word retrieval: neural correlates of switching during verbal fluency. *Neuropsychologia*, **44**(12), 2547–2557.

Hodges JR (1994). *Cognitive Assessment for Clinicians*. Oxford University Press, Oxford.

Hoerold D, Pender NP and Robertson IH (2013). Metacognitive and online error awareness deficits after prefrontal cortex lesions. *Neuropsychologia*, **51**(3), 385–391.

Hogan AM, Vargha-Khadem F, Saunders DE, Kirkham FJ and Baldeweg T (2006). Impact of frontal white matter lesions on performance monitoring: ERP evidence for cortical disconnection. *Brain*, **129**(8), 2177–2188.

Hooker CI, Paller KA, Gitelman DR, Parrish TB, Mesulam MM and Reber PJ (2003). Brain networks for analyzing eye gaze. *Brain Research. Cognitive Brain Research*, **17**(2), 406–418.

Hornak J, Rolls ET and Wade D (1996). Face and voice expression identification in patients with emotional and behavioural changes following ventral frontal lobe damage. *Neuropsychologia*, **34**(4), 247–261.

Hornak J, Bramham J, Rolls ET, Morris RG, O'Doherty J, Bullock PR and Polkey CE (2003). Changes in emotion after circumscribed surgical lesions of the orbitofrontal and cingulate cortices. *Brain*, **126**(7), 1691–1712.

Hornak J, O'Doherty, J, Bramham J, Rolls ET, Morris RG, Bullock PR and Polkey CE (2004). Reward-related reversal learning after surgical excisions in orbito-frontal or dorsolateral prefrontal cortex in humans. *Journal of Cognitive Neuroscience*, **16**(3), 463–478.

Hornberger M, Geng J and Hodges JR (2011). Convergent grey and white matter evidence of orbitofrontal cortex changes related to disinhibition in behavior variant frontotemporal dementia. *Brain*, **134**, 2502–2512.

Hoshi Y, Oda I, Wada Y, Ito Y, Yutaka Yamashita, Oda M, Ohta K, Yamada Y and Tamura M (2000). Visuospatial imagery is a fruitful strategy for the digit span backward task: a study with near-infrared optical tomography. *Brain Research. Cognitive Brain Research*, **9**(3), 339–342.

Hughes DL and Bryan J (2002). Adult age differences in strategy use during verbal fluency performance. *Journal of Clinical and Experimental Neuropsychology*, **24**(5), 642–654.

Hummert ML, Garstka TA, O'Brien LT, Greenwald AG and Mellott DS (2002). Using the implicit association test to measure age differences in implicit social cognitions. *Psychology and Aging*, **17**(3), 482–495.

Hunter EM, Phillips LH and MacPherson SE (2010). Effects of age on cross-modal emotion perception. *Psychology and Aging*, **25**(**4**), 779–787.

Hutchinson M, Schiffer W, Joseffer S, Liu A, Schlosser R, Dikshit S, Goldberg E and Brodie JD (1999). Task-specific deactivation patterns in functional magnetic resonance imaging. *Magnetic Resonance Imaging*, **17**(**10**), 1427–1436.

Hynes CA, Baird AA and Grafton ST (2006). Differential role of the orbital frontal lobe in emotional versus cognitive perspective-taking. *Neuropsychologia*, **44**(**3**), 374–383.

Iidaka T, Omori M, Murata T, Kosaka H, Yonekura Y, Okada T and Sadato N (2001). Neural interaction of the amygdala with the prefrontal and temporal cortices in the processing of facial expressions as revealed by fMRI. *Journal of Cognitive Neuroscience*, **13**(**8**), 1035–1047.

Imaizumi S, Mori K, Kiritani S, Kawashima R, Sugiura M, Fukuda H, Itoh K, Kato T, Nakamura A, Hatano K, Kojima S and Nakamura K (2001). Vocal identification of speaker and emotion activates different brain regions. *Neuroreport*, **8**(**12**), 2809–2812.

Isaacowitz DM, Löckenhoff CE, Lane RD, Wright R, Sechrest L, Riedel R and Costa PT (2007). Age differences in recognition of emotion in lexical stimuli and facial expressions. *Psychology and Aging*, **22**(**1**), 147–159.

Isingrini M and Vazou F (1997). Relation between fluid intelligence and frontal lobe functioning in older adults. *Journal of Aging and Human Development*, **45**(**2**), 99–109.

Jacobsen C (1935). Functions of frontal association area in primates. *Archives of Neurology and Psychiatry*, **33**(**3**), 558–569.

Jacobson SC, Blanchard M, Connolly CC, Cannon M and Garavan H (2011). An fMRI investigation of a novel analogue to the Trail-Making Test. *Brain and Cognition*, **77**(**1**), 60–70.

Jacoby LL (1991). A process dissociation framework: separating automatic from intentional uses of memory. *Journal of Memory and Language*, **30**, 513–541.

Jansma JM, Ramsey NF, Coppola R and Kahn RS (2000). Specific versus nonspecific brain activity in a parametric N-back task. *NeuroImage*, **12**(**6**), 688–697.

Jimura K, Yamashita K, Chikazoe J, Hirose S, Miyashita Y and Konishi S (2009). A critical component that activates the left inferior prefrontal cortex during interference resolution. *European Journal of Neuroscience*, **29**(**9**), 1915–1920.

Johnson MK, O'Connor M and Cantor J (1997). Confabulation, memory deficits, and frontal dysfunction. *Brain and Cognition*, **34**(**2**), 189–206.

Jonides J and Nee DE (2004). Resolving conflict in mind and brain. *American Psychological Association Science Briefs*, **18**.

Jonides J, Lacey SC and Nee DE (2005). Processes of working memory in mind and brain. *Current Directions in Psychological Science*, **14**(**1**), 2–5.

Juncos-Rabadan O, Pereiro AX and Facal D (2008). Cognitive interference and aging: insights from a spatial stimulus-response consistency task. *Acta Psychologica*, **127**(**2**), 237–246.

Jung HH, Kim CH, Chang JH, Park YG, Chung SS and Chang JW (2006). Bilateral anterior cingulotomy for refractory obsessive-compulsive disorder: long-term follow-up results. *Stereotactic and Functional Neurosurgery*, **84**(**4**), 184–189.

Just MA, Cherkassky VL, Keller TA, Kana RK and Minshew NJ (2007). Functional and anatomical cortical underconnectivity in autism: evidence from an FMRI study of an executive function task and corpus callosum morphometry. *Cerebral Cortex*, **17**(**4**), 951–961.

Kahane G and Shackel N (2008). Do abnormal responses show utilitarian bias? *Nature*, **452**, E5.

Kahlaoui K, Sante GD, Barbeau J, Maheux M, Lesage F, Ska B and Joanette Y (2012). Contribution of NIRS to the study of prefrontal cortex for verbal fluency in aging. *Brain and Language*, **121**(**2**), 164–173.

Kalbe E, Grabenhorst F, Brand M, Kessler J, Hilker R and Markowitsch HJ (2007). Elevated emotional reactivity in affective but not cognitive components of theory of mind: a psychophysiological study. *Journal of Neuropsychology*, **1**(**1**), 27–38.

Kalbe E, Schlegel M, Sack AT, Nowak DA, Dafotakis M, Bangard C, Brand M, Shamay-Tsoory S, Onur OA and Kessler J (2010). Dissociating cognitive from affective theory of mind: a TMS study. *Cortex*, **46**(**6**), 769–780.

Kana RK, Keller TA, Cherkassky VL, Minshew NJ and Just MA (2009). Atypical frontal-posterior synchronization of Theory of Mind regions in autism during mental state attribution. *Social Neuroscience*, **4**(**2**), 135–152.

Kapur N, Hutchinson P, Berry E, Hawkins K, Llewellyn D and Wilson B (2009). Executive dysfunction in a case of transoral-frontal self-inflicted gunshot injury. *Brain Injury*, **23**(**12**), 985–989.

Kawasaki M and Yamaguchi Y (2013). Frontal theta and beta synchronizations for monetary reward increase visual working memory capacity. *Social Cognitive and Affective Neuroscience*, **8**(**5**), 523–530.

Kawashima R, Satoh K, Itoh H, Ono S, Furumoto S, Gotoh R, Koyama M, Yoshioka S, Takahashi T, Takahashi K, Yanagisawa T and Fukuda H (1996). Functional anatomy of GO/NO-GO discrimination and response selection—a PET study in man. *Brain Research*, **728**(**1**), 79–89.

Kean S (2014, May). Phineas Gage, Neuroscience's most famous patient. *Slate*. Available at: http://www.slate.com/articles/health_and_science/science/2014/05/phineas_gage_neuroscience_case_true_story_of_famous_frontal_lobe_patient.html.

Keane J, Calder AJ, Hodges JR and Young AW (2001). Face and emotion processing in frontal variant frontotemporal dementia. *Neuropsychologia*, **40**(**6**), 655–665.

Keifer E (2010). Performance of patients with ventromedial prefrontal, dorsolateral prefrontal, and non-frontal lesions on the Delis–Kaplan Executive Function System. Doctoral Dissertation, University of Iowa.

Keightley ML, Winocur G, Graham SJ, Mayberg HS, Hevenor SJ and Grady CL (2003). An fMRI study investigating cognitive modulation of brain regions associated with emotional processing of visual stimuli. *Neuropsychologia*, **41**(**5**), 585–596.

Keightley ML, Winocur G, Burianova H, Hongwanishkul D and Grady CL (2006). Age effects on social cognition: faces tell a different story. *Psychology and Aging*, **21**(**3**), 5585–5572.

Keightley ML, Chiew KS, Winocur G and Grady CL (2007). Age-related differences in brain activity underlying identification of emotional expressions in faces. *Social Cognitive and Affective Neuroscience*, **2**(**4**), 292–302.

Kelly AMC, Hester R, Murphy K, Javitt DC, Foxe JJ and Garavan J (2004). Prefrontal-subcortical dissociations underlying inhibitory control revealed by event-related fMRI. *European Journal of Neuroscience*, **19**, 3105–3112.

Kemp J, Després O, Sellal F and Dufour A (2012). Theory of Mind in normal ageing and neurodegenerative pathologies. *Ageing Research Reviews*, **11**(2), 199–219.

Kemper S and Sumner A (2001). The structure of verbal abilities in young and older adults. *Psychology and Aging*, **16**(2), 312–322.

Kempler D, Teng EL, Dick M, Taussig I and Davis DS (1998). The effects of age, education, and ethnicity on verbal fluency. *Journal of the International Neuropsychological Society*, **4**(6), 531–538.

Kennedy KM and Raz N (2009). Aging white matter and cognition: differential effects of regional variations in diffusion properties on memory, executive functions, and speed. *Neuropsychologia*, **47**(3), 916–927.

Kerns JG (2006). Anterior cingulate and prefrontal cortex activity in an fMRI study of trial-to-trial adjustments on the Simon task. *NeuroImage*, 33, 399–405.

Kerns JG, Cohen JD, MacDonald III AW, Cho RY, Stenger VA and Carter CS (2004). Anterior cingulate conflict monitoring and adjustments in control. *Science*, **303**, 1023–1026.

Kiefer M, Marzinzik F, Weisbrod M, Scherg M and Spitzer M (1998). The time course of brain activations during response inhibition: evidence from event-related potentials in a go/no go task. *Neuroreport*, **9**(4), 765–770.

Kiehl KA, Liddle PF and Hopfinger JB (2000). Error processing and the rostral anterior cingulate: an event-related fMRI study. *Psychophysiology*, **37**(2), 216–223.

Killgore WD and Yurgelun-Todd DA (2004). Activation of the amygdala and anterior cingulate during nonconscious processing of sad versus happy faces. *NeuroImage*, **21**(4), 1215–1223.

Kilts CD, Egan G, Gideon DA, Ely TD and Hoffman JM (2003). Dissociable neural pathways are involved in the recognition of emotion in static and dynamic facial expressions. *NeuroImage*, **18**(1), 156–168.

Kimura HM, Hirose S, Kunimatsu A, Chikazoe J, Jimura K, Watanabe T, Abe O, Ohtomo K, Miyashita Y and Konishi S (2010). Differential temporo-parietal cortical networks that support relational and item-based recency judgments. *NeuroImage*, **49**(4), 3474–3480.

King JA, Korb, FM, von Cramon DY and Ullsperger M (2010). Post-error behavioural adjustments are facilitated by activation and suppression of task-relevant and task-irrelevant information processing. *Journal of Neuroscience*, **30**(38), 12759–12769.

Kircher T, Nagels A, Kirner-Veselinovic A and Krach S (2011). Neural correlates of rhyming vs. lexical and semantic fluency. *Brain Research*, 1391, 71–80.

Klein JC, Rushworth MFS, Behrens TEJ, Mackay CE, de Crespigny AJ, D'Arceuil H and Johansen-Berg H (2010). Topography of connections between human prefrontal cortex and mediodorsal thalamus studied with diffusion tractography. *NeuroImage*, **51**(2), 555–564.

Kliegel M, McDaniel MA and Einstein GO (2000). Plan formation, retention, and execution in prospective memory: a new approach and age-related effects. *Memory & Cognition*, **28**(6), 1041–1049.

Knight C, Alderman N and Burgess PW (2002). Development of a simplified version of the multiple errands test for use in hospital settings. *Neuropsychological Rehabilitation*, **12**(3), 231–255.

Knoch D, Pascual-Leone A, Meyer K, Treyer V and Fehr E (2006). Diminishing reciprocal fairness by disrupting the right prefrontal cortex. *Science*, **314**(5800), 829–832.

Knutson KM, Wood JN, Spampinato MV and Grafman J (2006). Politics on the brain: an FMRI investigation. *Social Neuroscience*, **1**(1), 25–40.

Knutson KM, Mah L, Manly CF and Grafman J (2007). Neural correlates of automatic beliefs about gender and race. *Human Brain Mapping*, **28**(10), 915–930.

Ko JH, Monchi O, Ptito A, Petrides M and Strafella AP (2008). Repetitive transcranial magnetic stimulation of dorsolateral prefrontal cortex affects performance of the Wisconsin Card Sorting Task during provision of feedback. *International Journal of Biomedical Imaging*, 2008, 143238.

Koechlin E, Basso G, Pietrini P, Panzer S and Grafman J (1999). The role of the anterior prefrontal cortex in human cognition. *Nature*, **399**(6732), 148–151.

Koechlin E, Ody C and Kouneiher F (2003). The architecture of cognitive control in the human prefrontal cortex. *Science*, **302**, 1181–1185.

Koenigs M and Tranel D (2007). Irrational economic decision-making after ventromedial prefrontal damage: evidence from the Ultimatum Game. *Journal of Neuroscience*, **27**(4), 951–956.

Koenigs M, Young L, Adolphs R, Tranel D, Cushman F, Hauser M and Damasio A (2007). Damage to the prefrontal cortex increases utilitarian moral judgements. *Nature*, **446**, 908–911.

Koenigs M, Kruepke M and Newman JP (2010). Economic decision-making in psychopathy: a comparison with ventromedial prefrontal lesion patients. *Neuropsychologia*, **48**(7), 2198–2204.

Kojima S and Goldman-Rakic P (1982). Delay-related activity of prefrontal neurons in rhesus monkeys performing delayed response. *Brain Research*, **248**, 43–49.

Konishi S, Nakajima K, Uchida I, Kameyama M, Nakahara K, Sekihara K and Miyashita Y (1998a). Transient activation of inferior prefrontal cortex during cognitive set shifting. *Nature Neuroscience*, **1**(1), 80–84.

Konishi S, Nakajima K, Uchida I, Sekihara K and Miyashita Y (1998b). No-go dominant brain activity in human inferior prefrontal cortex revealed by functional magnetic resonance imaging. *European Journal of Neuroscience*, **10**, 1209–1213.

Konishi S, Kawazu M, Uchida I, Kikyo H, Asakura I and Miyashita Y (1999a). Contributions of working memory to transient activation in human inferior prefrontal cortex during performance of the Wisconsin Card Sorting Task. *Cerebral Cortex*, **9**(7), 745–753.

Konishi S, Nakajima K, Uchida I, Kikyo H, Kameyama M and Miyashita Y (1999b). Common inhibitory mechanism in human inferior prefrontal cortex revealed by event-related functional MRI. *Brain*, **122**(5), 981–991.

Konishi S, Uchida I, Okuaki T, Machida T, Shirouzu I and Miyashita Y (2002). Neural correlates of recency judgment. *Journal of Neuroscience*, **22**(21), 9549–9555.

Konishi S, Hirose S, Jimura K, Chikazoe J, Watanabe T, Kimura HM and Miyashita Y (2010). Medial prefrontal activity during shifting under novel situations. *Neuroscience Letters*, **484**(3), 182–186.

Kopelman MD (1989). Remote and autobiographical memory, temporal context memory and frontal atrophy in Korsakoff and Alzheimer patients. *Neuropsychologia*, **27**(4), 437–460.

Kopelman MD, Stanhope N and Kingsley D (1997). Temporal and spatial context memory in patients with focal frontal, temporal lobe, and diencephalic lesions. *Neuropsychologia*, **35**(12), 1533–1545.

Kousaie S and Phillips NA (2012). Ageing and bilingualism: absence of a "bilingual advantage" in Stroop interference in a non-immigrant sample. *Quarterly Journal of Experimental Psychology*, **65**(2), 356–369.

Krajbich I, Adolphs R, Tranel D, Denburg NL, Camerer CF (2009). Economic games quantify diminished sense of guilt in patients with damage to the prefrontal cortex. *Journal of Neuroscience*, **29**(7), 2188–2192.

Krause L, Enticott PG, Zangen A and Fitzgerald PB (2012). The role of medial pre-frontal cortex in theory of mind: a deep rTMS study. *Behavioural Brain Research*, **228**(1), 87–90.

Krendl AC, Kensinger EA and Ambady N (2012). How does the brain regulate negative bias to stigma? *Social Cognitive and Affective Neuroscience*, **7**(6), 715–726.

Kril JJ and Halliday GM (2004). Clinicopathological staging of frontotemporal dementia severity: correlation with regional atrophy. *Dementia and Geriatric Cognitive Disorders*, **17**(4), 311–315.

Kringelbach ML and Rolls ET (2003). Neural correlates of rapid reversal learning in a sim-ple model of human social interaction. *NeuroImage*, **20**, 1371–1383.

Krueger F, Barbey AK, McCabe K, Strenziok M, Zamboni G, Solomon J, Raymont V and Grafman J (2009). The neural bases of key competencies of emotional intelligence. *Proceedings from the National Academy of Sciences of the USA*, **106**(52), 22486–22491.

LaBar KS, Gitelman DR, Parrish TB and Mesulam M (1999). Neuroanatomic overlap of working memory and spatial attention networks: a functional MRI comparison within subjects. *NeuroImage*, **10**(6), 695–704.

LaBar KS, Crupain MJ, Voyvodic JT and McCarthy G (2003). Dynamic perception of facial affect and identity in the human brain. *Cerebral Cortex*, **13**(10), 1023–1033.

Lai ZC, Moss MB, Killiany RJ and Herndon JG (1995). Executive system dysfunction in the aged monkey: spatial and object reversal learning. *Neurobiology of Aging*, **16**, 947–954.

Laiacona M, Inzaghi MG, De Tanti A and Capitani E (2000). Wisconsin card sorting test: a new global score, with Italian norms, and its relationship with the Weigl sorting test. *Neurological Sciences*, **21**(5), 279–291.

Lamar M and Resnick SM (2004). Aging and prefrontal functions: dissociating orbitofron-tal and dorsolateral abilities. *Neurobiology of Aging*, **25**(4), 553–558.

Lamar M, Yousem DM and Resnick SM (2004). Age differences in orbitofrontal activa-tion: an fMRI investigation of delayed match and nonmatch to sample. *NeuroImage*, **21**(4), 1368–1376.

Lambrecht L, Kreifelts B and Wildgruber D (2012). Age-related decrease in recognition of emotional facial and prosodic expressions. *Emotion*, **12**(3), 529–539.

Lange K, Williams LM, Young AW, Bullmore ET, Brammer MJ, Williams SC, Gray JA and Phillips ML (2003). Task instructions modulate neural responses to fearful facial expressions. *Biological Psychiatry*, **53**(3), 226–232.

Langenecker SA and Nielson KA (2003). Frontal recruitment during response inhibition in older adults replicated with fMRI. *Neuroimage*, **20**, 1384–1392.

Langenecker SA, Briceno EM, Hamid NM and Nielson KA (2007). An evaluation of dis-tinct volumetric and functional MRI contributions toward understanding age and task performance: a study in the basal ganglia. *Brain Research*, 1135(1), 58–68.

Larrabee GJ and Kane RL (1986). Reversed digit repetition involves visual and verbal processes. *International Journal of Neuroscience*, **30**, 11–15.

Latini B (around 1261–1266). *Il Tessoretto*. Translation available in JB Holloway (1981). *Il Tessoretto (The Little Treasure)*. Garland Publishing, Inc., New York.

Lauro LJ, Tettamanti M, Cappa SF and Papagno C (2008). Idiom comprehension: a prefrontal task? *Cerebral Cortex*, **18**(1), 162–170.

Law AS, Trawley SL, Brown LA, Stephens AN and Logie RH (2013). The impact of working memory load on task execution and online plan adjustment during multitasking in a virtual environment. *Quarterly Journal of Experimental Psychology*, **66**(6), 1241–1258.

Lawrence NS, Jollant F, O'Daly O, Zelaya F and Phillips ML (2009). Distinct roles of prefrontal cortical subregions in the Iowa Gambling Task. *Cerebral Cortex*, **19**(5), 1134–1143.

Lawrie SM, Buechel C, Whalley HC, Frith CD, Friston KJ and Johnstone EC (2002). Reduced frontotemporal functional connectivity in schizophrenia associated with auditory hallucinations. *Biological Psychiatry*, **51**, 1008–1011.

Lazeron RH, Rombouts SA, Machielsen WC, Scheltens P, Witter MP, Uylings HB and Barkhof F (2000). Visualizing brain activation during planning: the Tower of London test adapted for functional MR imaging. *American Journal of Neuroradiology*, **21**(8), 1407–1414.

Lazeron RH, Rombouts SA, Scheltens P, Polman CH and Barkhof F (2004). An fMRI study of planning-related brain activity in patients with moderately advanced multiple sclerosis. *Multiple Sclerosis*, **10**(5), 549–555.

Lee TM, Ip AK, Wang K, Xi CH, Hu PP, Mak HK, Han SH and Chan CC (2010). Faux pas deficits in people with medial frontal lesions as related to impaired understanding of a speaker's mental state. *Neuropsychologia*, **48**(6), 1670–1676.

Leibovici D, Ritchie K, Ledésert B and Touchon J (1996). Does education level determine the course of cognitive decline? *Age and Ageing*, **25**, 392–397.

Leimkuhler ME and Mesulam MM (1985). Reversible go-no go deficits in a case of frontal lobe tumor. *Annals of Neurology*, **18**(5), 617–619.

Leng NR and Parkin AJ (1988). Double dissociation of frontal dysfunction in organic amnesia. *British Journal of Clinical Psychology*, **27**, 359–362.

Lennox BR, Jacob R, Calder AJ, Lupson V and Bullmore ET (2004). Behavioural and neurocognitive responses to sad facial affect are attenuated in patients with mania. *Psychological Medicine*, **34**(5), 795–802.

Leopold A, Krueger F, dal Monte O, Pardini M, Pulaski SJ, Solomon J and Grafman J (2012). Damage to the left ventromedial prefrontal cortex impacts affective theory of mind. *Social Cognitive and Affective Neuroscience*, **7**(8), 871–880.

Leskelä M, Hietanen M, Kalska H, Ylikoski R, Pohjasvaara T, Mäntylä R and Erkinjuntti T (1999). Executive functions and speed of mental processing in elderly patients with frontal or nonfrontal ischemic stroke. *European Journal of Neurology*, **6**(6), 653–661.

Leung H, Gore J and Goldman-Rakic P (2002). Sustained mnemonic response in the human middle frontal gyrus during on-line storage of spatial memoranda. *Journal of Cognitive Neuroscience*, **14**(4), 659–671.

Leuret M (1839). *Anatomie Comparée du Système Nerveux, Considéré dans ses Rapports avec L'intelligence, Vol. 1*. Baillière, Paris.

Levine B, Stuss DT, Milberg WP, Alexander MP, Schwartz M and Macdonald R (1998). The effects of focal and diffuse brain damage on strategy application: evidence from focal lesions, traumatic brain injury and normal aging. *Journal of the International Neuropsychological Society*, **4**(**3**), 247–264.

Levinoff EJ, Phillips NA, Verret L, Babins L, Kelner N, Akerib V and Chertkow H (2006). Cognitive estimation impairment in Alzheimer disease and mild cognitive impairment. *Neuropsychology*, **20**, 123–132.

Lev-Ran S, Shamay-Tsoory SG, Zangen A and Levkovitz Y (2012). Transcranial magnetic stimulation of the ventromedial prefrontal cortex impairs theory of mind learning. *European Psychiatry*, **27**(**4**), 285–289.

Levy R and Goldman-Rakic PS (2000). Segregation of working memory functions within the dorsolateral prefrontal cortex. *Experimental Brain Research*, **133**(**1**), 23–32.

Lewis BL and O'Donnell P (2000). Ventral tegmental area afferents to the prefrontal cortex maintain membrane potential "up" states in pyramidal neurons via D(1) dopamine receptors. *Cerebral Cortex*, **10**(**12**), 1168–1175.

Lezak MD, Howieson DB and Loring DW (2004). *Neuropsychological assessment*, 4th edn. Oxford University Press, New York.

Lezak MD, Howieson DB, Bigler ED and Tranel D (2012). *Neuropsychological Assessment*, 5th edn. Oxford University Press, New York.

Li X, Lu Z-L, D'Argembeau A, Ng M and Bechara A (2010). The Iowa Gambling Task in fMRI images. *Human Brain Mapping*, **31**(**3**), 410–423.

Li X, Wang K, Wang F, Tao Q, Xie Y and Cheng Q (2012). Aging of theory of mind: the influence of educational level and cognitive processing. *International Journal of Psychology*, **48**(**4**), 715–727.

Liddle PF, Kiehl KA and Smith AM (2001). Event-related fMRI study of response inhibition. *Human Brain Mapping*, **12**(**2**), 100–109.

Lie CH, Specht K, Marshall JC and Fink GR (2006). Using fMRI to decompose the neural processes underlying the Wisconsin Card Sorting Test. *Neuroimage*, **30**(**3**), 1038–1049.

Lin C-H, Chiu Y-C, Lee P-L and Hsieh J-C (2007). Is deck B a disadvantageous deck in the Iowa Gambling Task? *Behavioral and Brain Functions*, **3**, 16–25.

Lin C-H, Chiu Y-C, Cheng C-M and Hsieh J-C (2008). Brain maps of Iowa gambling task. *BMC Neuroscience*, **9**, 72–86.

Lineweaver TT, Bondi MW, Thomas RG and Salmon DP (1999). A normative study of Nelson's (1976) modified version of the Wisconsin Card Sorting Test in healthy older adults. *The Clinical Neuropsychologist*, **13**(**3**), 328–347.

Linke J, Kirsch P, King AV, Gass A, Hennerici MH, Bongers A and Wessa M (2010). Motivational orientation modulates the neural response to reward. *NeuroImage*, **49**, 2618–2625.

Linnet J, Møller A, Peterson E, Gjedde A and Doudet D (2010). Dopamine release in ventral striatum during Iowa Gambling Task performance is associated with increased excitement levels in pathological gambling. *Addiction*, **106**(**2**), 383–390.

Liu J, Bai J and Zhang D (2008). Cognitive control explored by linear modelling behaviour and fMRI data during Stroop tasks. *Physiological Measurement*, **29**, 703–710.

Logan GD (1994). On the ability to inhibit thought and action: a users' guide to the stop signal paradigm. In D Dagenbach and TH Carr, eds, *Inhibitory Processes in Attention, Memory and Language*, pp. 189–239. Academic Press, San Diego.

Logie R, Law A, Trawley S and Nissan J (2010). Multitasking, working memory and remembering intentions. *Psychologica Belgica*, **50**(3&4), 309–326.

Logie RH and Maylor EA (2009). An Internet study of prospective memory across adulthood. *Psychology and Aging*, **24**(3), 767–774.

Loonstra S, Tarlow R and Sellers H (2001). COWAT metanorms across age, education, and gender. *Applied Neuropsychology*, **8**(3), 161–166.

LoPresti ML, Schon K, Tricarico MD, Swisher JD, Celone KA and Stern CE (2008). Working memory for social cues recruits orbitofrontal cortex and amygdala: a functional magnetic resonance imaging study of delayed matching to sample for emotional expressions. *Journal of Neuroscience*, **28**(14), 3718–3728.

Lough S and Hodges JR (2002). Measuring and modifying abnormal social cognition in frontal variant frontotemporal dementia. *Journal of Psychosomatic Research*, **53**(2), 639–646.

Lough S, Gregory C and Hodges JR (2001). Dissociation of social cognition and executive function in frontal variant frontotemporal dementia. *Neurocase*, **7**(2), 123–130.

Lu CH and Proctor RW (1995). The influence of irrelevant location information on performance: a review of the Simon and spatial Stroop effects. *Psychonomic Bulletin and Review*, **2**, 174–207.

Ludwig C, Borella E, Tettamanti M and de Ribaupierre A (2010). Adult age differences in the Color Stroop Test: a comparison between an item-by-item and a blocked version. *Archives of Gerontology and Geriatrics*, **51**(2), 135–142.

Luerding R, Weigand T, Bogdahn U and Schmidt-Wilcke T (2008). Working memory performance is correlated with local brain morphology in the medial frontal and anterior cingulate cortex in fibromyalgia patients: structural correlates of pain-cognition interaction. *Brain*, **131**(12), 3222–3231.

Lumme V, Aalto S, Ilonen T, Någren K and Hietala J (2007). Dopamine D2/D3 receptor binding in the anterior cingulate cortex and executive functioning. *Psychiatry Research*, **156**(1), 69–74.

Luo Q, Nakic M, Wheatley T, Richell R, Martin A and Blair RJ (2006). The neural basis of implicit moral attitude—an IAT study using event-related fMRI. *NeuroImage*, **30**(4), 1449–1457.

Luria AR (1966). *Higher Cortical Functions in Man*. Tavistock Publications, London.

Luria AR (1969). Frontal lobe syndromes in man. In P Vinken and G Bruyn, eds, *Handbook of Clinical Neurology*, Vol. 2, pp. 725–757. North-Holland, Amsterdam.

Luria AR (1973). *The Working Brain*. Basic Books: New York.

MacDonald AW, Cohen JD, Stenger VA and Carter CS (2000). Dissociating the role of the dorsolateral prefrontal and anterior cingulated cortex in cognitive control. *Science*, **288**, 1835–1838.

MacDonald AW, Pogue-Geile MF, Johnson MK and Carter CS (2003). A specific deficit in context processing in the unaffected siblings of patients with schizophrenia. *Archives of General Psychiatry*, **60**(1), 57–65.

MacDonald AW 3rd, Carter CS, Kerns JG, Ursu S, Barch DM, Holmes AJ, Stenger VA and Cohen JD (2005). Specificity of prefrontal dysfunction and context processing deficits to schizophrenia in never-medicated patients with first-episode psychosis. *American Journal of Psychiatry*, **162**, 475–484.

Machado TH, Fichman HC, Santos EL, Carvalho VA, Fialho PP, Koenig AM, Fernandes CS, Lourenço RA, de Paiva Paradela EM and Caramelli P (2009). Normative data for healthy elderly on the phonemic verbal fluency task—FAS. *Dementia & Neuropsychologia*, **3**(1), 55–60.

MacMillan M (2002). *An Odd Kind of Fame: Stories of Phineas Gage*. MIT Press, Cambridge, MA.

MacPherson S and Della Sala S (2001). Welcoming normative data for Wisconsin Card Sorting test. *Neurological Sciences*, **21**, 258–260.

MacPherson SE, Phillips LH and Della Sala S (2002). Age, executive function and social decision making: a dorsolateral prefrontal theory of cognitive aging. *Psychology and Aging*, **17**(4), 598–609.

MacPherson SE, Phillips LH and Della Sala S (2006). Age-related differences in the ability to perceive sad facial expressions. *Aging Clinical and Experimental Research*, **18**(5), 418–424.

MacPherson SE, Phillips LH, Della Sala S and Cantagallo A (2009). Iowa Gambling task impairment is not specific to ventromedial prefrontal lesions. *The Clinical Neuropsychologist*, **23**(3), 510–522.

MacPherson SE, Wagner GP, Murphy P, Bozzali M, Cipolotti L and Shallice T (2014). Bringing the cognitive estimation task into the 21st century: normative data on two new parallel forms. *PLoS One*, **9**(3), e92554.

Mah LW, Arnold MC and Grafman J (2005). Deficits in social knowledge following damage to ventromedial prefrontal cortex. *Journal of Neuropsychiatry and Clinical Neurosciences*, **17**(1), 66–74.

Maia TV and McClelland JL (2004). A reexamination of the evidence for the somatic marker hypothesis: what participants really know in the Iowa gambling task. *Proceedings of the National Academy of Sciences of the United States of America*, **101**(45), 16075–16080.

Maki PM, Zonderman AB and Weingartner H (1999). Age differences in implicit memory: fragmented object identification and category exemplar generation. *Psychology and Aging*, **14**, 284–294.

Malatesta CZ, Izard CE, Culver C and Nicolich M (1987). Emotion communication skills in young, middle-aged, and older women. *Psychology and Aging*, **2**, 193–203.

Malloy P, Bihrle A, Duffy J and Cimino C (1993). The orbitomedial frontal syndrome. *Archives of Clinical Neuropsychology*, **8**(3), 185–201.

Malmo R (1942). Interference factors in delayed response in monkeys after removal of frontal lobes. *Journal of Neurophysiology*, **5**, 295–308.

Manes F, Sahakian B, Clark L, Rogers R, Antoun N, Aitken M and Robbins T (2002). Decision-making processes following damage to the prefrontal cortex. *Brain*, **125**(3), 624–639.

Mani TM, Bedwell JS and Miller LS (2005). Age-related decrements in performance on a brief continuous performance test. *Archives of Clinical Neuropsychology*, **20**(5), 575–586.

Manly T, Hawkins K, Evans J, Woldt K and Robertson IH (2002). Rehabilitation of executive function: facilitation of effective goal management on complex tasks using periodic auditory alerts. *Neuropsychologia*, **40**(3), 271–281.

Marenco S, Coppola R, Daniel DG, Zigun JR and Weinberger DR (1993). Regional cerebral blood flow during the Wisconsin Card Sorting Test in normal subjects studied by xenon-133 dynamic SPECT: comparison of absolute values, percent distribution values, and covariance analysis. *Psychiatry Research*, **50**, 171–192.

Marschner A, Mell T, Wartenburger I, Villringer A, Reischies FM and Heekeren HR (2005). Reward-based decision-making and aging. *Brain Research Bulletin*, **67**, 382–390.

Martin A and Weisberg J (2003). Neural foundations for understanding social and mechanical concepts. *Cognitive Neuropsychology*, **20**(3–6), 575–587.

Mathalon DH, Whitfield SL and Ford JM (2003). Anatomy of an error: ERP and fMRI. *Biological Psychiatry*, **64**(1–2), 119–141.

Mathuranath PS, George A, Cherian PJ, Alexander A, Sarma SG and Sarma PS (2003). Effects of age, education and gender on verbal fluency. *Journal of Clinical and Experimental Neuropsychology*, **25**(8), 1057–1064.

Mattay VS, Fera F, Tessitore A, Hariri AR, Berman KF, Das S, Meyer-Lindenberg A, Goldberg TE, Callicott JH and Weinberger DR (2006). Neurophysiological correlates of age-related changes in working memory capacity. *Neuroscience Letters*, **392**(1–2), 32–37.

Mavaddat N, Sahakian BJ, Hutchinson PJ and Kirkpatrick PJ (1999). Cognition following subarachnoid hemorrhage from anterior communicating artery aneurysm: relation to timing of surgery. *Journal of Neurosurgery*, **91**(3), 402–407.

Mayda ABV, Westphal A, Carter CS and DeCarli C (2011). Late life cognitive control deficits are accentuated by white matter disease burden. *Brain*, **134**(6), 1673–1683.

Mayes AR and Daum I (1997). How specific are the memory and other cognitive deficits caused by frontal lobe lesions? In P Rabbitt, ed., *Methodology of Frontal and Executive Function*, pp. 155–176. Psychology Press, Hove.

Maylor EA, Moulson JM, Muncer A-M and Taylor LA (2002). Does performance on theory of mind tasks decline in old age? *British Journal of Psychology*, **93**(4), 465–485.

Mazza M, De Risio A, Sudan L, Roncone R and Casacchia M (2001). Selective impairments of theory of mind in people with schizophrenia. *Schizophrenia Research*, **47**, 299–308.

Mazza M, Costagliola C, Di Michele V, Magliani V, Pollice R, Ricci A, Di Giovanbattista E, Roncone R, Casacchia M and Galzio RJ (2007). Deficit of social cognition in subjects with surgically treated frontal lobe lesions and in subjects affected by schizophrenia. *European Archives of Psychiatry and Clinical Neurosciences*, **257**(1), 12–22.

McAlister C and Schmitter-Edgecombe M (2013). Naturalistic assessment of executive function and everyday multitasking in healthy older adults. *Neuropsychology, Development, and Cognition. Section B, Aging, Neuropsychology and Cognition*, **20**(6), 735–756.

McAllister TW, Saykin AJ, Flashman LA, Sparling MB, Johnson SC, Guerin SJ, Mamourian AC, Weaver JB and Yanofsky N (1999). Brain activation during working memory 1 month after mild traumatic brain injury: a functional MRI study. *Neurology*, **53**(6), 1300–1308.

McCarthy G, Blamire AM, Rothman DL, Gruetter R and Shulman RG (1993). Echo-planar magnetic resonance imaging studies of frontal cortex activation during word generation in humans. *Proceedings of the National Academy of Sciences of the USA*, **90**(11), 4952–4956.

McClure EB, Treland JE, Snow J, Schmajuk M, Dickstein DP, Towbin KE, Charney DS, Pine DS and Leibenluft E (2005). Deficits in social cognition and response flexibility in pediatric bipolar disorder. *American Journal of Psychiatry*, **162**(9), 1644–1651.

McCormack PD (1982). Temporal coding and study-phase retrieval in young and elderly adults. *Bulletin of the Psychonomic Society*, **20**(5), 242–244.

McDermott K and Knight RG (2004). The effects of aging on a measure of prospective remembering using naturalistic stimuli. *Applied Cognitive Psychology*, **18**(3), 349–362.

McDonald CR, Swartz BE, Halgren E, Patell A, Daimes R and Mandelkern M (2006). The relationship of regional frontal hypometabolism to executive function: a resting fluorodeoxyglucose PET study of patients with epilepsy and healthy controls. *Epilepsy & Behavior*, **9**(1), 58–67.

McDowd J, Hoffman L, Rozek E, Lyons KE, Pahwa R, Burns J and Kemper S (2011). Understanding verbal fluency in healthy aging, Alzheimer's disease, and Parkinson's disease. *Neuropsychology*, **25**(2), 210–225.

McFarland CP and Glisky EL (2009). Frontal lobe involvement in a task of time-based prospective memory. *Neuropsychologia*, **47**(7), 1660–1669.

McGeorge P, Phillips L, Crawford JR, Garden SE, Della Sala S and Milne AB (2001). Using virtual environments in the assessment of executive dysfunction. *Presence*, **10**(4), 375–383.

McGuire J, Langdon R, Coltheart M and Mackenzie C (2009). A reanalysis of the personal/impersonal distinction in moral psychology research. *Journal of Experimental Social Psychology*, **45**, 577–580.

McKinnon MC and Moscovitch M (2007). Domain-general contributions to social reasoning: theory of mind and deontic reasoning re-explored. *Cognition*, **102**(2), 179–218.

McLaughlin NCR, Moore DW, Fulwiler C, Bhadelia R and Gansler DA (2009). Differential contributions of lateral prefrontal cortex regions to visual memory processes. *Brain Imaging and Behavior*, **3**, 202–211.

McNab F, Leroux G, Strand F, Thorell L, Bergman S and Klingberg T (2008). Common and unique components of inhibition and working memory: an fMRI, within-subjects investigation. *Neuropsychologia*, **46**(11), 2668–2682.

Meguro K, Shimada M, Yamaguchi S, Ishizaki J, Ishii H, Shimada Y, Sato M, Yamadori A and Sekita Y (2001). Cognitive function and frontal lobe atrophy in normal elderly adults: implications for dementia not as aging-related disorders and the reserve hypothesis. *Psychiatry and Clinical Neurosciences*, **55**(6), 565–572.

Meinzer M, Flaisch T, Wilser L, Eulitz C, Rockstroh B, Conway T, Rothi LJG and Crosson B (2009). Neural signatures of semantic and phonemic fluency in young and old adults. *Journal of Cognitive Neuroscience*, **21**(10), 2007–2018.

Meinzer M, Seeds L, Flaisch T, Harnish S, Cohen ML, McGregor K, Conway T, Benjamin M and Crosson B (2012). Impact of changed positive and negative task-related brain activity on word-retrieval in aging. *Neurobiology of Aging*, **33**(4), 656–669.

Mell T, Heekeren HR, Marschner A, Wartenburger I, Villringer A and Reischies FM (2005). Effect of aging on stimulus-reward association learning. *Neuropsychologia*, **43**(4), 554–563.

Melrose RJ, Poulin RM and Stern CE (2007). An fMRI investigation of the role of the basal ganglia in reasoning. *Brain Research*, **1142**, 146–158.

Menon V, Adleman NE, White CD, Glover GH and Reiss AL (2001). Error-related brain activation during a Go/NoGo response inhibition task. *Human Brain Mapping*, **12**(3), 131–143.

Mesulam MM (1986). Frontal cortex and behavior. *Annals of Neurology*, **19**(4), 320–325.

Metzler C and Parkin AJ (2000). Reversed negative priming following frontal lobe lesions. *Neuropsychologia*, **38**, 363–379.

Milham MP, Erickson KI, Banich MT, Kramer AF, Webb A, Wszalek T and Cohen NJ (2002). Attentional control in the aging brain: insights from an fMRI study of the Stroop task. *Brain & Cognition*, **49**(3), 277–296.

Mill A, Allik J, Realo A and Valk R (2009). Age-related differences in emotion recognition ability: a cross-sectional study. *Emotion*, **9**(5), 619–630.

Miller EK and Cohen JD (2001). An integrative theory of prefrontal cortex function. *Annual Review of Neuroscience*, **24**, 167–202.

Milne E and Grafman J (2001). Ventromedial prefrontal cortex lesions in humans eliminate implicit gender stereotyping. *Journal of Neuroscience*, **21**(12), RC150.

Milner B (1963). Effects of different brain lesions on card sorting: the role of the frontal lobes. *Archives of Neurology*, **9**, 100–110.

Milner B, Corsi P and Leonard G (1991). Frontal-lobe contribution to recency judgements. *Neuropsychologia*, **29**(6), 601–618.

Minzenberg MJ, Laird AR, Thelen S, Carter CS and Glahn DC (2009). Meta-analysis of 41 functional neuroimaging studies of executive function in schizophrenia. *Archives of General Psychiatry*, **66**(8), 811–822.

Mioshi E, Dawson K, Mitchell J, Arnold R and Hodges JR (2006). The Addenbrooke's Cognitive Examination Revised (ACE-R): a brief cognitive test battery for dementia screening. *International Journal of Geriatric Psychiatry*, **21**, 1078–1085.

Mishkin M (1957). Effects of small frontal lesions on delayed alternation in monkeys. *Journal of Neurophysiology*, **20**(6), 615–622.

Mishkin M and Delacour J (1975). An analysis of short-term visual memory in the monkey. *Journal of Experimental Psychology. Animal Behavior Processes*, **1**(4), 326–334.

Mitchell DG, Fine C, Richell RA, Newman C, Lumsden J, Blair KS and Blair RJ (2006). Instrumental learning and relearning in individuals with psychopathy and in patients with lesions involving the amygdala or orbitofrontal cortex. *Neuropsychology*, **20**(3), 280–289.

Mittenberg W, Seidenburg M, O'Leary DS and DiGiulio DV (1989). Changes in cerebral functioning associated with normal aging. *Journal of Clinical and Experimental Neuropsychology*, **11**, 918–932.

Mok WP and Hraba J (1991). Age and gambling behavior: a declining and shifting pattern of participation. *Journal of Gambling Studies*, **7**(4), 313–335.

Moll J, de Oliveira-Souza R, Bramati IE and Grafman J (2002a). Functional networks in emotional moral and nonmoral social judgements. *NeuroImage*, **16**, 696–703.

Moll J, de Oliveira-Souza R, Eslinger PJ, Bramati IE, Mourao-Miranda J, Andreiuolo PA and Pessoa L (2002b). The neural correlates of moral sensitivity: a functional magnetic resonance imaging investigation of basic and moral emotions. *The Journal of Neuroscience*, **22**, 2730–2736.

Moll J, de Oliveira-Souza R, Moll FT, Bramati IE and Andreiuolo PA. (2002c). The cerebral correlates of set-shifting: an fMRI study of the trail making test. *Arquivos de Neuropsiquiatra*, **60**(4), 900–905.

Monchi O, Petrides M, Petre V, Worsley K and Dagher A (2001). Wisconsin Card Sorting revisited: distinct neural circuits participating in different stages of the task identified by event-related functional magnetic resonance imaging. *Journal of Neuroscience*, **21**(19), 7733–7741.

Moniz E (1936). *Tentatives Opératoires dans le Traitement de Certaines Psychoses.* Masson, Paris.

Montepare J, Koff E, Zaitchik D and Albert M (1999). The use of body movements and gestures as cues to emotions in younger and older adults. *Journal of Nonverbal Behavior*, **23**, 133–152.

Moor BG, de Macks ZAO, Güroğlu B, Rombouts SA, Van der Molen MW and Crone EA (2012). Neurodevelopmental changes of reading the mind in the eyes. *Social Cognitive and Affective Neuroscience*, **7**(1), 44–52.

Moran JM, Wig GS, Adams RB Jr, Janata P and Kelley WM (2004). Neural correlates of humor detection and appreciation. *NeuroImage*, **21**(3), 1055–1060.

Moran JM, Jolly E and Mitchell JP (2012). Social-cognitive deficits in normal aging. *Journal of Neuroscience*, **32**(16), 5553–5561.

Moreno C, Borod JC, Welkowitz J and Alpert M. (1993). The perception of facial emotion across the adult life span. *Developmental Neuropsychology*, **9**, 305–314.

Moretti L, Dragone D and di Pellegrino G (2009). Reward and social valuation deficits following ventromedial prefrontal damage. *Journal of Cognitive Neuroscience*, **21**(1), 128–140.

Morris JS, Friston KJ, Büchel C, Frith CD, Young AW, Calder AJ and Dolan RJ (1998). A neuromodulatory role for the human amygdala in processing emotional facial expressions. *Brain*, **121**(1), 47–57.

Morris RG, Downes JJ, Sahakian BJ, Evenden JL, Heald A and Robbins TW (1988). Planning and spatial working memory in Parkinson's disease. *Journal of Neurology, Neurosurgery & Psychiatry*, **51**, 757–766.

Morris RG, Kotitsa M, Bramham J, Brooks B and Rose FD (2002). Virtual reality investigation of strategy formation, rule breaking and prospective memory in patients with focal prefrontal neurosurgical lesions. *Proceedings from the 4th International Conference on Disability, Virtual Reality and Associated Technologies*, pp. 101–108. University of Reading, Reading, UK.

Moscovitch M and Winocur G (1995). Frontal lobes, memory, and aging. *Annals of the New York Academy of Sciences*, **769**, 119–150.

Mostofsky SH, Schafer JG, Abrams MT, Goldberg MC, Flower AA, Boyce A, Courtney SM, Calhoun VD, Kraut MA, Denckla MB and Pekar JJ (2003). fMRI evidence that the neural basis of response inhibition is task-dependent. *Brain Research. Cognitive Brain Research*, **17**(2), 419–430.

Mufson EJ and Pandya DN (1984). Some observations on the course and composition of the cingulum bundle in the rhesus monkey. *Journal of Comparative Neurology*, **225**, 31–43.

Muller F, Simion A, Reviriego E, Galera C, Mazaux J-M, Barat M and Joseph P-A (2010). Exploring theory of mind after severe traumatic brain injury. *Cortex*, **46**(9), 1088–1099.

Müller NG, Machado L and Knight RT (2002). Contributions of subregions of the prefrontal cortex to working memory: evidence from brain lesions in humans. *Journal of Cognitive Neuroscience*, **14**(5), 673–686.

Mummery CJ, Patterson K, Hodges JR and Wise RJ (1996). Generating "tiger" as an animal name or a word beginning with T: differences in brain activation. *Proceedings of the Royal Society of London, Series B, Biological Sciences*, **263**(1373), 989–995.

Murphy FC, Nimmo-Smith I and Lawrence AD (2003). Functional neuroanatomy of emotions: a meta-analysis. *Cognitive, Affective & Behavioral Neuroscience*, 3(3), 207–233.

Murphy P, Shallice T, Robinson G, MacPherson SE, Turner M, Woollett K, Bozzali M and Cipolotti L (2013). Impairments in proverb interpretation following focal frontal lobe lesions. *Neuropsychologia*, 51(11), 2075–2086.

Mutter SA, Naylor JC and Patterson ER (2005). The effects of age and task context on Stroop task performance. *Memory & Cognition*, 33(3), 514–530.

Nagahama Y, Fukuyama H, Yamauchi H, Matsuzaki S, Konishi J, Shibasaki H and Kimura J (1996). Cerebral activation during performance of a card sorting test. *Brain*, 119(5), 1667–1675.

Nagahama Y, Fukuyama H, Yamauchi H, Katsumi Y, Magata Y, Shibasaki H and Kimura J (1997). Age-related changes in cerebral blood flow activation during a Card Sorting Test. *Experimental Brain Research*, 114(3), 571–577.

Nagahama Y, Okina T, Suzuki N, Nabatame H and Matsuda M (2005). The cerebral correlates of different types of perseveration in the Wisconsin Card Sorting Test. *Journal of Neurology, Neurosurgery, and Psychiatry*, 76, 169–175.

Nagel IE, Chicherio C, Li SC, von Oertzen T, Sander T, Villringer A, Heekeren HR, Bäckman L and Lindenberger U (2008). Human aging magnifies genetic effects on executive functioning and working memory. *Frontiers in Human Neuroscience*, 2, 1.

Nakamura K, Kawashima R, Ito K, Sugiura M, Kato T, Nakamura A, Hatano K, Nagumo S, Kubota K, Fukuda H and Kojima S (1999). Activation of the right inferior frontal cortex during assessment of facial emotion. *Journal of Neurophysiology*, 82(3), 1610–1614.

Narumoto J, Yamada H, Iidaka T, Sadato N, Fukui K, Itoh H and Yonekura Y. (2000). Brain regions involved in verbal or nonverbal aspects of facial emotion recognition. *NeuroReport*, 11, 2571–2576.

Nathaniel-James DA, Fletcher P and Frith CD (1997). The function anatomy of verbal initiation and suppression using the Hayling Test. *Neuropsychologia*, 35(4), 559–566.

Nee DE, Wager TD and Jonides J (2007). Interference resolution: insights from a meta-analysis of neuroimaging tasks. *Cognitive, Affective and Behavioural Neuroscience*, 7(1), 1–17.

Nelson HE (1976). A modified card sorting test sensitive to frontal lobe defects. *Cortex*, 12(4), 313–324.

Nelson HE (1982). *National Adult Reading Test: Test Manual.* NFER-Nelson, Windsor, Berks.

Neubert FX, Mars RB, Thomas AG, Sallet J and Rushworth MF (2014). Comparison of human ventral frontal cortex areas for cognitive control and language with areas in monkey frontal cortex. *Neuron*, 81(3), 700–713.

Newcombe F (1987). Psychometric and behavioral evidence: scope, limitations, and ecological validity. In HS Levin, J Grafman and HM Eisenberg, eds, *Neurobehavioral Recovery from Head Injury*, pp. 129–145. Oxford University Press, New York.

Newman LM, Trivedi MA, Bendlin BB, Ries ML and Johnson SC (2007). The relationship between gray matter morphometry and neuropsychological performance in a large sample of cognitive healthy adults. *Brain Imaging and Behaviour*, 1, 3–10.

Newman MC, Allen JJB and Kaszniak AW (2001). Tasks for assessing memory for temporal order versus memory for items in aging. *Aging, Neuropsychology, and Cognition*, 8(1), 72–78.

Newman SD, Carpenter PA, Varma S and Just MA (2003). Frontal and parietal participation in problem solving in the Tower of London: fMRI and computational modeling of planning and high-level perception. *Neuropsychologia*, **41**, 1668–1682.

Newman SD, Greco JA and Lee D (2009). An fMRI study of the Tower of London: a look at problem structure differences. *Brain Research*, 1286, 123–132.

Nguyen CM, Koenigs M, Yamada TH, Teo SH, Cavanaugh JE, Tranel D and Denburg NL (2011). Trustworthiness and negative affect predict economic decision making. Trustworthiness and negative affect predict economic decision making. *Journal of Cognitive Psychology*, **23**(6), 748–759.

Nielson KA, Langenecker SA and Garavan H (2002). Differences in the functional neuroanatomy of inhibitory control across the adult lifespan. *Psychology and Aging*, **17**, 56–71.

Nieuwenhuis S, Ridderinkhof KR, De Jong R, Kok A and van der Molen MW (2000). Inhibitory inefficiency and failures of intention activation: age-related decline in the control of saccadic eye movements. *Psychology and Aging*, **15**, 635–647.

Nieuwenhuis S, Yeung N, van den Wildenberg W and Ridderinkhof KR (2003). Electrophysiological correlates of anterior cingulate function in a go/no-go task: effects of response conflict and trial type frequency. *Cognitive, Affective & Behavioral Neuroscience*, **3**(1), 17–26.

Nieuwenhuis S, Broerse A, Nielen MMA and De Jong R (2004). A goal activation approach to the study of executive function: an application to antisaccade tasks. *Brain and Cognition*, **56**, 198–214.

Niki H and Watanabe M (1976). Prefrontal unit activity and delayed response: relation to cue location versus direction of response. *Brain Research*, **105**, 79–88.

Nippold MA, Uhden LD and Schwarz IE (1997). Proverb explanation through the lifespan: a developmental study of adolescents and adults. *Journal of Speech, Language and Hearing Research*, **40**(2), 245–253.

Nitrini R, Caramelli P, Herrera Júnior E, Porto CS, Charchat-Fichman H, Carthery MT, Takada LT and Lima EP (2004). Performance of illiterate and literate nondemented elderly subjects in two tests of long-term memory. *Journal of the International Neuropsychological Society*, **10**, 634–638.

Norman DA and Shallice T (1980). Attention to action: willed and automatic control of behaviour. Center for Human Information Processing (Technical Report No. 99). University of California, San Diego.

Norman DA and Shallice T (1986). Attention to action: willed and automatic control of behaviour. In RJ Davidson, GE Schwartz and D Shapiro, eds, *Consciousness and Self-Regulation: Advances in Research and Theory*, pp. 1–18. Plenum Press, New York.

Northoff G, Grimm S, Boeker H, Schmidt C, Bermpohl F, Heinzel A, Hell D and Boesiger P (2006). Affective judgment and beneficial decision making: ventromedial prefrontal activity correlates with performance in the Iowa Gambling Task. *Human Brain Mapping*, **27**(7), 572–587.

Nosek BA, Banaji MR and Greenwald AG (2002). Harvesting implicit group attitudes and beliefs from a demonstration web site. *Group Dynamics: Theory, Research and Practice*, **6**(1), 101–115.

Nowak MA, Page KM and Sigmund K (2000). Fairness versus reason in the ultimatum game. *Science*, **289**(5485), 1773–1775.

Nyberg L, McIntosh AR, Cabeza R, Habib R, Houle S and Tulving E (1996). General and specific brain regions involved in encoding and retrieval of events: what, where, and when. *Proceedings of the National Academy of Sciences of the USA*, **93**(20), 11280–11285.

O'Carroll R, Egan V and MacKenzie DM (1994). Assessing cognitive estimation. *British Journal of Clinical Psychology*, **33**, 193–197.

Ochsner KN, Kosslyn SM, Cosgrove GR, Cassem EH, Price BH, Nierenberg AA and Rauch SL (2001). Deficits in visual cognition and attention following bilateral anterior cingulotomy. *Neuropsychologia*, **39**, 219–230.

O'Doherty J, Kringelbach ML and Rolls ET, Hornak J and Andrews C (2001). Abstract reward and punishment representations in the human orbitofrontal cortex. *Nature Neuroscience*, **4**(1), 95–102.

Ohrmann P, Kugel H, Bauer J, Siegmund A, Kölkebeck K, Suslow T, Wiedl KH, Rothermundt M, Arolt V and Pedersen A (2008). Learning potential on the WCST in schizophrenia is related to the neuronal integrity of the anterior cingulate cortex as measured by proton magnetic resonance spectroscopy. *Schizophrenia Research*, **106**(2–3), 156–163.

Okada G, Okamoto Y, Morinobu S, Yamawaki S and Yokota N (2003). Attenuated left prefrontal activation during a verbal fluency task in patients with depression. *Neuropsychobiology*, **47**(1), 21–26.

Okada G, Okamoto Y, Yamashita H, Ueda K, Takami H and Yamawaki S (2009). Attenuated prefrontal activation during a verbal fluency task in remitted major depression. *Psychiatry and Clinical Neurosciences*, **63**(3), 423–425.

O'Leary DS, Flaum M, Kesler ML, Flashman LA, Arndt S and Andreasen NC (2000). Cognitive correlates of the negative, disorganized, and psychotic symptom dimensions of schizophrenia. *Journal of Neuropsychiatry and Clinical Neurosciences*, **12**(1), 4–15.

Olsen RK, Nichols EA, Chen J, Hunt JF, Glover GH, Gabrieli JDE and Wagner AD (2009). Performance-related sustained and anticipatory activity in human medial temporal lobe during delayed match-to-sample. *Journal of Neuroscience*, **29**(38), 11880–11890.

Ongür D and Price JL (2000). The organization of networks within the orbital and medial prefrontal cortex of rats, monkeys and humans. *Cerebral Cortex*, **10**(3), 206–219.

Orbach J and Fischer GJ (1959). Bilateral resections of frontal granular Cortex. *A.M.A. Archives of Neurology*, **1**, 78–86.

Orr JM and Banich MT (2014). The neural mechanisms underlying internally and externally guided task selection. *NeuroImage*, **84**, 191–205.

Orgeta V and Phillips LH (2008). Effects of age and emotional intensity on the recognition of facial emotion. *Experimental Aging Research*, **34**(1), 63–79.

Oscar-Berman M (1975). The effects of dorsolateral-frontal and ventrolateral-orbitofrontal lesions on spatial discrimination learning and delayed response in two modalities. *Neuropsychologia*, **13**, 237–246.

Oscar-Berman M, Hancock M, Mildworf B, Hutner N and Weber DA (1990). Emotional perception and memory in alcoholism and aging. *Alcoholism, Clinical and Experimental Research*, **14**(3), 383–393.

Ostrosky F, Ardila A, Rosselli M, Lopez-Arango G and Uriel-Mendoza V (1998). Neuropsychological test performance in illiterate subjects. *Archives of Clinical Neuropsychology*, **13**(7), 645–660.

Ostrosky F, Ardila A and Rosselli M (1999). Neuropsi: a brief neuropsychological test battery in Spanish with norms by age and educational level. *Journal of the International Neuropsychological Society*, 5, 413–433.

O'Sullivan M, Jones DK, Summers PE, Morris RG, Williams SC and Markus HS (2001). Evidence for cortical "disconnection" as a mechanism of age-related cognitive decline. *Neurology*, 57(4), 632–638.

O'Sullivan M, Barrick TR, Morris RG, Clark CA and Markus HS (2005). Damage within a network of white matter regions underlies executive dysfunction in CADASIL. *Neurology*, 65(10), 1584–1590.

Overman W, Graham L, Redmond A, Eubank R, Boettcher L, Samplawski O and Walsh K (2006). Contemplation of moral dilemmas eliminates sex differences on the Iowa gambling task. *Behavioral Neuroscience*, 120(4), 817–825.

Owen AM (1997a). Cognitive planning in humans: neuropsychological, neuroanatomical and neuropharmacological perspectives. *Progress in Neurobiology*, 53, 431–450.

Owen AM (1997b). The functional organization of working memory processes within the human lateral frontal cortex: the contribution of functional neuroimaging. *European Journal of Neuroscience*, 9, 1329–1339.

Owen AM, Downes JJ, Sahakian BJ, Polkey CE and Robbins TW (1990). Planning and spatial working memory following frontal lobe lesions in man. *Neuropsychologia* 28(10), 1021–1034.

Owen AM, Sahakian BJ, Hodges JR, Summers BA, Polkey CE and Robbins TW (1995). Dopamine-dependent frontostriatal planning deficits in early Parkinson's disease. *Neuropsychology*, 9(1), 126–140.

Owen AM, Doyon J, Petrides M and Evans AC (1996a). Planning and spatial working memory: a positron emission tomography study in humans. *European Journal of Neuroscience, 8*, 353–364.

Owen AM, Evans AC and Petrides M (1996b). Evidence for a two-stage model of spatial working memory processing within the lateral frontal cortex: a positron emission tomography study. *Cerebral Cortex*, 6(1), 31–38.

Owen AM, Doyon J, Dagher A, Sadikot A and Evans AC (1998a). Abnormal basal ganglia outflow in Parkinson's disease identified with PET. Implications for higher cortical functions. *Brain*, 121(5), 949–965.

Owen AM, Stern CE, Look RB, Tracey I, Rosen BR and Petrides M (1998b). Functional organization of spatial and nonspatial working memory processing within the human lateral frontal cortex. *Proceedings of the National Academy of Sciences of the USA*, 95(13), 7721–7726.

Owen AM, Herrod NJ, Menon DK, Clark JC, Downey SP, Carpenter TA, Minhas PS, Turkheimer FE, Williams EJ, Robbins TW, Sahakian BJ, Petrides M and Pickard JD (1999). Redefining the functional organization of working memory processes within human lateral prefrontal cortex. *European Journal of Neuroscience*, 11(2), 567–574.

Owen AM, Lee ACH and Williams EJ (2000). Dissociating aspects of verbal working memory within the human frontal lobe: further evidence for a "process-specific" model of lateral frontal organization. *Psychobiology*, 28(2), 146–155.

Oztekin I, McElree B, Staresina BP and Davachi L (2008). Working memory retrieval: contributions of the left prefrontal cortex, the left posterior parietal cortex, and the hippocampus. *Journal of Cognitive Neuroscience*, 21(3), 581–593.

Pa J, Possin KL, Wilson SM, Quitania LC, Kramer JH, Boxer AL, Weiner MW and Johnson JK (2010). Gray matter correlates of set-shifting among neurodegenerative disease, mild cognitive impairment, and healthy older adults. *Journal of the International Neuropsychological Society*, **16**(4), 640–650.

Pandya DN and Yeterian EH (1996). Comparison of prefrontal architecture and connections. *Philosophical Transactions of the Royal Society of London, Series B: Biological Sciences*, **351**, 1423–1432.

Pardini M and Nichelli PF (2009). Age-related decline in mentalizing skills across adult life span. *Experimental Aging Research*, **35**(1), 98–106.

Park DC and Reuter-Lorenz P (2009). The adaptive brain: aging and neurocognitive scaffolding. *Annual Review of Psychology*, **60**, 173–196.

Park DC, Lautenschlager G, Hedden T, Davidson NS, Smith AD and Smith PK (2002). Models of visuospatial and verbal memory across the adult life span. *Psychology and Aging*, **17**(2), 299–320.

Parkin J and Java RI (1999). Deterioration of frontal lobe function in normal aging: influences of fluid intelligence versus perceptual speed. *Neuropsychology*, **13**(4), 539–545.

Parkin AJ, Walter BM and Hunkin NM (1995). Relationships between normal aging, frontal lobe function, and memory for temporal and spatial information. *Neuropsychology*, **9**(3), 304–312.

Parkin AJ, Bindschaedler C, Harsent L and Metzler C (1996). Pathological false alarm rates following damage to the left frontal cortex. *Brain and Cognition*, **32**(1), 14–27.

Partiot A, Vérin M, Pillon B, Teixeira-Ferreira C, Agid Y and Dubois B (1996). Delayed response tasks in basal ganglia lesions in man: further evidence for a striato-frontal cooperation in behavioural adaptation. *Neuropsychologia*, **34**(7), 709–721.

Pascual-Leone A and Hallett M (1994). Induction of errors in a delayed response task by repetitive transcranial magnetic stimulation of the dorsolateral prefrontal cortex. *Neuroreport*, **5**, 2517–2520.

Paulesu E, Goldacre B, Scifo P, Cappa SF, Gilardi MC, Castiglioni I, Perani D and Ca FF (1997). Functional heterogeneity of left inferior frontal cortex as revealed by fMRI. *Neuroreport*, **8**(8), 2011–2016.

Paus T, Petrides M, Evans AC and Meyer E (1993). Role of the human anterior cingulate cortex in the control of oculomotor, manual, and speech responses: a positron emission tomography study. *Journal of Neurophysiology*, **70**, 453–469.

Paxton JL, Barch DM, Racine CA and Braver TS (2008). Cognitive control, goal maintenance, and prefrontal function in healthy aging. *Cerebral Cortex*, **18**(5), 1010–1028.

Penetar DM and McDonough JH (1983). Effects of cholinergic drugs on delayed match-to-sample performance of rhesus monkeys. *Pharmacology, Biochemistry, and Behavior*, **19**(6), 963–967.

Perani D, Cappa SF, Tettamanti M, Rosa M, Scifo P, Miozzo A, Basso A and Fazio F (2003). A fMRI study of word retrieval in aphasia. *Brain and Language*, **85**(3), 357–368.

Pereira JB, Junqué C, Bartrés-Faz D, Martí MJ, Sala-Llonch R, Compta Y, Falcón C, Vendrell P, Pascual-Leone A, Valls-Solé J and Tolosa E (2013). Modulation of verbal fluency networks by transcranial direct current stimulation (tDCS) in Parkinson's disease. *Brain Stimulation*, **6**(1), 16–24.

Pérez-Alvarez F, Timoneda, C and Reixach J (2006). An fMRI study of emotional engagement in decision-making. *Transaction Advanced Research*, **2**, 45–51.

Periáñez JA, Maestú F, Barceló F, Fernández A, Amo C and Ortiz Alonso T (2004). Spatiotemporal brain dynamics during preparatory set shifting: MEG evidence. *NeuroImage*, **21**(2), 687–695.

Periáñez JA, Ríos-Lago M, Rodríguez-Sánchez JM, Adrover-Roig D, Sánchez-Cubillo I, Crespo-Facorro B, Quemada JI and Barceló F (2007). Trail Making Test in traumatic brain injury, schizophrenia, and normal ageing: sample comparisons and normative data. *Archives of Clinical Neuropsychology*, **22**(4), 433–447.

Perlmutter M, Metzger R, Nezworski T and Miller K (1981). Spatial and temporal memory in 20 to 60 year olds. *Journal of Gerontology*, **36**(1), 59–65.

Perner J and Wimmer H (1985). "John thinks that Mary thinks that …": attribution of second-order beliefs by 5- to 10-year-old children. *Journal Experimental Child Psychology*, **39**, 437–471.

Perret E (1974). The left frontal lobe of man and the suppression of habitual responses in verbal categorical behaviour. *Neuropsychologia*, **12**, 323–330.

Petersen SE, Fox PT, Posner MI, Mintun M and Rachle ME (1988). Positron emission tomographic studies of the cortical anatomy of single-word processing. *Nature*, **331**, 585–589.

Peterson BS, Skudlarski P, Zhang H, Gatenby JC, Anderson AW and Gore JC (1999). An fMRI study of Stroop word-colour interference: evidence for the cingulate subregions subserving multiple distributed attentional systems. *Biological Psychiatry*, **45**, 1237–1258.

Peterson BS, Kane MJ, Alexander GM, Lacadie C, Skudlarski P, Leung H-C, May J and Gore JC (2002). An event-related functional MRI study comparing interference effects in the Simon and Stroop tasks. *Cognitive Brain Research*, **13**, 427–440.

Petrides M (1991). Monitoring of selections of visual stimuli and the primate frontal cortex. *Proceedings of the Royal Society of London, Series B, Biological Sciences*, **246**, 293–298.

Petrides M (1994). Frontal lobes and working memory: evidence from investigations of the effects of cortical excisions in nonhuman primates. In F Boller, H Spinnler and JA Hendler, eds, *Handbook of Neuropsychology*, Vol. 9, pp. 59–82. Elseveir Science B.V., Amsterdam.

Petrides M (1995). Impairments on nonspatial self-ordered and externally ordered working memory tasks after lesions of mid-dorsal part of the lateral frontal cortex in the monkey. *Journal of Neuroscience*, **15**, 359–375.

Petrides M (2000a). Mapping prefrontal cortical systems for the control of cognition. In AW Toga and JC Mazziotta, eds, *Brain Mapping: The Systems*, 159–176. Academic Press, San Diego.

Petrides M (2000b). Dissociable roles of mid-dorsolateral prefrontal and anterior inferotemporal cortex in visual working memory. *Journal of Neuroscience*, **20**(19), 7496–7503.

Petrides M and Milner B (1982). Deficits on Subject-Ordered Tasks After Frontal- and Temporal-Lobe Lesions in Man. *Neuropsychologia*, **20**(3), 249–262.

Petrides M and Pandya DN (1994). Comparative architectonic analysis of the human and the macaque frontal cortex. In J Grafman and F Boller, eds, *Handbook of Neuropsychology*, Vol. 9, pp. 17–58. Elsevier, Amsterdam.

Petrides M and Pandya DN (2004). The frontal cortex. In G Paxinos and JK Mai, eds, *The Human Nervous System*, pp. 950–972. Elsevier/Academic Press, San Diego.

Petrides M, Alivisatos B, Evans AC and Meyer E (1993a). Dissociation of human mid-dorsolateral from posterior dorsolateral frontal cortex in memory processing. *Proceedings of the National Academy of Sciences of the USA*, **90**, 873–877.

Petrides M, Alivisatos B, Meyer E and Evans AC (1993b). Functional activation of the human frontal cortex during the performance of verbal working memory tasks. *Proceedings of the National Academy of Sciences of the USA*, **90**, 878–882.

Petrides M, Tomaiuolo F, Yeterian EH and Pandya DN (2012). The prefrontal cortex: comparative architectonic organization in the human and the macaque monkey brains. *Cortex*, **48**(1), 46–57.

Pfefferbaum A and Ford JM (1998). ERPs to stimuli requiring response production and inhibition: effects of age, probability and visual noise. *Electroencephalography and Clinical Neurophysiology*, **71**(1), 55–63.

Pfeifer B (1910). Psychiatrische störungen bei hirntumoren. *Archiv für Psychologie und Nervenkrankheiten*, **47**, 558–569.

Phan KL, Wager T, Taylor SF and Liberzon I (2002). Functional neuroanatomy of emotion: a meta-analysis of emotion activation studies in PET and fMRI. *NeuroImage*, **16**, 331–348.

Phelps EA, Hyder F, Blamire AM and Shulman RG (1997). FMRI of the prefrontal cortex during overt verbal fluency. *Neuroreport*, **8**(2), 561–565.

Phelps EA, O'Connor KJ, Cunningham WA, Funayama ES, Gatenby JC, Gore JC and Banaji MR (2000). Performance on indirect measures of race evaluation predicts amygdala activation. *Journal of Cognitive Neuroscience*, **12**(5), 729–738.

Phillips LH (1997). Do "frontal tests" measure executive function? Issues of assessment and evidence from fluency tests. In P Rabbitt, ed., *Methodology of Frontal and Executive Function*, pp. 191–214. Psychology Press, Hove.

Phillips LH (1999). Age and individual differences in letter fluency. *Developmental Neuropsychology*, **15**(2), 249–267.

Phillips LH, Della Sala S and Trivelli C (1996). Fluency deficits in patients with Alzheimer's disease and frontal lobe lesions. *European Journal of Neurology*, **3**, 102–108.

Phillips L, Wynn V, Gilhooly KJ, Della Sala S and Logie RH (1999). The role of memory in the Tower of London task. *Memory*, **7**, 209–231.

Phillips LH, Wynn VE, McPherson S and Gilhooly KJ (2001). Mental planning and the Tower of London task. *Quarterly Journal of Experimental Psychology, A*, **54**(2), 579–597.

Phillips LH, MacLean RDJ and Allen R (2002a). Age and the understanding of emotions: neuropsychological and sociocognitive perspectives. *Journals of Gerontology, Series B, Psychological Sciences and Social Sciences*, **57**(6), P526–P530.

Phillips LH, MacPherson SE and Della Sala S (2002b). Age, cognition, and emotion: the role of anatomical segregation in the frontal lobes. In J Grafman, ed., *Handbook of Neuropsychology*, 2nd edn, pp. 73–97. Elsevier, Amsterdam.

Phillips LH, Gilhooly KJ, Logie RH, Della Sala S and Wynn VE (2003). Age, working memory, and the Tower of London task. *European Journal of Cognitive Psychology*, **15**, 291–312.

Phillips LH, Kliegel M and Martin M (2006). Age and planning tasks: the influence of ecological validity. *International Journal of Aging and Human Development*, **62**, 175–184.

Phillips ML, Young AW, Senior C, Brammer M, Andrew C, Calder AJ, Bullmore ET, Perrett DI, Rowland D, Williams SC, Gray JA and David AS (1997). A specific neural substrate for perceiving facial expressions of disgust. *Nature*, **389**, 495–498.

Platek SM, Keenan JP, Gallup GG and Mohamed FB (2004). Where am I? The neurological correlates of self and other. *Brain Research. Cognitive Brain Research*, **19**(2), 114–122.

Prehn K, Wartenburger I, Mériau K, Scheibe C, Goodenough OR, Villringer A, van der Meer E and Heekeren HR (2008). Individual differences in moral judgement competence influence neural correlates of socio-normative judgements. *Social Cognitive and Affective Neuroscience*, **3**, 33–46.

Price BH, Daffner KR, Stowe RM and Mesulam MM (1990). The comportmental learning disabilities of early frontal lobe damage. *Brain*, **113**(5), 1383–1393.

Provost JS, Petrides M, Simard F and Monchi O (2012). Investigating the long-lasting residual effect of a set shift on frontostriatal activity. *Cerebral Cortex*, **22**(12), 2811–2819.

Ptak R and Schnider A (2004). Disorganised memory after right dorsolateral prefrontal damage. *Neurocase*, **10**(1), 52–59.

Pujol J, Vendrell P, Deus J, Junqué C, Bello J, Martí-Vilalta JL and Capdevila A (2001). The effect of medial frontal and posterior parietal demyelinating lesions on stroop interference. *NeuroImage*, **13**, 68–75.

Pujol J, Reixach J, Harrison BJ, Timoneda-Gallart C, Vilanova JC and Pérez-Alvarez F (2008). Posterior cingulate activation during moral dilemma in adolescents. *Human Brain Mapping*, **29**, 910–921.

Quadflieg S, Turk DJ, Waiter GD, Mitchell JP, Jenkins AC and Macrae CN (2009). Exploring the neural correlates of social stereotyping. *Journal of Cognitive Neuroscience*, **21**(8), 1560–1570.

Quintana J and Fuster JM (1999). From perception to action: temporal integrative functions of prefrontal and parietal neurons. *Cerebral Cortex*, **9**(3), 213–221.

Rabbitt P (1997). Introduction: methodologies and models in the study of executive function. In P Rabbit, ed., *Methodology of Frontal and Executive Function*, pp. 1–38. Psychology Press, Hove.

Rabbit PMA (1966). Errors and error correction in choice-response tasks. *Journal of Experimental Psychology*, **71**, 264–272.

Rahman S, Sahakian BJ, Hodges JR, Rogers RD and Robbins TW (1999). Specific cognitive deficits in mild frontal variant frontotemporal dementia. *Brain*, **122**(8), 1469–1493.

Rajah MN, Ames B and D'Esposito M (2008). Prefrontal contributions to domain-general executive control processes during temporal context retrieval. *Neuropsychologia*, **46**(4), 1088–1103.

Rajah MN, Languay R and Valiquette L (2010). Age-related changes in prefrontal cortex activity are associated with behavioural deficits in both temporal and spatial context memory retrieval in older adults. Cortex, **46**(4), 535–549.

Rajah MN, Crane D, Maillet D and Floden D (2011). Similarities in the patterns of prefrontal cortex activity during spatial and temporal context memory retrieval after equating task structure and performance. *NeuroImage*, **54**, 1549–1564.

Rajah MN and McIntosh AR (2006). Dissociating prefrontal contributions during a recency memory task. *Neuropsychologia*, **44**(3), 350–364.

Rajah MN and McIntosh AR (2008). Age-related differences in brain activity during verbal recency memory. *Brain Research*, 1199, 111–125.

Rajkowska G and Goldman-Rakic PS (1995). Cytoarchitectonic definition of prefrontal areas in the normal human cortex: II. Variability in locations of areas 9 and 46 and relationship to the Talairach Coordinate System. *Cerebral Cortex*, 5(4), 323–337.

Rakoczy H, Harder-Kasten A and Sturm L (2012). The decline of theory of mind in old age is (partly) mediated by developmental changes in domain-general abilities. *British Journal of Psychology*, 103(1), 58–72.

Ramnani N and Owen AM (2004). Anterior prefrontal cortex: insights into function from anatomy and neuroimaging. *Nature Reviews Neuroscience*, 5, 184–194.

Rand D, Basha-Abu Rukan S, Weiss PLT and Katz N (2009). Validation of the Virtual MET as an assessment tool for executive functions. *Neuropsychological Rehabilitation*, 19(4), 583–602.

Rapp AM, Leube DT, Erb M, Grodd W and Kircher TTJ (2004). Neural correlates of metaphor processing. *Cognitive Brain Research*, 20(3), 395–402.

Rapp PR (1990). Visual discrimination and reversal learning in the aged monkey (*Macaca mulatta*). *Behavioural Neuroscience*, 104, 876–884.

Rasmusson XD, Zonderman AB, Kawas C and Resnick SM (1998). Effects of age and dementia on the Trail Making Test. *The Clinical Neuropsychologist*, 12(2), 169–178.

Rasser PE, Johnston P, Lagopoulos J, Ward PB, Schall U, Thienel R, Bender S, Toga AW and Thompson PM (2005). Functional MRI BOLD response to Tower of London performance of first-episode schizophrenia patients using cortical pattern matching. *Neuroimage*, 26(3), 941–951.

Ravdin LD, Katzen HL, Agrawal P and Relkin NR (2003). Letter and semantic fluency in older adults: effects of mild depressive symptoms and age-stratified normative data. *The Clinical Neuropsychologist*, 17(2), 195–202.

Raven JC (1958). *Standard Progressive Matrices*. H. K. Lewis, London.

Raven J, Raven JC and Court JH (1998). *Manual for Raven's Progressive Matrices and Vocabulary Scales*. Harcourt Assessment, San Antonio, TX.

Ravnkilde B, Videbech P, Rosenberg R, Gjedde A and Gade A (2002). Putative tests of frontal lobe function: a PET-study of brain activation during Stroop's Test and verbal fluency. *Journal of Clinical and Experimental Neuropsychology*, 24(4), 534–547.

Raz M (2013). *The Lobotomy Letters: The Making of American Psychosurgery*. University of Rochester Press, Rochester, New York.

Raz N, Briggs SD, Marks W and Acker JD (1999). Age-related deficits in generation and manipulation of mental images: II. The role of the dorsolateral prefrontal cortex. *Psychology and Aging*, 14(3), 436–444.

Raz N, Lindenberger U, Rodrigue KM, Kennedy KM, Head D, Williamson A, Dahle C, Gerstorf D and Acker JD (2005). Regional brain changes in aging healthy adults: general trends, individual differences and modifiers. *Cerebral Cortex*, 15(11), 1676–1689.

Raz N, Ghisletta P, Rodrigue KM, Kennedy KM and Lindenberger U (2010). Trajectories of brain aging in middle-aged and older adults: regional and individual differences. *NeuroImage*, 51(2), 501–511.

Reitan RM and Wolfson D (1985). *The Halstead–Reitan Neuropsychological Test Battery: Therapy and Clinical Interpretation*. Neuropsychological Press, Tucson, AZ.

Reitan RM and Wolfson D (1993). *The Halstead-Reitan Neuropsychological Test Battery: Theory and Clinical Interpretation*, 2nd edn. Neuropsychology Press, Tucson, AZ.

Reitan RM and Wolfson D (1994). A selective and critical review of neuropsychological deficits and the frontal lobes. *Neuropsychology Review*, **4**, 161–198.

Remijnse PL, Nielen MMA, Uylings HBM and Veltman DJ (2005). Neural correlates of a reversal learning task with an affectively neutral baseline: an event-related fMRI study. *NeuroImage*, **26**, 609–618.

Resnick SM, Pham DL, Kraut MA, Zonderman AB and Davatzikos C (2003). Longitudinal magnetic resonance imaging studies of older adults: a shrinking brain. *The Journal of Neuroscience*, **23**(8), 3295–3301.

Resnick SM, Lamar M and Driscoll I (2007). Vulnerability of the orbitofrontal cortex to age-associated structural and functional brain changes. *Annals of the New York Academy of Sciences*, 1121, 562–575.

Reuter-Lorenz PA, Stanczak L and Miller AC (1999). Neural recruitment and cognitive aging: two hemispheres are better than one, especially as you age. *Psychological Science*, **10**, 494–500.

Reverberi C, Lavaroni A, Gigli GL, Skrap M and Shallice T (2005a). Specific impairments of rule induction in different frontal lobe subgroups. *Neuropsychologia*, **43**(3), 460–472.

Reverberi C, Toraldo A, D'Agostini S and Skrap M (2005b). Better without (lateral) frontal cortex? Insight problems solved by frontal patients. *Brain*, **128**(12), 2882–2890.

Rezai K, Andreasen NC, Alliger R, Cohen G, Swayze II V and O'Leary DS (1993). The neuropsychology of the prefrontal cortex. *Archives of Neurology*, **50**, 636–642.

Rhodes MG (2004). Age-related differences in performance on the Wisconsin card sorting test: a meta-analytic review. *Psychology and Aging*, **19**(3), 482–494.

Riccio CA, Reynolds CR, Lowe P and Moore JJ (2002). The continuous performance test: a window on the neural substrates for attention? *Archives of Clinical Neuropsychology*, **17**(3), 235–272.

Richer F, Décary A, Lapierre M-F, Rouleau I, Bouvier G and Saint-Hilaire J-M (1993). Target detection deficits in frontal lobectomy. *Brain and Cognition*, **21**, 203–211.

Richeson JA, Baird AA, Gordon HL, Heatherton TF, Wyland CL, Trawalter S and Shelton JN (2003). An fMRI investigation of the impact of interracial contact on executive function. *Nature Neuroscience*, **6**(12), 1323–1328.

Ridderinkhof KR, Span MM and van der Molen MW (2002). Perseverative behavior and adaptive control in older adults: performance monitoring, rule induction, and set shifting. *Brain and Cognition*, **49**(3), 382–401.

Rieger M, Gauggel S and Burmeister K (2003). Inhibition of ongoing responses following frontal, nonfrontal, and basal ganglia lesions. *Neuropsychology*, **17**(2), 272–282.

Riley JD, Moore S, Cramer SC and Lin JJ (2011). Caudate atrophy and impaired frontostriatal connections are linked to executive dysfunction in temporal lobe epilepsy. *Epilepsy Behavior*, **21**(1), 80–87.

Rilling JK, Sanfey AG, Aronson JA, Nystrom LE and Cohen JD (2004). The neural correlates of theory of mind within interpersonal interactions. *Neuroimage*, **22**(4), 1694–703.

Ringholz G (1989). *Inconsistent Attention in Chronic Survivors of Severe Closed Head Injury*. Unpublished doctoral dissertation. University of Houston, Houston, TX.

Rizzo S, Sandrini M and Papagno C (2007). The dorsolateral prefrontal cortex in idiom interpretation: an rTMS study. *Brain Research Bulletin*, **71**(5), 523–528.

Roalf DR, Mitchell SH, Harbaugh WT and Janowsky JS (2012). Risk, reward and economic decision-making in aging. *Journals of Gerontology, Series B, Psychological Sciences and Social Sciences*, **67**(3), 289–298.

Robbins TW (1996). Dissociating executive functions of the prefrontal cortex. *Philosophical Transactions of the Royal Society of London, Series B: Biological Sciences*, **351**(1346), 1463–1470.

Robbins TW, James M, Owen AM, Sahakian BJ, McInnes L and Rabbitt P (1994). Cambridge Neuropsychological Test Automated Battery (CANTAB): a factor analytic study of a large sample of normal elderly volunteers. *Dementia*, **5**(5), 266–281.

Robbins TW, James M, Owen AM, Sahakian BJ, Lawrence AD, McInnes L and Rabbitt PMA (1998). A study of performance on tests from the CANTAB battery sensitive to frontal lobe dysfunction in a large sample of normal volunteers: implications for theories of executive functioning and cognitive aging. *Journal of the International Neuropsychological Society*, **4**, 474–490.

Roberts KL and Hall DA (2008). Examining a supramodal network for conflict processing: a systematic review and novel functional magnetic resonance imaging data for related visual and auditory Stroop tasks. *Journal of Cognitive Neuroscience*, **20**(6), 1063–1078.

Roberts LE, Rau H, Lutzenberger W and Birbaumer N (1994). Mapping P300 waves onto inhibition: Go/No-Go discrimination. *Electroencephalography and Clinical Neurophysiology*, **92**(1), 44–55.

Robinson G, Shallice T, Bozzali M and Cipolotti L (2012). The differing roles of the frontal cortex in fluency tests. *Brain*, **135**, 2202–2214.

Robinson JL, Bearden CE, Monkul ES, Tordesillas-Gutiérrez D, Velligan DI, Frangou S and Glahn DC (2009). Fronto-temporal dysregulation in remitted bipolar patients: an fMRI delayed-non-match-to-sample (DNMS) study. *Bipolar Disorders*, **11**(4), 351–360.

Roca M, Parr A, Thompson R, Woolgar A, Torralva T, Antoun N, Manes F and Duncan J (2010). Executive function and fluid intelligence after frontal lobe lesions. *Brain*, **133**(1), 234–247.

Roca M, Torralva T, Gleichgerrcht E, Woolgar A, Thompson R, Duncan J and Manes F (2011). The role of Area 10 (BA10) in human multitasking and in social cognition: a lesion study. *Neuropsychologia*, **49**(13), 3525–3531.

Rodríguez-Aranda C (2003). Reduced writing and reading speed and age-related changes in verbal fluency tasks. *The Clinical Neuropsychologist*, **17**(2), 203–215.

Rodriguez-Aranda C and Martinussen M (2006). Age-related differences in performance of phonemic verbal fluency measured by Controlled Oral Word Association Task (COWAT): a meta-analytic study. *Developmental Neuropsychology*, **30**(2), 697–717.

Roefs A and Jansen A (2002). Implicit and explicit attitudes toward high-fat foods in obesity. *Journal of Abnormal Psychology*, **111**(3), 517–521.

Rogers RD, Owen AM, Middleton HC, Williams EJ, Pickard JD, Sahakian BJ and Robbins TW (1999). Choosing between small, likely rewards and large, unlikely rewards activates inferior and orbital prefrontal cortex. *Journal of Neuroscience*, **19**(20), 9029–9038.

Rolls ET (1996). The orbitofrontal cortex. *Philosophical Transactions of the Royal Society of London, Series B: Biological Sciences*, **351**, 1433–1444.

Rolls ET (1999). The functions of the orbitofrontal cortex. *Neurocase*, **5**, 301–312.

Rolls ET (2014a). *Emotion and Decision Making Explained*. Oxford University Press, Oxford.

Rolls ET (2014b). Emotion and decision making explained: précis. *Cortex* **59**, 185–193.

Rolls ET, Hornak J, Wade D and McGrath J (1994). Emotion-related learning in patients with social and emotional changes associated with frontal lobe damage. *Journal of Neurology, Neurosurgery, and Psychiatry*, **57**, 1525–1527.

Rolls ET, Critchley HD, Mason R and Wakeman EA (1996). Orbitofrontal cortex neurons: role in olfactory and visual association learning. *Journal of Neurophysiology*, **75**, 1970–1981.

Rosen VM and Engle RW (1997). The role of working memory capacity in retrieval. *Journal of Experimental Psychology: General*, **126**(3), 211–227.

Rosenbaum RS, Furey ML, Horwitz B and Grady CL (2010). Altered connectivity among emotion-related brain regions during short-term memory in Alzheimer's disease. *Neurobiology of Aging*, **31**(5), 780–786.

Rosselli M, Ardila A and Rosas P (1990). Neuropsychological assessment in illiterates. II: Language and praxic abilities. *Brain and Cognition*, **12**, 281–296.

Rosvold HE, Mirsky AF, Sarason I, Bransome ED and Beck LH (1956). A continuous performance test of brain damage. *Journal of Consulting Psychology*, **20**(5), 343–50.

Rowe JB, Toni I, Josephs O, Frackowiak RS and Passingham RE (2000). The prefrontal cortex: response selection or maintenance within working memory? *Science*, **288**(5471), 1656–1660.

Rowe JB, Owen AM, Johnsrude IS and Passingham RE (2001). Imaging the mental components of a planning task. *Neuropsychologia*, **39**(3), 315–327.

Royer A, Schneider FCG, Grosselin A, Pellet J, Barral F-G, Laurent B, Brouillet D and Lang F (2009). Brain activation during executive processes in schizophrenia. *Psychiatry Research*, **173**(3), 170–176.

Rubia K, Russell T, Overmeyer S, Brammer MJ, Bullmore ET, Sharma T, Simmons A, Williams SC, Giampietro V, Andrew CM and Taylor E (2001). Mapping motor inhibition: conjunctive brain activations across different versions of go/no-go and stop tasks. *NeuroImage*, **13**(2), 250–261.

Rubia K, Smith AB, Brammer MJ and Taylor E (2003). Right inferior prefrontal cortex mediates response inhibition while mesial prefrontal cortex is responsible for error detection. *NeuroImage*, **20**(1), 351–358.

Rudebeck PH, Bannerman DM and Rushworth MF (2008). The contribution of distinct subregions of the ventromedial frontal cortex to emotion, social behavior, and decision making. *Cognitive, Affective & Behavioral Neuroscience*, **8**(4), 485–497.

Rudman LA, Greenwald AG and McGhee DE (2001). Implicit self-concept and evaluative implicit gender stereotypes: self and ingroup share desirable traits. *Personality and Social Psychology Bulletin*, **27**, 1164–1178.

Ruffman T, Henry JD, Livingstone V and Phillips LH (2008). A meta-analytic review of emotion recognition and aging: implications for neuropsychological models of aging. *Neuroscience and Biobehavioral Reviews*, **32**(4), 863–881.

Rugg MD (1997). *Cognitive Neuroscience*. MIT Press, Cambridge, MA.

Rush BK, Barch DM and Braver TS (2006). Accounting for cognitive aging: context processing, inhibition or processing speed? *Neuropsychology, Development, and Cognition, Section B: Aging, Neuropsychology, and Cognition*, 13(3–4), 588–610.

Rushworth MFS and Behrens TEJ (2008). Choice, uncertainty and value in prefrontal and cingulate cortex. *Nature Neuroscience*, 11(4), 389–397.

Rushworth MF, Walton ME, Kennerley SW and Bannerman DM (2004). Action sets and decisions in the medial frontal cortex. *Trends in Cognitive Sciences*, 8(9), 410–417.

Russell TA, Rubia K, Bullmore ET, Soni W, Suckling J, Brammer MJ, Simmons A, Williams SCR and Sharma T (2000). Exploring the social brain in schizophrenia: left prefrontal underactivation during mental state attribution. *American Journal of Psychiatry*, 157(12), 2040–2042.

Rypma B, Prabhakaran V, Desmond JE, Glover GH and Gabrieli JD (1999). Load-dependent roles of frontal brain regions in the maintenance of working memory. *NeuroImage*, 9(2), 216–226.

Sabatinelli D, Fortune EE, Li Q, Siddiqui A, Krafft C, Oliver WT, Beck S and Jeffries J (2011). Emotional perception: meta-analyses of face and natural scene processing. *NeuroImage*, 54(3), 2524–2533.

Sabbagh MA (2004). Understanding orbitofrontal contributions to theory-of-mind reasoning: implications for autism. Brain and Cognition, 55(1), 209–219.

Sabbagh MA and Taylor M (2000). Neural correlates of theory-of-mind reasoning: an event-related potential study. *Psychological Science*, 11(1), 46–50.

Sabbagh MA, Moulson MC and Harkness KL (2004). Neural correlates of mental state decoding in human adults: an event-related potential study. *Journal of Cognitive Neuroscience*, 16(3), 415–426.

Sahakian BJ, Morris RG, Evenden JL, Heald AL, Levy R, Philpot M and Robbins TW (1988). A comparative study of visuospatial memory and learning in Alzheimer-Type dementia and Parkinson's disease. *Brain*, 111(3), 695–718.

St Jacques P, Rubin DC, LaBar KS and Cabeza R (2008). The short and long of it: neural correlates of temporal-order memory for autobiographical events. *Journal of Cognitive Neuroscience*, 20(7), 1327–1341.

Sakatani K, Lichty W, Xie Y, Li S and Zuo H (1999). Effects of aging on language-activated cerebral blood oxygenation changes of the left prefrontal cortex: near infrared spectroscopy study. *Journal of Stroke and Cerebrovascular Diseases*, 8(6), 398–403.

Salat DH, Kaye JA and Janowsky JS (2002). Greater orbital prefrontal volume selectively predicts worse working memory performance in older adults. *Cerebral Cortex*, 12(5), 494–505.

Salloum JB, Ramchandani VA, Bodurka J, Rawlings R, Momenan R, George D and Hommer DW (2007). Blunted rostral anterior cingulate response during a simplified decoding task of negative emotional facial expressions in alcoholic patients. *Alcoholism, Clinical and Experimental Research*, 31(9), 1490–1504.

Salthouse TA (1991). *Theoretical Perspectives on Cognitive Aging*. Erlbaum, Hillsdale, NJ.

Salthouse TA (1994). The aging of working memory. *Neuropsychology*, 8(4), 535–543.

Salthouse T (2005). Relations between cognitive abilities and measures of executive functioning. *Neuropsychology*, 19(4), 532–545.

Salthouse TA and Meinz EJ (1995). Aging, inhibition, working memory, and speed. *Journal of Gerontology: Psychological Sciences*, **50B**, P297–P306.

Salthouse TA, Atkinson TM and Berish DE (2003). Executive functioning as a potential mediator of age-related cognitive decline in normal adults. *Journal of Experimental Psychology: General*, **132**(4), 566–594.

Salvatierra JL and Roseelii M (2011). The effect of bilingualism and age on inhibitory control. *International Journal of Bilingualism*, **15**(1), 26–37.

Saltzman J, Strauss E, Hunter M and Archibald S (2000). Theory of mind and executive functions in normal human aging and Parkinson's disease. *Journal of the International Neuropsychological Society*, **6**(7), 781–788.

Samson AC, Zysset S and Huber O (2008). Cognitive humor processing: different logical mechanisms in nonverbal cartoons—an fMRI study. *Social Neuroscience*, **3**(2), 125–140.

Sanfey AG, Rilling JK, Aronson JA, Nystrom LE and Cohen JD (2003). The neural basis of economic decision-making in the Ultimatum Game. *Science*, **300**(5626), 1755–1758.

Sarazin M, Pillon B, Giannakopoulos P, Rancurel G, Samson Y and Dubois B (1998). Clinicometabolic dissociation of cognitive functions and social behavior in frontal lobe lesions. *Neurology*, **51**(1), 142–148.

Sarfati Y, Hardy-Baylé MC, Besche C and Widlöcher D (1997). Attribution of intentions to others in people with schizophrenia: a non-verbal exploration with comic strips. *Schizophrenia Research*, **25**(3), 199–209.

Sasaki K, Gemba H, Nambu A and Matsuzaki R (1993). No-go activity in the frontal association cortex of human subjects. *Neuroscience Research*, **18**(3), 249–252.

Sato W, Kochiyama T, Yoshikawa S, Naito E and Matsumura M (2004). Enhanced neural activity in response to dynamic facial expressions of emotion: an fMRI study. *Brain Research. Cognitive Brain Research*, **20**(1), 81–91.

Saxe R and Kanwisher N (2003). People thinking about thinking people. The role of the temporo-parietal junction in "theory of mind". *NeuroImage*, **19**, 1835–1842.

Schall U, Johnston P, Lagopoulos J, Jüptner M, Jentzen W, Thienel R, Dittmann-Balçar A, Bender S and Ward PB (2003). Functional brain maps of Tower of London performance: a positron emission tomography and functional magnetic resonance imaging study. *Neuroimage*, **20**(2), 1154–1161.

Schaufelberger M, Senhorini MC, Barreiros MA, Amaro E Jr, Menezes PR, Scazufca M, Castro CC, Ayres AM, Murray RM, McGuire PK and Busatto GF (2005). Frontal and anterior cingulate activation during overt verbal fluency in patients with first episode psychosis. *Revista Brasileira de Psiquiatria*, **27**(3), 228–232.

Schlösser R, Hutchinson M, Joseffer S, Rusinek H, Saarimaki A, Stevenson J, Dewey SL and Brodie JD (1998). Functional magnetic resonance imaging of human brain activity in a verbal fluency task. *Journal of Neurology, Neurosurgery & Psychiatry*, **64**(4), 492–498.

Schmiedek F, Li S-C and Lindenberger U (2009). Interference and facilitation in spatial working memory: age-associated differences in lure effects in the n-back paradigm. *Psychology and Aging*, **24**(1), 203–210.

Schnyer DM, Verfaellie M, Alexander MP, LaFleche G, Nicholls L and Kaszniak AW (2004). A role for right medial prefontal cortex in accurate feeling-of-knowing judgements: evidence from patients with lesions to frontal cortex. *Neuropsychologia*, **42**(7), 957–966.

Schoenbaum G, Nugent S, Saddoris MP and Gallagher M (2002). Teaching old rats new tricks: age-related impairments in olfactory reversal learning. *Neurobiology of Aging*, **23**, 555–564.

Schon K, Tinaz S, Somers D and Stern C (2008). Delayed match to object or place: an event-related fMRI study of short-term stimulus maintenance and the role of stimulus pre-exposure. *NeuroImage*, **39**(2), 857–872.

Schott BH, Niehaus L, Wittmann BC, Schutze H, Seidenbecher CI, Heinze HJ and Duzel E (2007). Ageing and early-stage Parkinson's disease affect separable neural mechanisms of mesolimbic reward processing. *Brain*, **130**, 2412–2424.

Schroder HS and Infantolino ZP (2013). Distinguishing between types of errors and adjustments. *Journal of Neuroscience*, **33**(47), 18356–18357.

Schwartz S, Baldo J, Graves RE and Brugger P (2003). Pervasive influence of semantics in letter and category fluency: a multidimensional approach. *Brain and Language*, **87**, 400–411.

Sebastian CL, Fontaine NM, Bird G, Blakemore SJ, Brito SA, McCrory EJ and Viding E (2011). Neural processing associated with cognitive and affective Theory of Mind in adolescents and adults. *Social Cognitive and Affective Neuroscience*, **7**(1), 53–63.

Semendeferi K, Armstrong E, Schleicher A, Zilles K and Van Hoesen GW (2001). Prefrontal cortex in humans and apes: a comparative study of area 10. *American Journal of Physical Anthropology*, **114**(3), 224–241.

Senhorini MC, Cerqueira CT, Schaufelberger MS, Almeida JC, Amaro E, Sato JR, Barreiros MA, Ayres AM, Castro CC, Scazufca M, Menezes PR and Busatto GF (2011). Brain activity patterns during phonological verbal fluency performance with varying levels of difficulty: a functional magnetic resonance imaging study in Portuguese-speaking healthy individuals. *Journal of Clinical and Experimental Neuropsychology*, **33**(8), 864–873.

Seo EH, Lee DY, Kim KW, Lee JH, Jhoo JH, Youn JC, Choo IH, Ha J and Woo JI (2006). A normative study of the Trail Making Test in Korean elders. *International Journal of Geriatric Psychiatry*, **21**(9), 844–852.

Shallice T (1982). Specific impairments of planning. *Philosophical Transactions of the Royal Society of London, Series B*, **298**, 199–209.

Shallice T (2002). Fractionation of the supervisory system. In DT Stuss and R Knight, eds, *Principles of Frontal Lobe Functions*, pp. 261–277. Oxford University Press, New York.

Shallice T and Burgess PW (1991a). Higher-order cognitive impairments and frontal lobe lesions in man. In HS Levin, HM Eisenberg and AL Benton, eds, *Frontal Lobe Function and Dysfunction*, pp. 125–138. Oxford University Press, New York.

Shallice T and Burgess PW (1991b). Deficits in strategy application following frontal lobe damage in man. *Brain*, **114**, 727–741.

Shallice T and Burgess PW (1993). Supervisory control of action and thought selection. In A Baddeley and L Weiskrantz, eds, *Attention: Selection, Awareness and Control: A Tribute to Donald Broadbent*, pp. 171–187. Clarendon Press, Oxford.

Shallice T and Burgess PW (1996). The domain of supervisory processes and the temporal organisation of behaviour. *Philosophical Transactions of the Royal Society of London B*, **351**, 1405–1412.

Shallice T and Cooper RP (2011). *The Organisation of Mind*. Oxford University Press, Oxford.

Shallice T and Evans ME (1978). The involvement of the frontal lobes in cognitive estimation. *Cortex*, **14**, 294–303.

Shallice T, Stuss DT, Picton TW, Alexander MP and Gillingham S (2008). Mapping task switching in frontal cortex through neuropsychological group studies. *Frontiers in Neuroscience*, **2**(1), 79–85.

Shamay-Tsoory SG and Aharon-Peretz J (2007). Dissociable prefrontal networks for cognitive and affective theory of mind: a lesion study. *Neuropsychologia*, **45**(13), 3054–3067.

Shamay-Tsoory SG, Tomer R, Berger BD and Aharon-Peretz J (2003). Characterization of empathy deficits following prefrontal brain damage: the role of the right ventromedial prefrontal cortex. *Journal of Cognitive Neuroscience*, **15**(3), 324–337.

Shamay-Tsoory SG, Tomer R and Aharon-Peretz J (2005a). The neuroanatomical basis of understanding sarcasm and its relationship to social cognition. *Neuropsychology*, **19**(3), 288–300.

Shamay-Tsoory SG, Tomer R, Berger BD, Goldsher D and Aharon-Peretz J (2005b). Impaired "affective theory of mind" is associated with right ventromedial prefrontal damage. *Cognitive and Behavioral Neurology*, **18**(1), 55–67.

Shamay-Tsoory SG, Aharon-Peretz J and Levkovitz Y (2007). The neuroanatomical basis of affective mentalizing in schizophrenia: comparison of patients with schizophrenia and patients with localized prefrontal lesions. *Schizophrenia Research*, **90**(1–3), 274–283.

Shamay-Tsoory SG, Harari H, Aharon-Peretz A and Levkovitz Y (2010). The role of the orbitofrontal cortex in affective theory of mind deficits in criminal offenders with psychopathic tendencies. *Cortex*, **46**, 668–677.

Shammi P and Stuss DT (1999). Humour appreciation: a role of the right frontal lobe. *Brain*, **122**(4), 657–666.

Shaw P, Bramham J, Lawrence EJ, Morris R, Baron-Cohen S and David AS (2005). Differential effects of lesions of the amygdala and prefrontal cortex on recognizing facial expressions of complex emotions. *Journal of Cognitive Neuroscience*, **17**(9), 1410–1419.

Shaw P, Lawrence E, Bramham J, Brierley B, Radbourne C and David AS (2007). A prospective study of the effects of anterior temporal lobectomy on emotion recognition and theory of mind. *Neuropsychologia*, **45**(12), 2783–2790.

Shenhav A and Greene JD (2010). Moral judgements recruit domain-general valuation mechanisms to integrate representations of probability and magnitude. *Neuron*, **67**, 667–677.

Shibata T, Shimoyama I, Ito T, Abla D, Iwasa H, Koseki K, Yamanouchi N, Sato T and Nakajima Y (1997). The time course of interhemispheric EEG coherence during a GO/NO-GO task in humans. *Neuroscience Letters*, **233**(2–3), 117–120.

Shimamura AP (2002). Muybridge in motion: travels in art, psychology, and neurology. *History of Photography*, **26**, 341–350.

Shimamura AP and Jurica PJ (1994). Memory interference effects and aging: findings from a test of frontal lobe functions. *Neuropsychology*, **8**, 408–412.

Shoqeirat MA, Mayes A, MacDonald C, Meudell P and Pickering A (1990). Performance on tests sensitive to frontal lobe lesions by patients with organic amnesia: Leng & Parkin revisited. *British Journal of Clinical Psychology*, **29**, 401–408.

Silberstein RB, Line P, Pipingas A, Copolov D and Harris P (2000). Steady-state visually evoked potential topography during the continuous performance task in normal controls and schizophrenia. *Clinical Neurophysiology*, **111**(5), 850–857.

Silveri MC, Di Betta AM, Filippini V, Leggio MG and Molinari M (1998). Verbal short-term store-rehearsal system and the cerebellum. Evidence from a patient with a right cerebellar lesion. *Brain*, **121**(11), 2175–2187.

Simmonds DJ, Pekar JJ and Mostofsky SH (2008). Meta-analysis of Go/No-go tasks demonstrating that fMRI activation associated with response inhibition is task-dependent. *Neuropsychologia*, **46**, 224–232.

Simon HA (1969/1974). *La Science des Systèmes/Science de l'artificiel*. Epi, Paris. Translation in JL Le Moigne, *The Sciences of the Artificial*. MIT Press, London.

Sivan AB (1992). *Benton Visual Retention Test Manual—Fifth Edition*. The Psychological Corporation, San Antonio, TX.

Slessor G, Phillips LH and Bull R (2007). Exploring the specificity of age-related differences in theory of mind tasks. *Psychology and Aging*, **22**(3), 639–643.

Smith EE, Jonides J, Koeppe RA, Awh E, Schumacher EH and Minoshima S (1995). Spatial versus object working memory: PET investigations. *Journal of Cognitive Neuroscience*, **7**(3), 337–356.

Smith EE, Jonides J and Koeppe R (1996). Dissociating verbal and spatial working memory using PET. *Cerebral Cortex*, **6**, 11–20.

Snowden JS, Gibbons ZC, Blackshaw A, Doubleday E, Thompson J, Craufurd D, Foster J, Happé F and Neary D (2003). Social cognition in frontotemporal dementia and Huntington's disease. *Neuropsychologia*, **41**(6), 688–701.

Specht K, Lie CH, Shah NJ and Fink GR (2009). Disentangling the prefrontal network for rule selection by means of a non-verbal variant of the Wisconsin Card Sorting Test. *Human Brain Mapping*, **30**(5), 1734–1743.

Spinnler H and Tognoni G (1987). Standardizzazione e taratura italiana di test neuropsicologici. *Italian Journal of Neurological Sciences, Supplement*, **8**, issue 6.

Sprengelmeyer R, Rausch M, Eysel UT and Przuntek H (1998). Neural structures associated with recognition of facial expressions of basic emotions. *Proceedings of the Royal Society of London, Series B, Biological Sciences*, **265**, 1927–1931.

Stanhope N, Guinan E and Kopelman MD (1998). Frequency judgements of abstract designs by patients with diencephalic, temporal lobe or frontal lobe lesions. *Neuropsychologia*, **36**, 1387–1396.

Steele VR, Claus ED, Aharoni E, Harenski C, Calhoun VD, Pearlson G and Kiehl KA. (2014). A large scale (N=102) functional neuroimaging study of error processing in a Go/NoGo task. *Behavioural Brain Research*, **268**, 127–138.

Steiner VAG, Mansur LL, Brucki SMD and Nitrini R (2008). Phonemic verbal fluency and age: a preliminary study. *Dementia & Neuropsychologia*, **2**(4), 328–332.

Stern ER, Gonzalez R, Welsh RC and Taylor SF (2010). Updating beliefs for a decision: neural correlates of uncertainty and underconfidence. *Journal of Neuroscience*, **30**(23), 8032–8041.

Stewart BD, von Hippel W and Radvansky GA (2009). Age, race, and implicit prejudice: using process dissociation to separate the underlying components. *Psychological Science*, **20**(2), 164–168.

Stone VE, Baron-Cohen S and Knight RT (1998). Frontal lobe contributions to theory of mind. *Journal of Cognitive Neuroscience*, **10**(5), 640–656.

Strauss E, Sherman EMS and Spreen O (2006). *A Compendium of Neuropsychological Tests: Administration, Norms, and Commentary.* Oxford University Press, New York.

Streit M, Dammers J, Simsek-Kraues S, Brinkmeyer J, Wölwer W and Ioannides A (2003). Time course of regional brain activations during facial emotion recognition in humans. *Neuroscience Letters*, **342**(1–2), 101–104.

Stretton J and Thompson PJ (2012). Frontal lobe function in temporal lobe epilepsy. *Epilepsy Research*, **98**(1), 1–13.

Stringaris AK, Medford N, Giora R, Giampietro VC, Brammer MJ and David AS (2006). How metaphors influence semantic relatedness judgments: the role of the right frontal cortex. *NeuroImage*, **33**(2), 784–793.

Stroop JR (1935). Studies of interference in serial verbal reactions. *Journal of Experimental Psychology*, **18**, 643–661.

Stuss DT (2006). Frontal lobes and attention: processes and networks, fractionation and integration. *Journal of the International Neuropsychological Society*, **12**, 261–271.

Stuss DT and Alexander MP (2000). Executive functions and the frontal lobes: a conceptual view. *Psychological Research*, **63**(3–4), 289–298.

Stuss DT and Alexander MP (2007). Is there a dysexecutive syndrome? In J Driver, P Haggard and T Shallice, eds, *Mental Processes in the Human Brain*, pp. 225–248. Oxford University Press, New York.

Stuss DT and Alexander MP (2009). Frontal lobe syndrome. In L Squire, ed., *Encyclopedia of Neuroscience*, pp. 375–381. Academic Press, Oxford.

Stuss DT and Benson DF (1986). *The Frontal Lobes.* Raven Press, New York.

Stuss DT and Knight RT (2002). *Principles of Frontal Lobe Function.* Oxford University Press, New York.

Stuss DT and Knight RT (2013). *Principles of Frontal Lobe Function*, 2nd edn. Oxford University Press, New York.

Stuss DT, Shallice T, Alexander MP and Picton TW (1995). A multidisciplinary approach to anterior attentional functions. *Annals of the New York Academy of Sciences*, **769**, 191–211.

Stuss DT, Alexander MP, Hamer L, Palumbo C, Dempster R, Binns M, Levine B and Izukawa D (1998). The effects of focal anterior and posterior brain lesions on verbal fluency. *Journal of the International Neuropsychological Society*, **4**(3), 265–278.

Stuss DT, Levine B, Alexander MP, Hong J, Palumbo C, Hamer L, Murphy KJ and Izukawa D (2000). Wisconsin Card Sorting Test performance in patients with focal frontal and posterior brain damage: effects of lesion location and test structure on separable cognitive processes. *Neuropsychologia*, **38**(4), 388–402.

Stuss DT, Bisschop SM, Alexander MP, Levine B, Katz D and Izukawa D (2001a). The Trail Making Test: a study in focal lesion patients, *Psychological Assessment*, **13**, 230–239.

Stuss DT, Floden D, Alexander MP, Levine B and Katz D (2001b). Stroop performance in focal lesion patients: dissociation of processes and frontal lobe lesion location. *Neuropsychologia*, **39**, 771–786.

Stuss DT, Alexander MP, Floden D, Binns MA, Levine B, McIntosh AR, Rajah N and Hevenor SJ (2002). Fractionation and localization of distinct frontal lobe processes: evidence from focal lesions in humans. In DT Stuss and R Knight, eds, *Principles of Frontal Lobe Functions*, pp. 261–277. Oxford University Press, New York.

Stuss DT, Alexander MP, Shallice T, Picton TW, Binns MA, Macdonald R, Borowiec A and Katz DI (2005). Multiple frontal systems controlling response speed. *Neuropsychologia*, **43**, 396–417.

Suhr J and Hammers D (2010). Who fails the Iowa Gambling Test (IGT)? Personality, neuropsychological, and near-infrared spectroscopy findings in healthy young controls. *Archives of Clinical Neuropsychology*, **25**(4), 293–302.

Sullivan EV and Pfefferbaum A (2007). Neuroradiological characterization of normal adult ageing. *British Journal of Radiology*, **80**(2), S99–108.

Sullivan S and Ruffman T (2004a). Social understanding: how does it fare with advancing years? *British Journal of Psychology*, **95**(1), 1–18.

Sullivan S and Ruffman T (2004b). Emotion recognition deficits in the elderly. *International Journal of Neuroscience*, **114**(3), 403–432.

Sun X, Zhang X, Chen X, Zhang P, Bao M, Zhang D, Chen J, He S and Hu X (2005). Age-dependent brain activation during forward and backward digit recall revealed by fMRI. *NeuroImage*, **26**(1), 36–47.

Suzuki A, Hoshino T, Shigemasu K and Kawamura M (2007). Decline or improvement? Age-related differences in facial expression recognition. *Biological Psychology*, **74**(1), 75–84.

Suzuki M, Fujii T, Tsukiura T, Okuda J, Umetsu A, Nagasaka T, Mugikura S, Yanagawa I, Takahashi S and Yamadori A (2002). Neural basis of temporal context memory: a functional MRI study. *NeuroImage*, **17**(4), 1790–1796.

Swick D and Jovanovic J (2002). Anterior cingulate cortex and the Stroop task: neuropsychological evidence for topographic specificity. *Neuropsychologia*, **40**, 1240–1253.

Swick D and Turken U (2002). Dissociation between conflict detection and error monitoring in the human anterior cingulate cortex. *Proceeding of the National Academy of Sciences of the USA*, **99**(25), 16354–16359.

Swick D, Ashley V and Turken AU (2008). Left inferior frontal gyrus is critical for response inhibition. *BMC Neuroscience*, **9**, 102.

Szatkowska I, Grabowska A and Szymańska O (2000). Phonological and semantic fluencies are mediated by different regions of the prefrontal cortex. *Acta Neurobiologiae Experimentalis*, **60**(4), 503–508.

Szatkowska I, Szymanska O, Bojarskie P and Grabowska A (2007). Cognitive inhibition in patients with medial orbitofrontal damage. *Experimental Brain Research*, **181**, 109–115.

Tabibnia G, Satpute AB and Lieberman MD (2008). The sunny side of fairness. *Psychological Science*, **19**(4), 339–347.

Tamez E, Myerson J, Morris L, White DA, Baum C and Connor LT (2011). Assessing executive abilities following acute stroke with the trail making test and digit span. *Behavioural Neurology*, **24**(3), 177–185.

Taylor R and O'Carroll R (1995). Cognitive estimation in neurological disorders. *British Journal of Clinical Psychology*, **34**(2), 223–228.

Teixeira-Ferreira C, Vérin M, Pillon B, Levy R, Dubois B and Agid Y (1998). Spatio-temporal working memory and frontal lesions in man. *Cortex*, **34**(1), 83–98.

Telling AL, Meyer AS and Humphreys GW (2010). Distracted by relatives: effects of frontal lobe damage on semantic distraction. *Brain and Cognition*, **73**(3), 203–214.

Teuber H-L (2009). The riddle of frontal lobe function in man. *Neuropsychology Review*, **19**(**1**), 25–46.

Théodoridou ZD and Triarhou LC (2012). Challenging the supremacy of the frontal lobe: early views (1906–1909) of Christfried Jakob on the human cerebral cortex. *Cortex*, **48**(**1**), 15–25.

Thiebaut de Schotten M, Dell'Acqua F, Valabregue R and Catani M (2012). Monkey to human comparative anatomy of the frontal lobe association tracts. *Cortex*, **48**(**1**), 82–96.

Thorpe SJ, Rolls ET and Maddison S (1983). The orbitofrontal cortex: neuronal activity in the behaving monkey. *Experimental Brain Research*, **49**(**1**), 93–115.

Tomb I, Hauser M, Deldin P and Caramazza A (2002). Do somatic markers mediate decisions on the gambling task? *Nature Neuroscience*, **5**(**11**), 1103–1104.

Tombaugh TN, Kozak J and Rees L (1999). Normative data stratified by age and education for two measures of verbal fluency: FAS and animal naming. *Archives of Clinical Neuropsychology*, **14**(**2**), 167–177.

Tomer R and Levin BE (1993). Differential effects of aging on two verbal fluency tasks. *Perceptual and Motor Skills*, **76**(**2**), 465–466.

Toone BK, Okocha CI, Sivakumar K and Syed GM (2000). Changes in regional cerebral blood flow due to cognitive activation among patients with schizophrenia. *British Journal of Psychiatry*, **177**, 222–228.

Torralva T, Kipps CM, Hodges JR, Clark L, Bekinschtein T, Roca M, Calcagno ML and Manes F (2007). The relationship between affective decision-making and theory of mind in the frontal variant of fronto-temporal dementia. *Neuropsychologia*, **45**(**2**), 342–349.

Torralva T, Roca M, Gleichgerrcht E, Lopez P and Manes F (2009a). INECO Frontal Screening (IFS): an efficient, sensitive, and specific tool to assess executive functions in dementia. *Journal of the International Neuropsychological Society*, **15**, 777–786.

Torralva T, Roca M, Gleichgerrcht E, Bekinschtein T and Manes F (2009b). A neuropsychological battery to detect specific executive and social cognitive impairments in early frontotemporal dementia. *Brain*, **132**(**5**), 1299–1309.

Tranel D, Bechara A and Denburg NL (2002). Asymmetric functional roles of right and left ventromedial prefrontal cortices in social conduct, decision-making, and emotional processing. *Cortex*, **38**(**4**), 589–612.

Tranel D, Hathaway-Nepple J and Anderson SW (2007). Impaired behavior on real-world tasks following damage to the ventromedial prefrontal cortex. *Journal of Clinical and Experimental Neuropsychology*, **29**(**3**), 319–332.

Troyer A (2000). Normative data for clustering and switching on verbal fluency tasks. *Journal of Clinical and Experimental Neuropsychology*, **22**, 370–378.

Troyer K, Moscovitch M and Winocur G (1997). Clustering and switching as two components of verbal fluency: evidence from younger and older healthy adults. *Neuropsychology*, **11**(**1**), 138–146.

Troyer K, Moscovitch M, Winocur G, Alexander MP and Stuss D (1998). Clustering and switching on verbal fluency: the effects of focal frontal- and temporal-lobe lesions. *Neuropsychologia*, **36**(**6**), 499–504.

Tsuchida A and Fellows LK (2009). Lesion evidence that two distinct regions within prefrontal cortex are critical for n-back performance in humans. *Journal of Cognitive Neuroscience*, **21**(**12**), 2263–2275.

Tsujimoto S, Genovesio A and Wise SP (2011). Frontal pole cortex: encoding ends at the end of the endbrain. *Trends in Cognitive Sciences*, **15**(4), 169–176.

Turken AU and Swick D (1999). Response selection in the human anterior cingulate cortex. *Nature Neuroscience*, **2**(10), 920–924.

Turken AU and Swick D (2008). The effect of orbitofrontal lesions on the error-related negativity. *Neuroscience Letters*, **441**(1), 7–10.

Turnbull OH, Berry H and Bowman CH (2003). Direct versus indirect emotional consequences on the Iowa Gambling Task. *Brain and Cognition*, **53**(2), 389–392.

Uekermann J, Thoma P and Daum I (2008). Proverb interpretation changes in aging. *Brain and Cognition*, **67**(1), 51–57.

Ullsperger M and von Cramon DY (2001). Subprocesses of performance monitoring: a dissociation of error processing and response competition revealed by event-related fMRI and ERPs. *NeuroImage*, **14**(6), 1387–1401.

Ullsperger M and von Cramon DY (2004). Neuroimaging of performance monitoring: error detection and beyond. *Cortex*, **40**(4–5), 593–604.

Ungerleider LG, Courtney SM and Haxby JV (1998). A neural system for human visual working memory. *Proceedings of the National Academy of Sciences of the USA*, **95**(3), 883–890.

Unterrainer JM, Rahm B, Kaller CP, Ruff CC, Spreer J, Krause BJ, Schwarzwald R, Hautzel H and Halsband U (2004). When planning fails: individual differences and error-related brain activity in problem solving. *Cerebral Cortex*, **14**(12), 1390–1397.

Unterrainer JM, Ruff CC, Rahm B, Kaller CP, Spreer J, Schwarzwald R and Halsband U (2005). The influence of sex differences and individual task performance on brain activation during planning. *Neuroimage*, **24**(2), 586–590.

Uylings HBM and van Enden CG (1990). Qualitative and quantitative comparison of the prefrontal cortex in rat and in primates, including humans. *Progress in Brain Research*, **85**, 31–62.

Uylings HBM, Rajkowska G, Sanz-Arigita E, Amunts K and Zilles K (2005). Consequences of large interindividual variability for human brain atlases: Converging macroscopical imaging and microscopical neuroanatomy. *Anatomy and Embryology*, **210**(5–6), 423–431.

Uylings HBM, Sanz-Arigita EJ, de Vos K, Pool CW, Evers P and Rajkowska G (2010). 3-D cytoarchitectonic parcellation of human orbitofrontal cortex correlation with postmortem MRI. *Psychiatry Research*, **183**(1), 1–20.

Valenstein ES (1986). *Great and Desperate Cures!: Rise and Decline of Psychosurgery and Other Radical Treatments for Mental Illness*. Basic Books, New York.

Valentin GG (1841). Hirn- und Nervenlehre. In ST Soemmerrin, ed., *Vom Baue des Menschlichen*. Korpers, Leipzig.

Van den Berg E, Nys GM, Brands AM, Ruis C, van Zandvoort MJ and Kessels RP (2009). The Brixton Spatial Anticipation Test as a test for executive function: validity in patient groups and norms for older adults. *Journal of the International Neuropsychological Society*, **15**(5), 695–703.

Van den Bos R, Houx BB and Spruijt BM (2006). The effect of reward magnitude differences on choosing disadvantageous decks in the Iowa Gambling Task. *Biological Psychology*, **71**(2), 155–161.

van den Heuvel OA, Groenewegen HJ, Barkhof F, Lazeron RH, van Dyck R and Veltman DJ (2003). Frontostriatal system in planning complexity: a parametric functional magnetic resonance version of Tower of London task. *Neuroimage*, **18**(2), 367–374.

van den Heuvel OA, Veltman DJ, Groenewegen HJ, Cath DC, van Balkom AJ, van Hartskamp J, Barkhof F and van Dyck R (2005). Frontal-striatal dysfunction during planning in obsessive-compulsive disorder. *Archives of General Psychiatry*, **62**(3), 301–309.

Van Der Elst W, Van Boxtel MPJ, Van Breukelen GJP and Jolles J (2006a). The Stroop Color-Word Test: Influence of age, sex, and education; and normative data for a large sample across the adult age range. *Assessment*, **13**(1), 62–79.

Van der Elst W, Van Boxtel MPJ, Van Breukelen GJP and Jolles J (2006b). Normative data for the Animal, Profession and Letter M Naming verbal fluency tests for Dutch speaking participants and the effects of age, education, and sex. *Journal of the International Neuropsychological Society*, **12**(1), 80–89.

Van Der Lubbe RHJ and Verleger R (2002). Aging and the Simon task. *Psychophysiology*, **39**, 100–110.

Van Der Werf YD, Weerts JG, Jolles J, Witter MP, Lindeboom J and Scheltens P (1999). Neuropsychological correlates of a right unilateral lacunar thalamic infarction. *Journal of Neurology, Neurosurgery, & Psychiatry*, **66**(1), 36–42.

Vannorsdall TD, Schretlen DJ, Andrejczuk M, Ledoux K, Bosley LV, Weaver JR, Skolasky RL and Gordon B (2012). Altering automatic verbal processes with transcranial direct current stimulation. *Frontiers in Psychiatry*, **3**, 1–6.

Van Overwalle F (2009). Social cognition and the brain: a meta-analysis. *Human Brain Mapping*, **30**(3), 829–858.

van't Wout M, Kahn RS, Sanfey AG and Aleman A (2005). Repetitive transcranial magnetic stimulation over the right dorsolateral prefrontal cortex affects strategic decision-making. *Neuroreport*, **16**(16), 1849–1852.

Van Veen V and Carter CS (2002). The anterior cingulate as a conflict monitor: fMRI and ERP studies. *Physiology & Behaviour*, **77**(4–5), 477–482.

Vendrell P, Junqué C, Pujol J, Jurado MA, Molet J and Grafman J (1995). The role of prefrontal regions in the stroop task. *Neuropsychologia*, **33**, 341–352.

Verfaellie M and Heilman KM (1987). Response preparation and response inhibition after lesions of the medial frontal lobe. *Archives of Neurology*, **44**(12), 1265–1271.

Verhaeghen P and De Meersman L (1998). Aging and the Stroop effect: a meta-analysis. *Psychology & Aging*, **13**(1), 120–126.

Verhaeghen P, Marcoen A and Goossens L (1993). Facts and fictions about memory aging: a quantitative integration of research findings. *Journal of Gerontology: Psychological Sciences*, **48**, P157–P171.

Vérin M, Partiot A, Pillon B, Malapani C, Agid Y and Dubois B (1993). Delayed response tasks and prefrontal lesions in man—evidence for self-generated patterns of behaviour with poor environmental modulation. *Neuropsychologia*, **31**(12), 1379–1396.

Vicq d'Azyr and Moreau de la Sarthe JL (1805). *Oeuvres de Vicq d'Azyr. Recueillies et publiees avec des notes et un discours sur sa vie et ses ouvrages*. De l'imprimerie de Baudoin, Paris.

Vijayashankar N and Brody H (1979). A quantitative study of the pigmented neurons in the nuclei locus coeruleus and subcoeruleus in man as related to aging. *Journal of Neuropathology & Experimental Neurology*, **38**(5), 490–497.

Villardita C, Cultrera S, Cupone V and Mejìa R (1985). Neuropsychological test performances and normal aging. *Archives of Gerontology and Geriatrics*, **4**(4), 311–319.

Vogeley K, Bussfeld P, Newen A, Herrmann S, Happé F, Falkai P, Maier W, Shah NJ, Fink GR and Zilles K (2001). Mind reading: neural mechanisms of theory of mind and self-perspective. *NeuroImage*, **14**(1), 170–181.

Vogt C and Vogt O (1919). Allgemeinere ergebnisse unserer hirnforschung. *Journal für Psychologie und Neurologie*, **25**, 279–461.

Volle E, de Lacy Costello A, Coates LM, McGuire C, Towgood K, Gilbert S, Kinkingnehun S, McNeil JE, Greenwood R, Papps B, van den Broeck M and Burgess PW (2012). Dissociation between verbal response initiation and suppression after prefrontal lesions. *Cerebral Cortex*, **22**, 2428–2440.

Völlm BA, Taylor AN, Richardson P, Corcoran R, Stirling J, McKie S, Deakin JF and Elliott R (2006). Neuronal correlates of theory of mind and empathy: a functional magnetic resonance imaging study in a nonverbal task. *NeuroImage*, **29**(1), 90–98.

Von Economo C, Koskinas GN (1925). *Die Cytoarchitektonik der Hirnrinde des Erwachsenen Menschen. Textband und Atlas*. Springer, Wien.

Voytko ML (1999). Impairments in acquisition and reversals of two-choice discriminations by aged rhesus monkeys. *Neurobiology of Aging*, **20**, 617–627.

Wager TD, Sylvester C-YC, Lacey SC, Nee DE, Franklin M and Jonides J (2005). Common and unique components of response inhibition revealed by fMRI. *NeuroImage*, **27**, 323–340.

Wagner G, Koch K, Reichenbach JR, Sauer H and Schlösser RG (2006a). The special involvement of the rostrolateral prefrontal cortex in planning abilities: an event-related fMRI study with the Tower of London paradigm. *Neuropsychologia*, **44**(12), 2337–2347.

Wagner M, Rihs TA, Mosimann UP, Fisch HU and Schlaepfer TE (2006b). Repetitive transcranial magnetic stimulation of the dorsolateral prefrontal cortex affects divided attention immediately after cessation of stimulation. *Journal of Psychiatric Research*, **40**(4), 315–321.

Wagner S, Sebastian A, Lieb K, Tüscher O and Tadi A (2014). A coordinate-based ALE functional MRI meta-analysis of brain activation during verbal fluency tasks in healthy control subjects. *BMC Neuroscience*, **15**(1), 19.

Wallesch CW, Kornhuber HH, Köllner C, Haas HC and Hufnagl JM (1983). Language and cognitive deficits resulting from medial and dorsolateral frontal lobe lesions. *Archiv für Psychiatrie und Nervenkrankheiten*, **233**(4), 279–296.

Walter H, Adenzato M and Ciaromidaro A (2004). Understanding intentions in social interaction: the role of the anterior paracingulate cortex. *Journal of Cognitive. Neuroscience*, **16**, 1854–1863.

Wang Y and Su Y (2006). Theory of mind in old adults: the performance on Happé's stories and faux pas stories. *Psychologia*, **49**(4), 228–237.

Wang Y and Su Y (2013). Age-related differences in the performance of theory of mind in older adults: a dissociation of cognitive and affective components. *Psychology and Aging*, **28**(1), 284–291.

Warburton E, Wise RJ, Price CJ, Weiller C, Hadar U, Ramsay S and Frackowiak RS (1996). Noun and verb retrieval by normal subjects Studies with PET. *Brain*, **119**(1), 159–179.

Warkentin S, Risberg J, Nilsson A, Karlson S and Graae E (1991). Cortical activity during speech production: a study of regional cerebral blood flow in normal subjects performing a word fluency task. *Neuropsychiatry, Neuropsychology and Behavioral Neurology*, **4**(**4**), 305–316.

Watanabe J, Sugiura M, Sato K, Sato Y, Maeda Y, Matsue Y, Fukuda H and Kawashima R (2002). The human prefrontal and parietal association cortices are involved in NO-GO performances: an event-related fMRI study. *NeuroImage*, **17**(3), 1207–1216.

Wechsler D (1997a). *Wechsler Memory Scale—Third Edition (WMS-III)*. The Psychological Corporation, San Antonio, TX.

Wechsler D (1997b). *Wechsler Adult Intelligence Scale—Third Edition (WAIS-III)*. Harcourt Assessment, San Antonio, TX.

Wechsler D (1981). *Manual for the Wechsler Adult Intelligence Scale—Revised*. Psychological Corporation, New York.

Wechsler D (1984). *Wechsler Memory Scale—Revised*. Psychological Corporation, New York.

Wechsler D (2008). *Wechsler Adult Intelligence Scale—Fourth Edition (WAIS-IV)*. Pearson, San Antonio, TX.

Wecker NS, Kramer JH, Wisniewski A, Delis DC and Kaplan E (2000). Age effects on executive ability. *Neuropsychology*, **14**, 409–414.

Wegesin DJ, Jacobs DM, Zubin NR, Ventura PR and Stern Y (2000). Source memory and encoding strategy in normal aging. *Journal of the Clinical and Experimental Neuropsychology*, **22**(4), 455–464.

Weigl E (1927). Zur Psychologie sogenannter Abstraktionsprozesse. I. Untersuchungen über das "Ordnen". / On the psychology of the so-called processes of abstraction. I. Investigations on "arranging in order". *Zeitschrift für Psychologie*, **103**, 1–45.

Weiler JA, Bellebaum C and Daum I (2008). Aging effect acquisition and reversal of reward-based associative learning. *Learning and Memory*, **15**, 190–197.

Weiss EM, Siedentopf C, Hofer A, Deisenhammer EA, Hoptman MJ, Kremser C, Golaszewski S, Felber S, Fleischhacker WW and Delazer M (2003). Brain activation pattern during a verbal fluency test in healthy male and female volunteers: a functional magnetic resonance imaging study. *Neuroscience Letters*, **352**, 191–194.

West R and Alain C (2000). Age-related decline in inhibitory control contributes to the increased Stroop effect observed in older adults. *Psychophysiology*, **37**(2), 179–189.

West R and Bell MA (1997). Stroop color-word interference and electroencephalo-gram activation: evidence for age-related decline of the anterior attention system. *Neuropsychology*, **11**(3), 421–427.

West R and Moore K (2005). Adjustments of cognitive control in younger and older adults. *Cortex*, **41**, 570–581.

West R and Travers S (2008). Tracking the temporal dynamics of updating cognitive control: An examination of error processing. *Cerebral Cortex*, **18**, 1112–1124.

West R, McNerney MW and Krauss I (2007). Impaired strategic monitoring as the locus of a focal prospective memory deficit. *Neurocase*, **13**(2), 115–126.

West RL, Ergis AM, Winocur G and Saint-Cyr J (1998). The contribution of impaired working memory monitoring to performance of the Self-Ordered Pointing Task in normal aging and Parkinson's disease. *Neuropsychology*, **12**, 546–554.

Whalley HC, Simonotto E, Flett S, Marshall I, Ebmeier KP, Owens DGC, Goddard NH, Johnstone EC and Lawrie SM (2004). fMRI correlates of state and trait effects in subjects at genetically enhanced risk of schizophrenia. *Brain*, **127**(3), 478–490.

Wheeler EZ and Fellows LK (2008). The human ventromedial frontal lobe is critical for learning from negative feedback. *Brain*, **131**, 1323–1331.

Whitney C, Weis S, Krings T, Huber W, Grossman M and Kircher T (2009). Task-dependent modulations of prefrontal and hippocampal activity during intrinsic word production. *Journal of Cognitive Neuroscience*, **21**(4), 697–712.

Wiegersma S, van der Scheer E and Human R (1990). Subjective ordering, short-term memory, and the frontal lobes. *Neuropsychologia*, **28**(1), 95–98.

Wildgruber D, Riecker A, Hertrich I, Erb M, Grodd W, Ethofer T and Ackermann H (2005). Identification of emotional intonation evaluated by fMRI. *NeuroImage*, **24**(4), 1233–1241.

Wild-Wall N, Falkenstein M and Hohnsbein J (2008). Flanker interference in young and older participants as reflected in event-related potentials. *Brain Research*, **1211**, 72–84

Williams JH, Waiter GD, Perra O, Perrett DI and Whiten A (2005). An fMRI study of joint attention experience. *NeuroImage*, **25**(1), 133–140.

Williams T (1958). *Suddenly, Last Summer*. New Directions, New York.

Williams ZM, Bush G, Rauch SL, Cosgrove GR and Eskandar EN (2004). Human anterior cingulate neurons and the integration of monetary reward with motor responses. *Nature Neuroscience*, **7**(12), 1370–1375.

Wilmsmeier A, Ohrmann P, Suslow T, Siegmund A, Koelkebeck K, Rothermundt M, Kugel H, Arolt V, Bauer J and Pedersen A (2010). Neural correlates of set-shifting: decomposing executive functions in schizophrenia. *Journal of Psychiatry & Neuroscience*, **35**(5), 321–329.

Wilson BA, Alderman N, Burgess P, Emslie H and Evans J (1996). *Behavioural Assessment of the Dysexecutive Syndrome*. Thames Valley Test Company, Bury St Edmunds.

Wimmer H and Perner J (1983). Beliefs about beliefs: representation and constraining function of wrong beliefs in young children's understanding of deception. *Cognition*, **13**, 103–128.

Wittfoth M, Kustermann E, Fahle M and Herrmann M (2008). The influence of response conflict on error processing: evidence from event-related fMRI. *Brain Research*, **1194**, 118–129.

Wong B, Cronin-Golomb A and Neargarder S (2005). Patterns of visual scanning as predictors of emotion identification in normal aging. *Neuropsychology*, **19**(6), 739–749.

Wood S, Busemeyer J, Koling A, Cox CR and Davis H (2005). Older adults as adaptive decision makers: evidence from the Iowa Gambling Task. *Psychology and Aging*, **20**(2), 220–225.

Woodward TS, Ruff CC, Thornton AE, Moritz S and Liddle PF (2003). Methodological considerations regarding the association of Stroop and verbal fluency performance with the symptoms of schizophrenia. *Schizophrenia Research*, **61**(2–3), 207–214.

Woolgar A, Thompson R, Bor D and Duncan J (2011). Multi-voxel coding of stimuli, rules, and responses in human frontoparietal cortex. *NeuroImage*, **56**, 744–752.

Yee LTS, Roe K and Courtney SM (2010). Selective involvement of superior frontal cortex during working memory for shapes. *Journal of Neurophysiology*, **103**(1), 557–563.

Yen C-P, Kuan C-Y, Sheehan J, Kung S-S, Wang C-C, Liu C-K and Kwan AL (2009). Impact of bilateral anterior cingulotomy on neurocognitive function in patients with intractable pain. *Journal of Clinical Neuroscience*, **16**, 214–219.

Yeterian EH, Pandya DN, Tomaiuolo F and Petrides M (2012). The cortical connectivity of the prefrontal cortex in the monkey brain. *Cortex*, **48**(1), 57–80.

Yeung N, Botvinick MM and Cohen JD (2004). The neural basis of error detection: conflict monitoring and the error-related negativity. *Psychological Review*, **111**(**4**), 931–959.

Yochim BP, Baldo JV, Kane KD and Delis DC (2009). D-KEFS Tower Test performance in patients with lateral prefrontal cortex lesions: the importance of error monitoring. *Journal of Clinical and Experimental Neuropsychology*, **31**(**6**), 658–663.

Yochim B, Baldo J, Nelson A and Delis DC (2007). D-KEFS Trail Making Test performance in patients with lateral prefrontal cortex lesions. *Journal of the International Neuropsychological Society*, **13**, 704–709.

Yoon JH, Minzenberg MJ, Ursu S, Ryan Walter BS, Wendelken C, Ragland JD and Carter CS (2008). Association of dorsolateral prefrontal cortex dysfunction with disrupted coordinated brain activity in schizophrenia: relationship with impaired cognition, behavioral disorganization, and global function. *American Journal of Psychiatry*, **165**(**8**), 1006–1014.

Young L, Bechara A, Tranel D, Damasio H, Hauser M and Damasio A (2010). Damage to ventromedial prefrontal cortex impairs judgment of harmful intent. *Neuron*, **65**, 845–851.

Young L, Cushman F, Hauser M and Saxe R (2007). The neural basis of the interaction between theory of mind and moral judgment. *Proceedings of the National Academy of Sciences of the USA*, **104**, 8235–8240.

Young L and Saxe R (2008a). The neural basis of belief encoding and integration in moral judgement. *NeuroImage*, **40**, 1912–1920.

Young L and Saxe R (2008b). An fMRI investigation of spontaneous mental state inference for moral judgement. *Journal of Cognitive Neuroscience*, **21**, 1396–1405.

Zaitchik D (1990). When representations conflict with reality—the preschoolers' problem with false beliefs and false photographs. *Cognition*, **35**, 41–68.

Zakzanis KK, Mraz R and Graham SJ (2005). An fMRI study of the Trail Making Test. *Neuropsychologia*, **43**, 1878–1886.

Zald DH (2007). Orbital versus dorsolateral prefrontal cortex: anatomical insights into content versus process differentiation models of the prefrontal cortex. *Annals of the New York Academy of Sciences*, **1121**, 395–406.

Zappalà G, Measso G, Cavarzeran F, Grigoletto F, Lebowitz B, Pirozzolo F, Amaducci L, Massari D and Crook T (1995). Aging and memory: corrections for age, sex and education for three widely used memory tests. *Italian Journal of Neurological Sciences*, **16**(**3**), 177–184.

Zeef EJ, Sonke CJ, Kok A, Buiten MM and Kenemans JL (1996). Perceptual factors affecting age-related differences in focused attention: performance and psychophysiological analyses. *Psychophysiology*, **33**(**5**), 555–565.

Zeigarnik B (1927). Über das Erhalten erledigter und unerledigter Handlungen. *Psychologische Forschung*, **9**, 1–85.

Zempleni M, Haverkort M, Renken R and Stowe LA (2007). Evidence for bilateral involvement in idiom comprehension: an fMRI study. *NeuroImage*, **34**(**3**), 1280–1291.

Zimmerman ME, Brickman AM, Paul RH, Grieve SM, Tate DF, Gunstad J, Cohen RA, Aloia MS, Williams LM, Clark CR, Whitford TJ and Gordon E (2006). The relationship between frontal gray matter volume and cognition varies across the healthy adult. *American Journal of Geriatric Psychiatry*, **14**(**10**), 823–833.

Zorrilla LT, Aguirre GK, Zarahn E, Cannon TD and D'Esposito M (1996). Activation of the prefrontal cortex during judgments of recency: a functional MRI study. *Neuroreport*, 7(15–17), 2803–2806.

Zysset S, Muller K, Lohmann G and von Cramon DY (2001). Color-word matching Stroop task: separating interference and response conflict. *Neuroimage*, **13**, 29–36.

Zysset S, Schroeter ML, Neumann J and von Cramon DY (2007). Stroop interference, hemodynamic response and aging: an event-related fMRI study. *Neurobiology of Aging*, **28**, 937–946.

Index

Page references to Figures, Photographs or Tables are in *italic* print.